# INDOOR AIR POLLUTION

THE JOHNS HOPKINS SERIES
IN ENVIRONMENTAL TOXICOLOGY
Zoltan Annau, series editor

*Neurobehavioral Toxicology*
edited by Zoltan Annau

*Monitoring the Worker for Exposure and Disease: Scientific, Legal, and Ethical
Considerations in the Use of Biomarkers*
Nicholas A. Ashford, Christine J. Spadafor, Dale B. Hattis,
and Charles C. Caldart

*Variations in Susceptibility to Inhaled Pollutants: Identification, Mechanisms,
and Policy Implications*
edited by Joseph D. Brain, Barbara D. Beck, A. Jane Warren,
and Rashid A. Shaikh

*Aging and Environmental Toxicology: Biological and Behavioral Perspectives*
edited by Ralph L. Cooper, Jerome M. Goldman, and Thomas J. Harbin

*The Toxicity of Methyl Mercury*
edited by Christine U. Eccles and Zoltan Annau

*Lead Toxicity: History and Environmental Impact*
edited by Richard Lansdown and William Yule

*Toxic Chemicals, Health, and the Environment*
edited by Lester B. Lave and Arthur C. Upton

# INDOOR
# AIR POLLUTION
*A Health Perspective*

Edited by

JONATHAN M. SAMET, M.D., M.S.
Professor of Medicine and Chief, Pulmonary Division
and New Mexico Tumor Registry
University of New Mexico School of Medicine

and

JOHN D. SPENGLER, PH.D., M.S.
Professor, Department of Environmental Science and Physiology
Harvard University School of Public Health

THE JOHNS HOPKINS UNIVERSITY PRESS
*Baltimore and London*

The Johns Hopkins University Press
701 West 40th Street
Baltimore, Maryland 21211-2190
The Johns Hopkins Press Ltd., London

The paper used in this book meets the minimum requirements of American
National Standards for Information Sciences—Permanence of Paper for
Printed Library Materials, ANSI Z39.48-1984.

Library of Congress Cataloging-in-Publication Data

Indoor air pollution : a health perspective / edited by Jonathan M.
   Samet and John D. Spengler.
      p.   cm. — (The Johns Hopkins series in environmental
   toxicology)
      Includes bibliographical references and index.
      ISBN 0-8018-4124-0. — ISBN 0-8018-4125-9 (pbk.)
      1. Indoor air pollution—Health aspects.   I. Samet, Jonathan M.
   II. Spengler, John D.   III. Series.
   RA577.5.I54   1991
   613′.5—dc20                                              90-49482
                                                                CIP

# CONTENTS

# CONTRIBUTORS

DAVID W. BEARG, M.S., president, Life Energy Associates, Concord, Mass.

HARRIET A. BURGE, Ph.D., associate research scientist, Division of Internal Medicine, Department of Allergy, University of Michigan

WILLIAM S. CAIN, Ph.D., fellow, John B. Pierce Foundation Laboratory; and professor of epidemiology and psychology, Yale University School of Medicine

DAVID B. COULTAS, M.D., assistant professor of medicine, University of New Mexico Medical Center and New Mexico Tumor Registry

JAMES C. FEELEY, Ph.D., president, Pathogen Control Associates, Tucker, Ga.

DAVID T. HARRJE, M.S., research engineer, Center for Energy and Environmental Studies, School of Engineering and Applied Science, Princeton University

LAURENCE S. KIRSCH, M.S., J.D., associate, Cadwalader, Whickersham and Taft, Washington, D.C.

ROBERT A. KRIEGER, Ph.D., director of environmental toxicology, Delta Environmental Consultants, St. Paul, Minn.

WILLIAM E. LAMBERT, Ph.D., research assistant professor, Department of Family, Community, and Emergency Medicine, University of New Mexico Medical Center and New Mexico Tumor Registry

BRIAN P. LEADERER, Ph.D., M.P.H., associate fellow, John B. Pierce Foundation Laboratory; and associate professor of epidemiology and environmental health, Yale University

JERRY F. LUDWIG, Ph.D., senior scientist, Environmental Health and Engineering, Inc., Newton, Mass.; and research associate, Physical Science and Engineering Program, Department of Environmental Science and Physiology, Harvard School of Public Health

MARIAN C. MARBURY, Sc.D., environmental epidemiologist, Minnesota Department of Health

JOHN F. McCARTHY, Sc.D., president, Environmental Health and Engineering, Inc., Newton, Mass.

P. BARRY RYAN, M.D., Ph.D., assistant professor, Department of Environmental Science and Physiology, Harvard School of Public Health

MARK R. SCHUYLER, M.D., chief, Medical Service, Veterans Administration Medical Center, Albuquerque; and professor and vice chairman, Department of Medicine, University of New Mexico School of Medicine

WILLIAM TURNER, M.S., manager, Building Air Quality Assessment Group, Harriman Associates, Auburn, Me.

LANCE A. WALLACE, Ph.D., environmental scientist, U.S. Environmental Protection Agency, Warrenton, Va.

DAVID N. WEISSMAN, M.D., Veterans Administration Medical Center, Albuquerque; and assistant professor of medicine, University of New Mexico School of Medicine

JAMES E. WOODS, JR., Ph.D., William E. Jamerson professor of building construction, College of Architecture and Urban Studies, Virginia Polytechnic Institute and State University

# PREFACE

This book provides a comprehensive review of the rapidly enlarging evidence on indoor air quality and health. The audience for this material continues to grow as the dimensions of the indoor air quality problem become more and more apparent. The issues surrounding indoor air quality are diverse, and the large numbers of specialists involved in the research include epidemiologists, risk assessors, experts in air monitoring, microbiologists, engineers, and psychologists. As the hazards posed by indoor air pollution have been recognized, the evidence on adverse health effects has become increasingly relevant for physicians and other health care providers. The dominant contributions of indoor sources to the total personal exposures for some pollutants have given the subject importance for local, state, and federal regulators. Adverse effects of indoor air pollution have also been the subject of litigation.

The impact of indoor air quality problems on property values and sales has been well demonstrated in the case of radon; it is likely that documentation of adequate indoor air quality for radon and other pollutants may eventually be required at the time of sale of all properties. Such a requirement will bring builders, real estate salespersons, and homeowners into the audience for information on indoor air quality. During the last two decades, outbreaks of illness related to work environments other than industrial settings have been reported with increasing frequency. These outbreaks, often referred to as the "sick-building syndrome" or "tight-building syndrome," have added the building operator and the employer to the list of those who should be concerned about indoor air quality.

A single volume cannot address the needs of so diverse an audience. The intent of this book is to provide a review for the health-oriented readership, and for policymakers, engineers, and lawyers. Unfortunately, the book will not serve the relatively small group of researchers who are directly involved with indoor air quality problems.

The structure of this book reflects the complexity of the problem of indoor air quality. The book begins with a perspective on outdoor and indoor air quality. Subsequent chapters address the sources of indoor air pollution, the levels of pollution in homes, the assessment of indoor air quality, and the operating characteristics of buildings. The major topic of the book is the health effects of indoor pollutants. Pollutants that are specifically considered include carbon monoxide, formaldehyde, other volatile organic compounds, environmental tobacco smoke, nitrogen dioxide, radon, and wood smoke. The effects of biologic agents are considered separately and include infectious agents and those agents that cause disease through immunologic mechanisms. Building-related illnesses are also considered in a separate chapter. The topical problem of indoor asbestos is covered in Chapter 2, but the health risks do not receive separate treatment. The occupational hazards of asbestos have been amply described, and direct evidence on the health risks of indoor asbestos is unavailable. The remaining chapters of the book address such other important dimensions of indoor air quality as the control of pollution and its legal aspects. Policy on indoor air is considered in the introductory chapter.

# ACKNOWLEDGMENTS

This book originated with an invitation from Reuben M. Cherniack, editor of the *American Review of Respiratory Disease,* to prepare a "state-of-art" review on indoor air pollution. We accepted and quickly discovered that the task was far larger than we had anticipated. Nevertheless, with our colleague Marian Marbury, we completed the review, which was published in December 1987 and January 1988. Discussions with Zoltan Annau led to an invitation to expand the review into a book for the Johns Hopkins Series in Environmental Toxicology.

During the preparation of this book, we both had support from numerous funding agencies, the availability of which facilitated our work. John D. Spengler derived support from the National Institute of Environmental Health Sciences, the Environmental Protection Agency, the Electric Power Research Institute, the Department of National Health and Welfare Canada, and the Gas Research Institute. Jonathan M. Samet was funded by the Department of Energy, the Health Effects Institute, and the National Heart, Lung, and Blood Institute. Portions of Chapters 2, 6, 7, 9, 10, and 15, in an earlier form, originally appeared in the *American Review of Respiratory Disease* and are reprinted with permission from *ARRD* 1987, Volume 136, and *ARRD* 1988, Volume 137. Portions of Chapter 6, in an earlier form, originally appeared in the *Annals of Sports Medicine* 4 (1988). Portions of Chapter 15, in an earlier form, originally appeared in the *Journal of the National Cancer Institute* 81 (1989). Chapter 17 is being published simultaneously in *Indoor Air Pollution: The Complete Resource Guide*, by the Bureau of National Affairs, Inc.

The contributions of many people were needed to complete this book. The authors worked hard in preparing their chapters and in revising them after review. Rebecca Mosher worked tirelessly in entering the material and preparing illustrations. Dorothy Warner also worked on the volume. Lee Fernando kept everyone organized. Rita Elliott edited the volume. Her diligence in assuring that the volume was readable and that the material was correct deserves special thanks. Wendy Harris remained supportive throughout preparation of the manuscript.

# INDOOR AIR POLLUTION

# 1

# A PERSPECTIVE ON INDOOR AND OUTDOOR AIR POLLUTION

John D. Spengler, Ph.D., M.S.
Jonathan M. Samet, M.D., M.S.

Pollution is one of the more pressing problems of our age. Pollution of the atmosphere has now reached a level that poses a potential threat not only to the health and well-being of entire populations but to the survival of life. Air pollution is not a new phenomenon, however; throughout the earth's history, gases have been released into the atmosphere by moltant volcanic activity, by the combustion of biomass, by the volatilization of organic compounds, and by the release of bioeffluents from living organisms. Similarly, particles have become suspended in the atmosphere by the abrasive action of surface winds, fires, wave action, and the fracture of crystalline aerosols, and by the natural biologic production of spores, fibers, and seeds. Even when generated by these natural processes, air pollution can have adverse effects upon the climate and the weather, upon agriculture, and upon mankind.

Human beings have long contributed to the pollution of the atmosphere. The black, sooted rock walls of Canyon duChelly in Arizona are vivid reminders that from earliest times the warmth and protection of fire have brought pollutants. When people built shelters for dwelling, they brought the pollutants into the indoor living space. However, smoke from cooking and heating fires was not the only pollution in earlier dwellings. The great castles of medieval Europe were cold and damp, and the smell of mildew lingers yet for modern-day tourists. Since the Dark Ages, and even today in countries in which primitive conditions still exist, peasants have shared squalid dirt-floored shelters with their domesticated beasts, and the benefits of shared warmth have been accompanied by exposure to diseases transmitted by pests and a plethora of microorganisms that flourish in such conditions.

And what of modern people with their scientific knowledge and advanced technology? Is the air of the modern home, public buildings, and cities cleaner and healthier than that in the past? In our more developed societies, we have designed structures to shield us from the natural elements and to provide comfort. But in the construction of these buildings and in the creation of the infrastructure and transportation that are part of the overall comfort design, we have released into the environment many of the by-products of industrialization. The same natural processes that occur over millennia have been accelerated into decades, as extraction of ores and burning of fossil fuels have released metals, sulfur dioxide ($SO_2$), carbon monoxide (CO), carbon dioxide ($CO_2$), nitrogen oxides ($NO_x$), and many other organic and inorganic constituents into the atmosphere.

Along with a growing population and expanding economies has come greater utilization of fuels and of agricultural and mineral resources. As a result, air pollution is no longer a local problem but affects large segments of the world's population. Both the nature and geographic scale of air pollution have expanded since organization of municipal smoke ordinances and smoke control districts and inspectors in the late nineteenth century. Air pollution is no longer considered just soot and annoying odors in industrial or urban areas. The broader definition for atmospheric pollution developed by the Commonwealth of Massachusetts's Department of Public Health in 1961 is appropriate for both indoor and outdoor air pollution today: "Atmospheric pollution is the presence in the ambient air space of one or more air contaminants or combination thereof in such quantities and of such duration as to (a) cause a nuisance; (b) be injurious or, on the basis of current information, be potentially injurious to human or animal life, to vegetation, or to property; or (c) unreasonably interfere with the comfortable enjoyment of life and property or the conduct of business."

By the end of the 1940s, air pollution in the United States obtained national recognition. President Truman directed the secretary of the interior to head the interdepartmental committee that organized the first U.S. Technical Conference on Air Pollution, held in May 1950. Five years later Congress enacted the first national legislation, the Air Pollution Control Act, which was passed with the strong support of the California delegation. The act authorized $3 million annually for five years for research, training, and technical assistance to states (Stern 1982). However, it was not until the Clean Air Act of 1963 that the federal government established its right over the states to legislate air pollution on the constitutional basis of interstate commerce. The secretary of health, education, and welfare, through the surgeon general and Public Health Service, struggled for seven years to abate interstate pollution problems through complicated and slow conference abatement procedures. However, during this time, Congress passed the Motor Vehicle Air Pollution Control Act of 1965, in which the process to establish national emission standards for new motor vehicles was established. By the late 1960s, it was clear that the Clean Air Act of 1963 and its 1967 amendments were not sufficient to mount an effective national effort. Financial incentives alone were not adequate to establish individual state legislation and pollution control programs. The Clean Air Act Amendments of 1970 and the establishment of the Environmental Protection Agency (EPA) radically changed the course of pollution

2   John D. Spengler and Jonathan M. Samet

control. The EPA was required to establish national ambient air, that is, outside air, quality standards and given enforcement authority. Congress imposed federal mobile source emission standards, and states had to establish air pollution implementation plans in compliance with federal criteria. The national ambient air quality standards (NAAQSs) currently in existence are listed in Table 1.1 along with those of some other nations.

The Clean Air Act has been amended several times since 1970. In 1977 among the issues addressed by Congress was the prevention of significant deterioration of air quality by unrestricted development in areas currently cleaner than the standards. Congress also expressed its concern about the potential for stratospheric ozone depletion, for hazardous air pollutants emitted from relatively few sources, and the revision of automobile standards and ambient air quality standards. Although slated for reauthorization during the 1980s, the Clean Air Act was not amended during the decade. However, in 1980 Congress created the national acid precipitation assessment program with statutory responsibility to prepare comprehensive scientific, technologic, and economic information relevant to developing policies for the control of acid deposition effects. Acid deposition, commonly referred to as *acid rain*, is a major environmental problem confronting the United States and Canada as well as other regions of the world. There is substantial evidence that the pollutants from fossil fuel combustion have damaged lakes, forests, and crops, reduced visibility, and perhaps have resulted in increased morbidity among exposed populations.

As we start the last decade of this century, policies and legislation to resolve the pressing environmental problems that are no longer local-scale issues have eluded us. Ironically, as we await further amendments to the Clean Air Act to address regional and global-scale air pollution concerns, we are beginning to recognize that air pollution is still very familiar to each of us in our schools, offices, and homes.

Atmospheric concentrations of contaminants depend on many factors, which in themselves vary temporally and spatially. The density and intensity of pollution sources in urbanized areas often result in higher exposures in cities than in more rural areas. Pollutants released into the atmosphere may be rapidly diluted, but mixing with the atmosphere may be suppressed by temperature inversion or modified by structures and terrain, which thereby increase surface-level pollution.

The atmosphere is never static. Contaminants are transported, diluted, and removed by surface reactions, precipitated, or disassociated into submolecular components by solar radiation. Reactive components can undergo transformation. A substantial fraction of the gaseous $SO_2$ and nitrogen oxide is transformed to particulate species, existing as sulfuric acid, nitric acid, or other acids (U.S. Congress, Office of Technology Assessment 1985). In the lower atmosphere, halogenated synthetic gases used as refrigerants, propellants, and biocides have reaction half-lives that are measured in decades. However, once these gases are diffused or mixed into the stratosphere by strong convective storms, they decompose in the unfiltered ultraviolet energy of incoming solar radiation, and the

Table 1.1   Air Quality Standards or Guidelines for Contaminants

| Pollutant | Relevant Concentration | Comments |
|-----------|------------------------|----------|
| Particles | 150 μg/m³ | Japanese indoor standard enforced in office buildings (<3.5 μm) |
| | 150 μg/m³ | U.S. EPA outdoor NAAQS for particles less than 10-μm diameter, 24-hour average |
| | 120 μg/m³ | European WHO ambient air quality guideline, 24-hour total suspended particulates |
| | 70 μg/m³ | European WHO ambient air quality guideline, 24-hour thoracic particles (<10 μm) |
| | 480 μg/m³ | Germany outdoor standard, 1 hour, for total particle concentration |
| Nitrogen dioxide | 50 ppb | NAAQS for $NO_2$ annual average set by EPA |
| | 75 ppb (150 μg/m³) | European WHO ambient air quality guideline, 24 hours |
| | 200 ppb (400 μg/m³) | European WHO ambient air quality guideline, 1 hour |
| Carbon monoxide | 9 ppm (10 mg/m³) | Germany and U.S. NAAQS for 8 hours, outdoors |
| | 35 ppm (40 mg/m³) | Germany and U.S. NAAQS for 1 hour, outdoors |
| | 3 ppm (30 mg/m³) | European WHO, 1 hour |
| | 55 ppm (60 mg/m³) | European WHO, 30 min not to be exceeded in 8 hours, outdoors |
| | 90 ppm (100 mg/m³) | European WHO, 15 min not to be exceeded in 8 hours, outdoors |
| Carbon dioxide | 5,000 ppm (9,000 mg/m³) | OSHA[a] standard, 8 hours |
| | 1,000 ppm (1,800 mg/m³) | Japanese indoor air quality standard not to be exceeded in office buildings; used as indicator of adequate building ventilation without other sources |
| | 650 ppm | Commonwealth of Massachusetts recommended value for indoors |
| | 350–450 ppm | Typical outdoor levels in urban areas |
| | 5,000 ppm | Indicates 2.25 cfm/person |
| | 3,000 ppm | Indicates ~4 cfm/person |
| | 1,000 ppm | Indicates ~15 cfm/person |
| | 500 ppm | Indicates ~50 cfm/person |

(*continued*)

4   John D. Spengler and Jonathan M. Samet

Table 1.1 (*Continued*)

| Pollutant | Relevant Concentration | Comments |
|---|---|---|
| | 1.25 ppm (1,500 μg/m$^3$) | ACGIH[b] occupational TLV (threshold limit value) |
| Formaldehyde | 1 ppm | OSHA, 8 hours, workplace |
| | 0.7 ppm | Sweden, maximum allowed in older buildings |
| | 0.4 ppm (480 μg/m$^3$) | Department of Housing and Urban Development limit for new mobile or manufactured housing |
| | 0.25 ppm | NRC[c] guide to safeguard against irritant effects for vast majority of public |
| | 0.1 ppm (120 μg/m$^3$) | Swedish limit for new homes; ASHRAE indoor guideline |
| | 0.08 ppm (100 μg/m$^3$) | European WHO 30-min outdoor guideline |
| Volatile organic compounds (VOCs) (e.g., benzene, styrene, chloroform, methylene chloride, ethylene oxide, tetrachloroethylene) | 2 mg/m$^3$ | Mixtures of VOCs commonly found indoors associated with symptoms and performance in Danish studies; several specific VOCs are known or suspected human carcinogens—EPA has developed cancer risk values; several VOCs have occupational standards |
| Styrene | 800 μg/m$^3$ | European WHO 2-hour outdoor guideline for non-cancer/odor effects |
| Tetrachloroethylene | 5 mg/m$^3$ | European WHO 24-hour outdoor guideline for non-cancer/odor effects |
| Toluene | 8 mg/m$^3$ | European WHO 24-hour outdoor guideline for non-cancer/odor effects |
| Trichloroethylene | 1 mg/m$^3$ | European WHO 24-hour outdoor guideline for non-cancer/odor effects |
| Semivolatile organics (e.g., chlorinated and brominated hydrocarbons used as insecticides, pesticides, fungicides; polycyclic and aromatic hydrocarbons from combustion, preservatives, transformer fluids) | 5 μg/m$^3$ | NRC guideline for chlordane concentration in residences; has also been applied to other termiticides <br> EPA has developed cancer risk values for several known or suspected human carcinogens <br> Occupational standards exist for many of these compounds <br> For general guideline, the indoor levels should not |

(*continued*)

Table 1.1 (*continued*)

| Pollutant | Relevant Concentration | Comments |
|-----------|------------------------|----------|
| | | exceed ambient levels, cause irritation, or contribute to a lifetime cancer risk $>10^{-5}$ |
| Asbestos fibers (e.g., chrysotile, crocidolite, and other amphiboles) | 0.2 fibers/cm³ | OSHA, 8-hour workplace average, fibers $>5$-μm length; |
| | 0.1 fibers/cm³ | OSHA action level requiring respiratory protection for workers |
| | Equal to or less than ambient fiber concentration | EPA reoccupancy requirements after removal by transmission electron microscopy; nonspecific to fiber type |
| Radon and radon decay products | 22 pCi/liter (400 Bcq/m³) | Swedish action level for required remediation |
| | 20 pCi/liter | Canadian Radiation Protection Bureau |
| | 11 pCi/liter | U.K. action level for existing dwellings |
| | 8 pCi/liter | National Council on Radiation Protection action level |
| | 5.5 pCi/liter | Sweden, design level for new buildings |
| | 5 pCi/liter | Bonneville Power Administration action level |
| | 4 pCi/liter | EPA limit for uranium-processing site homes; EPA action guideline |
| | 3 pCi/liter | U.K. new dwelling levels |
| | 2 pCi/liter | ASHRAE guidelines in *Standard 62-1981* |

[a]OSHA, Occupational Safety and Health Administration.
[b]ACGIH, American Conference of Governmental and Industrial Hygienists.
[c]NRC, National Research Council.

released atomic components of chlorine, bromine, and fluorine can react quickly to reduce the amount of stratospheric ozone.

In the potential danger that halogenated hydrocarbons pose to the ozone and radiative balance of the earth's atmosphere (Ember et al. 1986), we see an example of a process that sets human activity apart from the "natural" processes of atmospheric pollution. Not only have humans hastened the pollution process, we have also added to the polluting substances volatile and semivolatile organic molecules that are not produced by natural processes. Many of the polluting compounds are associated with toxic or hazardous air pollutants released from fuel additives, paint solvents, cleaners, degreasers, and insecticides. The pollutants are found outgasing from soils and water near industrial and municipal waste sites.

Perhaps more important from a human exposure perspective, they are emitted into our indoor environments from furnishings, structural components, and the many other products that modern society has developed.

As we examine air pollution in the world today, we see many reminders of the problems that accompanied urbanization in ancient Rome and the growing cities of Europe in the Middle Ages. Air pollution came from heating and cooking fires, from brick kilns, iron works, smelting, and burning garbage. In the seventeenth century, diarist John Evelyn wrote:

It is this horrid smoke, which obscures our churches and makes our palaces look old, which fouls our clothes and corrupts the water so that the very rain and refreshing dews which fall in the several seasons precipitate this impure vapor, which with its black and tenacious quality, spots and contaminates whatever is exposed to it. (Evelyn 1661)

Yet today, the primary emissions of sulfur oxides, nitrogen oxides, CO, particulates, and metals are severely polluting many cities of Asia, Africa, Latin America, and eastern Europe. Even in the nations that have addressed the problem of primary emissions from heavy industry, power plants, and automobiles, new problems are posed by toxic compounds from the newer, modern industries and a more subtle form of air pollution caused by the secondary formation of acids and ozone.

Understanding the changing nature of air pollution problems in the United States and developing countries is important to recognizing the relevance of indoor exposures. The contaminants in the outdoor air contribute to human exposures directly, and indirectly if they penetrate indoors. Indoor sources such as unvented combustion, evaporation of organic compounds, abrasion, release of microorganisms, and intrusion of radon, a soil gas, can be the predominant contributor to human exposures, particularly in locations with low ambient levels. However, for reactive air pollutants formed in the ambient air, human exposures are determined primarily by outdoor concentrations. Ozone and acidic aerosols are examples of outdoor reactive pollutants for which reduction of outdoor concentrations has been shown to reduce indoor concentrations.

The global environmental monitoring system (GEMS), a project sponsored by the World Health Organization (WHO) and the United Nations Environment Program (UNEP), was created in the early 1970s to monitor air quality in countries all over the world. Many urbanized areas in developing countries still have ambient $SO_2$ and particulate pollution levels that are ten to one hundred times the concentrations currently experienced in the United States and western Europe. In these situations, human exposures will be proportionally more influenced by ambient conditions. Exposure studies in Zagreb, Yugoslavia, demonstrated that the ratio between average personal exposure and respirable particle levels outdoors decreases with the increased outdoor concentration. Sega and Fugas (1982) implied that with outdoor pollution, personal exposures are approximated by the ambient concentrations.

In examining exposures and concentrations that can occur indoors, comparison with ambient air pollution levels is informative. In the United States and Canada, standardized ambient monitoring for several pollutants has been conducted since the 1950s by federal, state, local, and privately funded organizations. The monitoring sites have been established to determine compliance with standards, to make baseline regulatory measurements, to document trends in rural areas, and to accomplish other special purposes. Ambient monitoring has also been conducted throughout most of western Europe. However, methods and protocols vary, making the direct comparison of concentrations difficult. Comparisons of particle concentrations across countries are particularly difficult because particles vary by size, composition, and other attributes. Some instruments determine mass concentration gravimetrically, and others infer dust loadings by the indirect methods of transmission or reflectance. Comparison of particulate concentrations should, therefore, include a reference to the size fraction collected and the analytical methods.

In the United States and other countries with established air pollution control programs, the ambient concentrations of many contaminants have decreased. Soot-grimed cities, with visible emissions from factories, automobiles, and stacks on buildings, have almost disappeared. There has been a marked decrease in ambient concentrations of total suspended particulates (TSP), $SO_2$, lead and other metals, and CO (U.S. EPA 1989). Fossil fuel-related organic carbon compounds such as benzo[a]pyrene have also decreased substantially since the 1960s. These decreases reflect many factors, including industrial and automobile controls, new electrical power-generating facilities with taller stacks built away from the urban areas, the burning of cleaner fuels with lower sulfur content, and a decline in manufacturing-related industries.

The cleanup of ambient air pollution in the United States has been under way for two decades. As TSP decreased during the 1970s, so did many of the metals and organics included in the particulate matter. Many industrialized urban areas had concentrations of benzo[a]pyrene exceeding 10 $ng/m^3$ when coal was burned in homes, factories, and buildings; today, the annual concentrations are below 1 $ng/m^3$ (U.S. EPA 1982).

Sulfur dioxide concentrations in urban areas have decreased since the 1960s. A restriction to low-sulfur fuels for residential and commercial use has resulted in impressive improvements in air quality in many cities in colder climates. Presently, all major population centers are in compliance with the NAAQS for $SO_2$. Annual emissions of $SO_2$ have decreased by 15 percent from a 1970 high of more than thirty million tons per year.

Carbon monoxide is emitted primarily by vehicle sources. Federal emission control standards for new vehicles resulted in a 77 percent reduction of emissions between 1975 and 1981. This decline alone has been responsible for marked improvement in ambient CO levels. For example, Figure 1.1 shows trends of CO

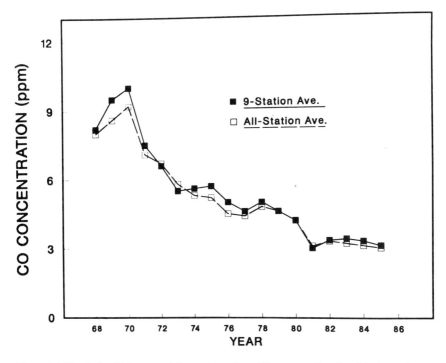

Figure 1.1. Trends for third-quarter daily maximum hour CO concentrations (ppm) in the south coast air basin, Los Angeles. *Source:* Kuntasal and Chang (1987), reprinted with permission.

in the south coast air basin of Los Angeles and Orange Counties; a downward trend in maximum hourly CO concentrations was measured during the third quarter of the year between 1968 and 1985 (Kuntasal and Chang 1987). Although similar progress has occurred in many urban areas, with the increase of vehicle miles traveled and congestion in localized "hot spots," the CO concentration still exceeds the NAAQS in many cities.

In contrast to the improvements in ambient concentrations of $SO_2$, TSP, and CO, levels of other pollutants have either shown no change or increased. As newer vehicles have complied with federal mobile source emission standards, the average model year hydrocarbon emissions have been reduced by 88 percent and emissions of nitrogen oxides by 50 percent between 1973 and 1982. These reductions are offset, in part, by increased vehicle miles traveled and a trend toward an aging fleet of cars. In terms of actual reductions in transportation-related emissions, only 38 percent hydrocarbon and 21 percent CO reductions have been realized (Walker 1985). However, both smog-chamber studies and careful analysis of data have revealed that ozone production from hydrocarbons becomes more efficient at lower concentrations (Altshuller 1983; Fox, Kamens, and Jeffries 1975). In certain areas of the country, population growth and urban sprawl have caused total automobile and stationary sources of ozone precursors to increase.

From the mid–1970s to the early 1980s, there was a 2.3 percent per year overall increase in ozone in Texas and a 7.8 percent per year increase in the number of hours during which ozone concentrations exceeded 120 ppb, the U.S. one-hour standard. In California, the number of hours exceeding 120 ppb decreased by 5.2 percent per year through the mid–1980s (Walker 1985). Other measures of ozone in California, such as the annual mean concentration, show little change. There has been a decrease in ozone in Los Angeles, as shown in Figure 1.2, and a noticeable reduction of "smog" days; however, high ozone exposures in the area do still occur.

Most of the U.S. population east of the Mississippi River experiences spring and summer ozone conditions that produce at least one hour exceeding 100 ppb. EPA estimates that 107 communities and 135 million people live in areas that exceed the NAAQS for ozone. In Europe, elevated ozone levels, with the associated drop in visibility and increase in forest damage, are now being recognized.

Ambient air pollution related to automobile and truck emissions is increasing in most developing countries. The growing population of automobiles without emission controls in many rapidly expanding urban areas in these countries has created serious ozone problems. Mexico City has perhaps the worst of these conditions. Because of the intense sunlight at high altitude and the congested traffic, Mexico

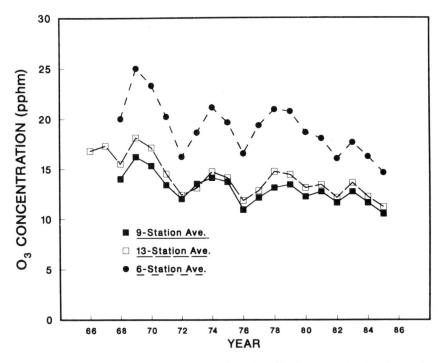

Figure 1.2. Trends for third-quarter daily maximum hour $O_3$ (oxidant) concentrations (ppm) across the south coast air basin in Los Angeles. *Source:* Kuntasal and Chang (1987), reprinted with permission.

John D. Spengler and Jonathan M. Samet

City is already experiencing ozone levels that routinely exceed 200 ppb.

Through complex chemical reactions, precursor gaseous emissions of nitrogen oxides and $SO_2$ can be converted to acidic gases and particles. Common acidic species include sulfuric acid, ammonia bisulfate, acidic particles, and nitrous and nitric acidic gases. The sulfate particulates are in the submicron size range and can serve as efficient condensation nuclei and efficiently scatter visible light. Because 80 percent of $SO_2$ emissions in the United States occurs in the eastern third of the nation, it is not surprising that sulfate particles are the most prominent fraction of the inhalable-size particles (U.S. EPA 1982).

Areas of the United States that experience sulfate exposures are shown in Figure 1.3, which plots the spatially averaged annual sulfate concentration ($\mu g/m^3$). The regions of highest sulfate concentration include portions of the states of West Virginia, Ohio, Maryland, Pennsylvania, and New York. Seasonally, sulfate concentrations are higher in spring and summer. Depending on atmospheric conditions and ammonia emissions, sulfate particles can be in the form of strong acids such as sulfuric or ammonia bisulfate.

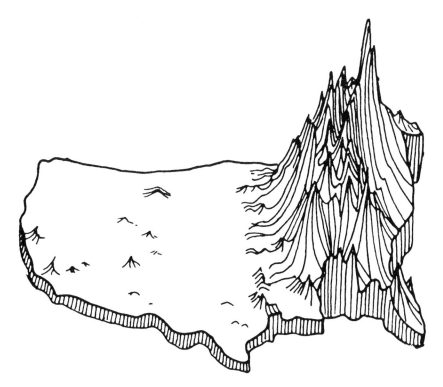

Figure 1.3. The relative annual sulfate particle concentrations ($\mu g/m^3$) spatially averaged across the United States. The highest concentrations are in eastern Ohio, western Pennsylvania, and northern West Virginia, of approximately 20–25 $\mu g/m^3$. *Source:* Adapted from Meyers et al. (1978) and Wilson et al. (1980), with permission.

Atmospheric concentrations of acidic aerosols and gases have not been measured on a routine basis in the United States. Monitoring has been done as a component of various research projects, using different methods and averaging times. Most of the published literature is summarized in the United States Environmental Protection Agency's Acid Aerosols Issue Paper (U.S. EPA 1989).

Acidic aerosol events can occur at any time during the year but are more intense and more frequent during the warmer months. Thus, the highest atmospheric acid concentrations occur at times when people are more likely to be outdoors. Measurements from the mid–United States indicate that daily acid particle concentrations can exceed 15 $\mu g/m^3$ $H_2SO_4$ equivalence (Spengler et al. 1989). More recent measurements during the summer of 1988 indicate that daily levels can exceed 20 $\mu g/m^3$ $H_2SO_4$. Spengler and co-workers (1989) documented an acid aerosol episode in southern Ontario. During this two-day event the highest hourly concentration approached 50 $\mu g/m^3$ $H_2SO_4$ equivalence. Other episodic acid events in the eastern United States have been shown to last a few hours to a few days in duration and result in substantial population exposures (Spengler et al. 1986).

Concern over ambient acid concentrations is recent in the United States. In London, however, daily measurements of sulfuric acid were made between 1963 and 1973. Unlike conditions in the United States, acidity increased during winter months, probably because of increased heating fuel use and adverse meteorologic conditions (Ito and Thurston 1987).

Other acid species besides sulfuric acid and ammonia bisulfate may be present in the atmosphere. In the Los Angeles basin of southern California, acidic gases and acidified fog are of concern. The acid species commonly identified include nitric, hydrochloric, acetic, formic, benzoic, and other organic acids. Hourly concentrations in the summer clearly show nitric acid increasing late in the morning to an afternoon maximum around 3 P.M. Nitric acid ($HNO_3$) dominates during the daytime, but there is a substantial amount of formic and acetic acids at night. The pattern is consistent with that of ozone and indicates the reactive chemistry of automobile-related hydrocarbon and nitrogen oxide emissions (Grosjean, Williams, and Van Neste 1982).

We have focused on only a few of the many ambient pollutants. Several monitoring programs have examined an array of trace elements and organic compounds in the air. The focus is not on the concentrations of each component but rather on the interpretation, to infer source contributions. Using a variety of multivariate techniques, the fractional contributions to ambient particulate pollution can be ascribed to a few dominant sources. These techniques have been applied in several areas in the United States which differ in local and distant source contributions (Gordon 1988). Morandi (1985) studied the sources of urban particulate pollution in three New Jersey cities (Figure 1.4). Secondary sulfates contributed the most mass to the measured concentrations of respirable particles at all three locations. Soil dust, automobile emissions, and oil burning contributed to ambient particle concentrations. The cities differed in the proportion contributed and in the presence of city-specific industrial sources. In contrast, similar work by Cooper, Watson, and Hunt-

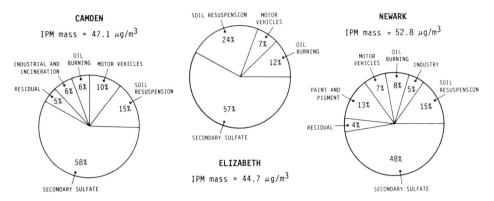

Figure 1.4. Source contributions (percent) to inhalable particulate matter (IMP) in three New Jersey urban areas. *Source:* From *Toxic Air Pollution: A Comprehensive Study of Non-Criteria Air Pollutants,* by Paul J. Lioy and Joan M. Daisey. Copyright 1987, Lewis Publishers, Inc., Chelsea, Mich. Used with permission

zicker (1979) in Portland showed less sulfate contribution and more impact from vegetative burning. Thus, there are substantial regional differences in sources. In the West, agricultural and domestic wood burning are noticeable sources, and the sulfur fraction is less important.

## AMBIENT AIR POLLUTION IN THE INTERNATIONAL SCENE

Many cities throughout the world have heavily contaminated air. Uncontrolled industry, growing automobile congestion, polluting cooking methods, and heating fuels cause cities of eastern Europe, Asia, Africa, and South America to resemble such cities as London, Pittsburgh, and New York thirty years ago. Since 1973 the WHO through its GEMS has been documenting total suspended particulate and $SO_2$ pollution. Beginning in 1978, $NO_2$ and lead have been monitored at traffic-related stations. By 1978, about 43 countries or areas with 170 monitoring stations were participating (WHO 1978). In a study of developing countries, Kirk Smith (1988) illustrated the relationship between pollution and national wealth by plotting urban particle air pollution against personal income (Figure 1.5). It is not uncommon for winter days in Beijing to be dark and gray because particle concentrations exceed 500 $\mu g/m^3$ (WHO EHE/EFP/85.5). Similarly, residential coal burning in the black townships of South Africa casts a thick morning pall of pollution in which particle concentrations can exceed 1,000 $\mu g/m^3$ (Kemeny, Ellerbeck, and Briggs 1988; Tshangwe, Kgamphe, and Annegarn 1988). In fact, regardless of whether or not indoor pollution sources exist, where the ambient air is heavily contaminated, human exposure can be dominated by the outdoor pollution.

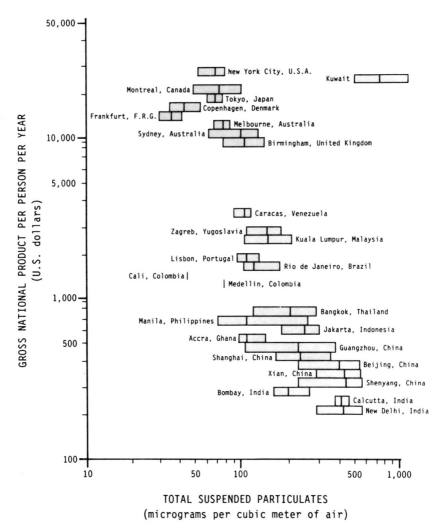

Figure 1.5. Total suspended particulate concentrations (μg/m³ in urban areas versus the gross national product per person [U.S. dollars]). *Source:* Smith (1988), reprinted with permission.

## INDOOR AIR POLLUTION IN THE INTERNATIONAL SCENE

Although ambient air pollution in developing countries is a problem mainly in urban areas, indoor air pollution can be quite high even in remote villages. Many of the world's poor people cook and heat their homes with biomass fuels of wood, crop residue, or dried animal dung. Some cultures use coal or briquettes made from powdered coal or charcoal. In his book *Biofuels, Air Pollution and Health: A Global Review* (1987), Kirk Smith asserted that exposure to emissions from biomass cooking and heating fuels is an important contributing factor to the incidence of early childhood respiratory infections and the development of chronic lung disease. Smith recounted that in numerous locations around the world the burning of wood, coal, charcoal, crop residue, and animal dung routinely produces indoor particle concentrations exceeding 1,000 $\mu g/m^3$, benzo[a]pyrene concentrations exceeding 1,000 $\mu g/m^3$, and CO concentrations exceeding 35 ppm, levels no longer encountered in developed countries with established ambient air pollution control programs. Concentrations in rural village huts, whose residents burn biomass fuels, exceed by factors of 10 to 100 the concentrations of particles and organic particulate matter in homes with modern cooking and heating appliances. Studies in India, Africa, China, and Nepal illustrate how universal these conditions are among poorer populations of developing countries (Smith 1987).

Human exposure to air pollutants is determined by concentrations outdoors and indoors. Although this book focuses on the health effects of indoor-generated contaminants, we deliberately set the perspective that contamination of outdoor air has important implications for human health and the earth's ecosystem. Most persons participate in outdoor activities and spend more time outdoors when the weather is good, thereby increasing their exposure to photochemically reactive pollutants like ozone, to acid sulfates, and to acid nitrate compounds. However, these and other less reactive pollutants are also brought into the indoor environment by natural and mechanical ventilation. The pollution of indoor air by ambient air can be minimized by reducing the air exchange, sealing the buildings, and by using filters, condensation coils, and duct work. With an effective ventilation system, contaminants that do penetrate to interior spaces go through several processes that speed removal. Most indoor environments have a large surface area compared with the volume; gases, vapors, and particles can be absorbed or can stick to these surfaces. Larger particles settle out because the indoor air currents are typically one-tenth to one-hundredth of the velocity of outdoor currents. Unless the air exchange is quite rapid, even nonreactive contaminants have lower integrated concentrations indoors than outdoors.

Most indoor living or working environments have air pollutant sources. Even people and pets can be sources of fibers, particles, organic vapors, and microbiologic material. Additional pollution comes from heating and cooking combustion sources, emissions from tobacco, abrasion of surfaces, outgasing of vapors, intrusion of soil gases, and a plethora of biologic sources; thus, it should not be surprising to find indoor environments that are substantially more polluted than the nearby outdoor air. High concentrations of pollution in indoor settings can, at times, dominate short- and long-term exposures and may be associated with discomfort, irritation, illness, and even death.

Human comfort has always been the primary focus of the design and operation of ventilation systems for buildings. The elements of comfort include, among other factors, temperature, temperature gradients, draftiness, humidity, noise, odors, and lighting. Subjective components also influence an occupant's perception of the environment. How comfortable, relaxed, or safe a person feels about an indoor space might depend on the furnishings, decorations, access to environmental controls, view of the exterior, neatness, cleanliness, and perception of hazards. Hodgson and co-workers (1987) added vibration to the elements that influence comfort. We do not yet have comprehensive data on the bounds for these factors which will lead to a judgment that indoor environmental quality is acceptable.

The American Society of Heating, Refrigerating, and Air-Conditioning Engineers (ASHRAE) developed consensus guidelines for ventilation requirements. Depending on the structure and use of the internal space, ASHRAE standards require different ventilation rates, measured as the cubic feet of outside air per minute per person. The current ventilation standards are published in a document entitled "Ventilation for Acceptable Indoor Air Quality," and are referred to as ASHRAE *Standard 62–1989*. This revised standard recommends 20 cfm/person as the minimum for offices and offers different requirements for other settings, although not less than 15 cfm/person in nonresidential buildings. The previous version (ASHRAE *Standard 62–1981*) advised 5 cfm/person as a minimum for nonsmoking environments and 25 cfm/person for areas with smoking permitted. At 15 cfm/person, $CO_2$ levels would be about 1,000 ppm in the absence of unvented combustion sources. In the presence of non-$CO_2$-producing sources, even 1,000 ppm of $CO_2$ might not be a valid indicator of adequate ventilation.

Table 1.2    Ventilation Standards and Guidelines for Residences[a]

| Region | Standard | Comment |
|---|---|---|
| Canada | 0.5 ACH[b] | Mechanical ventilation, mobile homes |
| California | 0.7 ACH | Standard for "tight" new residential buildings |
| Sweden | 0.5 ACH | All new structures with mechanical ventilation |
| France | 0.5 ACH | All new structures with mechanical ventilation |
| South Dakota | 0.5 ACH | All under consideration for mechanically and |
| Wisconsin | | naturally ventilated structures |
| Northwest Power Planning Council | | |
| ASHRAE | 0.35 ACH | Proposed in the new revised *ASHRAE Standard 62-1989* for living areas |
| | 15 cfm/person | ASHRAE *Standard 62-1989* |
| | 100 cfm | Installed mechanical exhaust capacity |

[a]Standards or guidelines for minimum air exchange or ventilation.
[b]Air exchanges per hour, 0.5 ACH indicates that one-half the volume of residence would be exchanged with outside air. In reality, it is applicable only with mechanical ventilation system. Minimum air exchange can not be guaranteed by construction alone.

Table 1.3 Ventilation Standards for Rooms within Residences

| | U.S. Standards | | |
| | ASHRAE *Standard 62-1973*; Single-Unit Dwellings (cfm/person) | | ANSI[a]/ASHRAE *Standard 62-1980*; Single or Multiple Units |
| Area | Minimum | Recommended | Minimum |
|---|---|---|---|
| General living areas and bedrooms | 5 | 7–10 | 15 cfm/person |
| Kitchens | 20 | 30–50 | 100 (intermittent exhaust capacity) 25 (continuous or windows) |
| Toilets, bathrooms | 20 | 30–50 | 50 (intermittent exhaust capacity) 25 (continuous or windows) |
| Basements, utility rooms | 5 | 5 | NA[b] |
| Garages (separate)[c] | | | 100 cfm/car space |
| Garages (common)[c] | | | 1.5 cfm/ft$^2$ |

| *Proposed Northern European Standards* | |
| Area | Minimum |
|---|---|
| General living areas | Minimum = 8 cfm/bed |
| | Continuous = 0.5 ACH[d] (measured in spring and autumn) |
| Kitchens | Continuous = 20 cfm, in addition to one of the following, depending upon stove type: |
| Electric stoves | |
| 2 rings | Minimum = 60-cfm capacity exhaust fan |
| >2 rings | Exhaust fan with capacity to remove 80% cooking fumes |
| Gas stoves | Exhaust fan with capacity to remove all combustion products |
| Toilets | Continuous = 20 cfm, in addition to either a 60 cfm-capacity exhaust fan or operable windows |

[a]ANSI, American National Standards Institute.
[b]NA, not applicable.
[c]Recommended by ASHRAE *Standard 62-1989*.
[d]Air changes per hour.

Tables 1.2 to 1.4 summarize some ventilation standards and guidelines for residences and commercial buildings.

In the absence of pollution sources, ventilation air serves three purposes. A minimum amount of fresh air is required to replace respired oxygen. Under most circumstances, less than 1 cfm/person is needed. About 2.5 cfm/person is needed to dilute $CO_2$, keeping concentrations below 5,000 ppm. Therefore, ventilation rates above the minimum of 2.5 cfm/person are required to dissipate odors, moisture, and heat. Few people would work without complaining in an environment that had only the minimum ventilation rate. Thus, ventilation is also needed

Table 1.4 Outdoor Air Requirements for Ventilation in Commercial Facilities

| Location | Estimated Occupancy (persons per 1,000-ft³ or 100-m² floor area) | Ventilation Requirement (cfm/person) | | |
|---|---|---|---|---|
| | | ASHRAE 62-1981 Smoking | Nonsmoking | ASHRAE 62-1989 |
| Food and beverage services | | | | |
| Dining rooms | 70 | 35 | 7 | 20 |
| Kitchens | 20 | | 10 | 15 |
| Cafeterias, fast food | 100 | 35 | 7 | 20 |
| Bars and lounges | 100 | 50 | 10 | 30 |
| Hotels, motels, resorts | | | | |
| Bedrooms | 5 | 30[a] | 15[a] | 30[a] |
| Bathrooms | | 50[a] | 25[a] | 35[a] |
| Lobbies | 30 | 15 | 5 | 15 |
| Conference rooms | 50 | 35 | 7 | 20 |
| Assembly rooms | 120 | 35 | 7 | 15 |
| Gambling casinos | 120 | 35 | 7 | 30 |
| Offices | | | | |
| Office spaces | 7 | 20 | 5 | 20 |
| Meeting and waiting | 60 | 35 | 7 | 20 |
| Smoking rooms | 70 | 50 | | 60 |
| Retail and shops | | | | |
| Sales floors | 30 | 25 | 5 | 15 |
| Malls/arcades | 20 | 10 | 5 | 20 |
| Barber and beauty | 25 | 35 | 20 | 25 |
| Health spas | 20 | | 15 | 20 |
| Sports and recreational | | | | |
| Discotheques | 100 | 35 | 7 | |
| Bowling alleys | 70 | 35 | 7 | 25 |
| Playing floors | 30 | | 20 | 20 |
| Spectator areas | 150 | 35 | 7 | 15 |
| Ice arenas[b] | | | | 0.5[c] |
| Swimming pools | | 0.5 | | 0.5[c] |
| Theaters | | | | |
| Lobbies and lounges | 150 | 35 | 7 | 20 |
| Auditoriums | | | | 15 |
| Transportation | | | | |
| Waiting rooms | 150 | 35 | 7 | 15 |
| Vehicles | 150 | | | 15 |
| Educational | | | | |
| Classrooms | 50 | 25 | 5 | 15 |
| Laboratories | 30 | | 10 | 20 |
| Training shops | 30 | 35 | 7 | 20 |
| Music rooms | 50 | 35 | 7 | 15 |
| Libraries | 20 | | 5 | 15 |
| Athletic lockers | | | | 0.5 |
| Corridors | | | | 0.1 |
| Hospitals, nursing and convalescent homes | | | | |
| Patient rooms | 10 | 35[d] | 7[d] | 25[d] |
| Medical procedure rooms | 10 | 35 | 7 | 15 |

(*continued*)

Table 1.4    (*Continued*)

| Location | Estimated Occupancy (persons per 1,000-ft$^3$ or 100-m$^2$ floor area) | Ventilation Requirement (cfm/person) | | |
|---|---|---|---|---|
| | | ASHRAE 62-1981 Smoking | Nonsmoking | ASHRAE 62-1989 |
| Operating rooms | 20 | | 40 | 30 |
| Recovery/intensive care units | 20 | | 15 | 15 |

*Source*: Adapted from ASHRAE *62-1981* and *62-1989*.
$^a$cfm/room.
$^b$If area has ice cleaner with internal combustion, add special ventilation.
$^c$cfm/ft$^2$ based on surface area of ice or pool.
$^d$cfm/bed

to reduce odors and maintain comfort. More than fifty years ago, Yaglou and co-workers (1936, 1937) investigated the acceptability of various ventilation rates. Most experiments were conducted in a chamber that was occupied by the experimental subjects, and the ventilation rate to the chamber was modified. Occupants and visitors were asked to smell the air and rate its acceptability. Through a series of experiments, Yaglou determined that a minimum of 10 cfm/person was required to provide an "odor-free" indoor environment. This approach assumes that the outdoor fresh air is odor free. Yaglou's experiments have been the primary reference for codes and standards for the last forty years.

Our appreciation of air involves more than just odor or a chemical sensation. We sense temperature. The sensation of heat is dependent upon the accompanying humidity and air motion. The relationship between temperature and humidity has led to the development of an "effective temperature" that relates to comfort. The definition of *effective temperature* is that temperature at which saturated air would provide the same sensation of comfort as does the actual temperature and humidity. Of course, the insulating property of clothing modifies the perception of comfort.

The concept of effective temperature has practical value. On a cold dry winter day, the relative humidity of a home typically might be 20 percent. With the heat set at 20°C (69°F), increasing the relative humidity to 70 percent would create the sensation of warming the air by close to 4°C, and the temperature would feel more like 75°F. In the summer, very low humidities make hot weather more bearable because of evaporative cooling of the skin.

Most people are familiar with the concept of wind chill. Skin exposed to wind and cold temperatures will have the sensation of lower temperature. Body heat is advected away more quickly with high wind speeds, causing more rapid cooling of heated surfaces. This phenomenon has applications to indoor environments. By the middle of one of the hottest summers on record for the northeastern United States (1988), fans were sold out in most commercial retail stores. Since blowing air across the body gives the sensation of cooling, the sensation of air movement in buildings, cars, and homes (drafts) is critical to comfort. Too little air movement can give the feeling of stuffiness, and too much draft can result in feeling chilled.

Even without pollution, comfort and acceptable indoor air quality are achieved with an appropriate balance among several factors, including temperature, relative humidity, odors, and airflow. Figure 1.6 describes a rather broad comfort and human tolerance zone. People feel most comfortable if the indoor air temperature is between 20 and 27°C (68 and 80°F) with relative humidities between 30 and 70 percent.

A broader definition of acceptable indoor air quality might also consider physical, chemical, and biologic contaminants. However, of the numerous contaminants that have been identified indoors, standards or guidelines have been published for only a few. In many instances, the standards and guidelines are based on ambient air quality or occupational standards. Some of these values have been modified in consideration of the differences between occupational settings and residences, public buildings, and offices. However, for most indoor contaminants, epidemiologic studies conducted on the exposed populations have not been done, and relevant guidelines have not been prepared. For example, we lack guidelines for most of the numerous volatile organic compounds identified in indoor air quality surveys.

There is no universally adopted comprehensive definition of acceptable indoor air quality. This is understandable given the diversity of sources and indoor environments. We have prepared a list of air quality standards and guidelines that have been applied to indoor environments (see Table 1.1). Some are standards promulgated by countries or states; others are suggested only as action levels and are not enforceable. Still other values are based on occupational standards or recommendations from professional organizations. The list is not comprehensive; we recognize that even suggesting a universal guideline for many of the indoor contaminants discussed in this book is unreasonable at this time. The levels set forth today may not prove adequate to protect the entire population against all long-term health effects. Presentation of these standards here does not imply endorsement by the authors; they are intended merely to serve as a guide to the reader.

Standards should recognize the functional use of the indoor space and characteristics of the occupants. It might be reasonable to have different values for the same contaminant in a preschool and in a nursing home. Contaminants with chronic effects might have limits appropriate for homes, for example, where we may spend two-thirds of our lives, but not for sports arenas. Even in homes, concerns about carcinogenic pollutants may be different for young children than for elderly residents. For example, the response to a slightly elevated radon concentration in the basement might depend on occupant ages and expected length of residency.

Subjective judgments about acceptable indoor environmental conditions are made daily. For comfort and irritation effects, nonsensitized individuals can tolerate a broad range of conditions. In part, tolerance of indoor environmental conditions reflects the perceived benefits derived from that space. Breathing passive

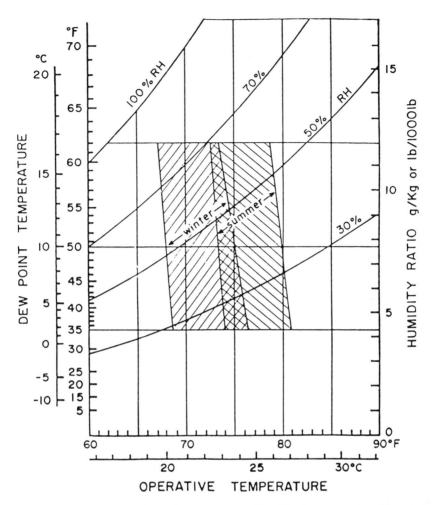

Figure 1.6. Acceptable ranges of operative temperature and humidity for a person clothed in typical summer and winter clothing engaged in light activity (mainly sedentary, ≤ 1.2 metabolic equivalents). *Source: ASHRAE Standard 55-1981.*

cigarette smoke at concentrations of a few hundred micrograms per cubic meter while in a nightclub might be acceptable for a few hours, especially during an enjoyable performance. However, these same levels at work might cause complaints.

In defining acceptable indoor air quality, it should be recognized that current knowledge is very limited. Undoubtedly, synergistic effects occur among pollutants in indoor air, but our understanding of the effects of mixtures is limited. The recent work of Molhave and his colleagues illustrates that exposures to mixtures of volatile organic compounds commonly found indoors evoke sensory and performance reactions at levels well below any known threshold limit value (Molhave, Busch, and Pedersen 1986). Berglund and Lindvall (1986) suggested that the response might be deeply rooted in man's psychological "fright-flight" response. They conjectured that with exposure to these mixtures of organic compounds we perceive an irritating chemical sensation. Subconsciously we wish to flee the sensations, but socially we have been conditioned to believe indoor environments are safe or that we must stay at work. Berglund and Lindvall (1986) argued that these conflicts create a series of stress-related symptoms. These experiments indicate the need for more studies of the effects of complex mixtures.

In developing indoor air quality guidelines, it must be recognized that a segment of the population may be particularly sensitive or reactive at very low concentrations. For example, prior exposure to biologic or chemical agents may lead to an immunologic response such as development of specific antibodies, and with additional exposure, even at low concentrations, the sensitized person might experience allergic reactions. Many individuals report immediate or delayed reactions to a wide variety of materials or indoor environments. Often, it is difficult to discern whether the person is displaying a physiologic response to a chemical, physical, or biologic agent, or a psychologically mediated response.

Thus, developing a definition of acceptable indoor air quality which addresses *all* determinants of comfort and health for *all* individuals seems impossible at present. Simply shifting definitions developed for outdoor air to indoor air is unsatisfactory. Definitions of outdoor air pollution (e.g., the Commonwealth of Massachusetts) emphasize not only health effects but also enjoyment and productivity. Because outdoor air is common property, pollution is controlled through statutory and legal means for the benefit of all persons. By contrast, indoor environments are maintained at direct cost by homeowners and building owners or operators. Shifting social and environmental contexts and changing costs for heating, cooling, and cleaning indoor air may affect concepts of acceptability.

Nevertheless, although a lasting definition of acceptable indoor air quality cannot be given, we suggest that health, comfort, productivity, and cost must all be considered. Even though some may consider the inclusion of cost as inappropriate, the specification of fiscally unachievable conditions would have little value. Achieving the proper balance between cost on the one hand and health, comfort, and productivity on the other may be difficult. Searching for consensus among building occupants may prove to be a successful approach. Occupants need information about the indoor air they breathe and the systems in place to maintain indoor air quality. Providing occupants with some control over indoor air quality may be needed to assure acceptability.

It is likely that the definition of acceptable indoor air quality will be debated well into the next century. However, guiding principles should be adopted now. Occupants need insight, information, and influence. Regardless of economic considerations, levels of contaminants cannot be allowed which cause or contribute to severe irritation, sensitization, or illness of any type.

In the United States and many other countries, regulations have been implemented with the goal of achieving clean outdoor air and thereby improving public health. Reductions in outdoor concentrations of many pollutants have been well documented, and obvious pollution episodes with attendant morbidity and mortality are now rare. As the outdoor air has become cleaner, the importance of indoor air in determining exposures to many inhaled pollutants has become increasingly evident. It is now clear that protection of public health requires satisfactory outdoor and indoor air quality. Moreover, the public also expects a degree of indoor air quality to assure comfort.

The Clean Air Act provides a regulatory framework for the United States which is designed to achieve and maintain lowered pollutant levels in outdoor air, meeting standards established to prevent the occurrence of adverse health effects. This complex legislation specifies that standards should be set for ambient air quality and provides a process for achieving clean outdoor air. The Clean Air Act is administered by the EPA, which has enforcement authority.

We lack a comparable comprehensive legal, regulatory, administrative and technical framework for approaching the problem of indoor air pollution. Indoor air quality problems may result from natural sources, poor building design, inadequate building maintenance, structural components and furnishings, consumer products, and occupant activities. Control of these diverse sources of pollution in the air of public and private buildings poses an unprecedented challenge—a challenge that we are only now recognizing.

The U.S. government has not yet established a framework to develop policies for indoor air as it has for outdoor air. Sexton and co-workers (Sexton 1986, 1987) addressed the sequence of steps which must be followed to evolve responsible and effective control strategies (Table 1.5). Scientific data are needed for the first steps of problem definition and health risk assessment. Sources and exposures must be characterized, not only for health risk assessment but also as a basis for the development of methods for control.

The concepts and terminology of health risk assessment were defined and described in a 1983 report by a committee of the National Research Council (NRC 1983). The concept of health risk assessment is uncomplicated. The first step is hazard identification; that is, agents that pose a risk to human health are identified through epidemiologic observations, animal bioassay, short-term *in vitro* tests, or other toxicologic evidence. Second, the dose-response relationships that quantify the risk per unit exposure to the agent are established. Third, the distribution of human exposure to the agent is determined. Fourth, by combining the dose-response relationship with the information on exposure, the magnitude of the human health problem is estimated.

Health risk assessment provides a useful approach for estimating the hazard posed to the population and for identifying uncertainties in the scientific evidence which may require resolution before policy can be evolved. It may also be used to

Table 1.5   Summary of the Major Steps in Addressing Indoor Air Quality Problems

| | |
|---|---|
| Problem definition | Resolution of policy issues |
|    Emission sources |    Building "publicness" |
|    Dilution |    Conservation benefits |
|    Indoor concentrations |    Voluntary versus nonvoluntary risks |
|    Activity patterns |    Importance of short-term/long-term health effects |
|    Exposures |    Public versus private responsibility |
|    Health consequences |    Local, state, or federal intervention |
| Health risk assessment |    Appropriate government responses |
|    Number of people exposed | Alternative government responses |
|    Severity of exposure |    No action |
|    Dose-response relationship |    More research |
| Applicability of mitigating measures |    Public information |
|    Ventilation |    Economic incentives |
|    Source removal |    Moral suasion |
|    Source modification |    Legal liability |
|    Air cleaning |    Guidelines |
|    Behavioral adjustment |    Rules/regulations |

compare the hazards posed by different pollutants as a basis for establishing priorities and to estimate the potential reduction in health risk which would follow intervention.

Sexton's third step is an assessment of the applicability of available measures for mitigation, which may be broadly classified as increased ventilation, source removal, source modification, air cleaning, and change in behavior. Selection of the optimal mitigation approach must balance technological feasibility, efficacy, cost, and acceptability.

Decisions in problem definition, health risk assessment, and applicability of mitigation measures are made primarily on the basis of scientific evidence. However, the answers to critical policy questions require a process that integrates government and private interests and responsibilities. The need to create an approach for dealing with these issues on indoor air quality is immediate. For example, radon is a well-documented cause of lung cancer, it has now been found to be present in all homes, and at high concentrations comparable to levels found in uranium mines in some homes (Samet and Nero 1989). Effective and relatively inexpensive methods are available for measuring radon in indoor air and for lowering concentrations to levels presently judged as acceptable. Yet, we have not evolved a national control strategy for radon which addresses satisfactorily the policy issues and options described by Sexton (Sexton 1986; Nero 1988; Samet and Nero 1989).

The government has diverse options for controlling an indoor air pollution problem, ranging from taking no action to implementing specific rules and regulations. The choice of option should maximize public health protection and acceptability to the population and acknowledge the responsibilities and liabilities of the involved parties. Although this broad basis for selection among options available to the government is evident, a systematic approach to decision making has not yet been developed. The federal government has so far pursued voluntary industry codes and standards for kerosene space heaters and has offered an "action guideline" for radon; it has also provided guidance on handling asbestos in schools and has now moved to begin eliminating new use of asbestos. Indoor air pollution by environmental tobacco smoke has been handled by some states and municipalities, and public education has been undertaken by governmental and nongovernmental agencies to alter behavior.

Existing statutory authorities do not provide a single federal agency with jurisdiction over indoor air (Table 1.6) (Sexton 1986). The EPA is responsible for ambient air through the Clean Air Act. Under the provisions of Title IV of the Superfund Amendments and Reauthorization Act of 1986, Radon and Indoor Air Quality Research, Congress directed the EPA to establish a research program to address radon and other indoor pollutants. The research program was mandated to address data gathering, to coordinate research activities, and to assess federal actions on mitigation of environmental and health risks associated with indoor air.

Table 1.6   Federal Laws Potentially Applicable to Indoor Air

National Environmental Policy Act: A broad act that establishes as a national goal "to assure for all Americans safe, healthful, productive, and aesthetically and culturally pleasing surroundings."
Clean Air Act: Gives EPA regulatory authority over outdoor air.
Toxic Substances Control Act: Provides EPA with authority to collect and develop data on the risks of chemicals and to restrict manufacturing, distribution, and use of toxic chemicals, including indoor air contaminants.
Federal Insecticides, Fungicide, and Rodenticide Act: Provides EPA with authority to collect data, to monitor, and to regulate pesticide use, including those used indoors.
Asbestos Hazard Emergency Response Act and the Asbestos School Hazard Detection and Control Act: Requires EPA to develop regulations detailing methods for handling asbestos in schools. The Detection and Control Act creates a task force for the problem.
Superfund Amendments and Reauthorization Act, Title IV: Radon Gas and Indoor Air Quality Research Act: Requires EPA to establish a research program.
Safe Drinking Water Act: Authorizes EPA to perform research on contaminants in drinking water. The regulatory authority extends to contaminants in public water supplies which have adverse effects through indoor air pollution.
Consumer Product Safety Act: Provides Consumer Product Safety Commission with authority to regulate consumer products causing injury.
Federal Hazardous Substance Act: Authorizes Consumer Product Safety Commission to require labeling for household products that are hazardous.
Occupational Safety and Health Act: As a national policy, "To assure as far as possible every working man and woman in the nation safe and healthy working conditions."
National Manufactured Housing Construction and Safety Standards Act of 1974: Directs the Department of Housing and Urban Development to establish standards for construction and safety of manufactured housing. Features related to indoor air pollution have been regulated.
Department of Energy Organization Act of 1977: Requires integration of national environmental protection goals in developing energy programs. Mandates research on energy technologies and programs.
Energy Reorganization Act of 1974: Charges Environmental Research and Development Administration (ERDA) with research on environmental, biomedical, physical, and safety research related to energy.
Atomic Energy Act: Authorizes research relevant to radon and nonionizing radiation.
Energy Conservation and Production Act: Has the goal of reducing energy demand, but Department of Energy must consider potential health consequences.

An implementation plan has now been prepared and reviewed by a committee of the agency's Science Advisory Board (U.S. EPA 1987).

In its 1987 report to Congress on indoor air quality, as mandated by Title IV, above, the EPA outlined policy objectives and strategy. Research was proposed to refine understanding of health effects; emphasis was placed on obtaining data for risk assessment. The agency also planned to identify and assess mitigation methods for high-priority problems. The proposed strategy for control was multifaceted and included regulating under existing authorities (Table 1.6), augmenting governmental and private capabilities to manage indoor air quality problems, referring problems to other federal agencies having regulatory authority, and requesting regulatory authority from Congress. The agency stated a clear preference for avoiding regulation and achieving its goals through research and development, dissemination of information, and technical assistance and training.

In addition to the EPA, other federal agencies are also involved in indoor air quality. The National Institute for Occupational Safety and Health conducts health hazard evaluations of workplaces considered to be unhealthy; large numbers of evaluations have been conducted in nonindustrial settings to evaluate problems related to indoor air quality. The Department of Energy oversees energy conservation activities, and it is charged with considering the health consequences of energy conservation programs; it also has its own research program in several areas, including radon. Under the Consumer Product Safety Act, the Consumer Product Safety Commission has authority to regulate products causing injury. The commission has addressed asbestos, urea-formaldehyde foam insulation, biologic dissemination from humidifiers, and unvented combustion appliances. The Department of Housing and Urban Development sets building standards for agency-funded projects and standards for materials for mobile homes. Federal activities on indoor air are coordinated through the congressionally mandated Interagency Committee on Indoor Air Quality.

The policy dilemma posed by indoor air pollution has become increasingly evident as the contributions of indoor air pollution to personal exposures have been described in research conducted during the 1970s and 1980s. The complex and expensive activities mandated by the Clean Air Act address only selected pollutants and only the outdoor contributions to personal exposures. The protection of public health will require substantial evolution of our approach to policy-making on indoor air quality.

## REFERENCES

Altshuller, A. P. 1983. Review: Natural volatile organic substances and their effect on air quality in the United States. *Atmos. Environ.* 17:2131–65.
American Society of Heating, Refrigerating, and Air-Conditioning Engineers. 1981. *ASHRAE Standard 55-1981: Thermal environmental conditions for human occupancy.* Atlanta, Ga.: ASHRAE.

American Society of Heating, Refrigerating, and Air-Conditioning Engineers. 1981. *ASHRAE Standard 62-1981: Ventilation for acceptable indoor air quality.* Atlanta, Ga.: ASHRAE.

American Society of Heating, Refrigerating, and Air-Conditioning Engineers. 1989. *ASHRAE Standard 62-1989: Ventilation for acceptable indoor air quality.* Atlanta, Ga.: ASHRAE.

Berglund, B., and Lindvall, T. 1986. Sensory reactions to "sick buildings." *Environ. Int.* 12:147–59.

Cooper, J. A.; Watson, J. G.; and Huntzicker, J. J. 1979. Summary of the Portland aerosol characterization study. Paper 79-24.4 presented at the seventy-second annual meeting of the Air Pollution Control Association, 24–29 June, Cincinnati, Ohio.

Ember, L. R., et al. 1986. Tending the global commons. *Chem. Eng. News* 64:14–15.

Evelyn, J. 1661. *Fumiogorum, or the inconvenience of the Aer and Smoake of London Dissipated. Together with some remedies humbly proposed.* 2d printing 1772, quoted in Lodge, J. P. 1969. *The Smoke of London: Two Prophecies.* Maxwell Reprint Co., Fairview Park, Elmsford, N.Y.

Fox, D. L.; Kamens, R.; and Jeffries, H. 1975. Photochemical smog system: Effect of dilution on ozone formation. *Science* 188:1113–14.

Gordon, G. 1988. Receptor models. *Environ. Sci. Technol.* 22:1132–52.

Grosjean, D.; Williams, E.; and Van Neste, A. 1982. Measurements of organic acids in the south coast air basin. *Final report A5-177-32 for California Air Resources Board.*

Hodgson, M. J., et al. 1987. Vibration as a cause of tight building syndrome symptoms. *Indoor air '87: Proceedings of the fourth international conference on indoor air quality and climate.* Ed. B. Seifert et al., 449–53. Berlin: Institute for Water, Soil, and Air Hygiene.

Ito, K., and Thurston, G. D. 1987. The estimation of London, England, aerosol exposure from historical visibility records. Paper 87-42.2, presented at the eightieth annual meeting of the Air Pollution Control Association, 21–26 June, New York.

Kemeny, E.; Ellerbeck, R. H.; and Briggs, A. B. 1988. An assessment of smoke pollution in Soweto: Residential air pollution. *Proceedings of the National Association for Clean Air,* 10–11 November, Pretoria, South Africa, 152–63. Available through NACA, P.O. Box 5777, Johannesburg 2000, South Africa.

Kuntasal, G., and Chang, T. Y. 1987. Trends and relationships of $O_3$, $NO_x$ and HC in the south coast air basin of California. *J. Air Pollut. Control Assoc.* 35:1158–63.

Meyers, R. E., et al. 1978. *Constraints on coal utilization with respect to air pollution production and transport over long distances: Summary.* Upton, N.Y.: Brookhaven National Laboratory Report.

Molhave, L.; Busch, B.; and Pedersen, O. F. 1986. Human reactions to low concentrations of volatile organic compounds. *Environ. Int.* 12:169–75.

Morandi, M. T. 1985. Development of source apportionment models for inhalable particulate matter and its extractable organic fractions in urban areas of New Jersey. New York University.

Morandi, M. T.; Daisey, J. M.; and Lioy, P. J. 1987. Inhalable particulate matter and extractable organic matter receptor source apportionment models for the ATEOS urban sites. In *Toxic air pollution: A comprehensive study of non-criteria air pollutants.* Ed. P. J. Lioy and J. M. Daisey, 228. Chelsea, Mich.: Lewis Publishers.

National Research Council. 1983. Committee on the Institutional Means for Assessment of

Risks to Public Health. *Risk Assessment in the Federal Government: Managing the Process.* Washington, D.C.: National Academy Press.

Nero, A. V., Jr. 1988. Controlling indoor air pollution. *Sci Am.* 258:42–48.

Samet, J. M., and Nero, A. V., Jr. 1989. Indoor radon and lung cancer: A strategy for control? *N. Engl. J. Med.* 320:591–94.

Sega, K., and Fugas, M. 1982. Personal exposure versus monitoring station data for respirable particles. *Environ. Int.* 8:259–63.

Sexton, K. 1986. Indoor air quality: An overview of policy and regulatory issues. *Sci. Technol. Human Values* 11:53–67.

Sexton, K. 1987. Public policy implications of exposure to indoor pollution. In *Indoor Air '87: Proceedings of the fourth international conference on indoor air quality and climate.* Ed. B. Seifert et al., Vol. 4, 105–16. Berlin: Institute for Water, Soil, and Air Hygiene.

Smith, K. 1987. *Biofuels, air pollution, and health.* New York: Plenum.

Smith, K. R. 1988. Air pollution: Assessing total exposure in developing countries. *Environment* 30:16.

Spengler, J. D., et al. 1986. Sulfuric acid and sulfate aerosol events in two U.S. cities. In *Aerosols.* Ed. S. D. Lee, et al., 107–20. Chelsea, Mich.: Lewis Publishers.

Spengler, J. D. et al. 1989. Exposures to acidic aerosols. *Environ. Health Perspect.* 79:43–51.

Stern, A. C. 1982. History of air pollution legislation in the United States. *J. Air Pollut. Control Assoc.* 32:44–61.

Tshangwe, H. T.; Kgamphe, J. S.; and Annegarn, H. J. 1988. Indoor-outdoor air particulate study in a Soweto home: Residential air pollution. *Proceedings of the National Association for Clean Air,* 10–11. November, Pretoria, South Africa, 164–75. Available through NACA, P.O. Box 5777, Johannesburg 2000, South Africa.

U.S. Congress. Office of Technology Assessment. 1985. *Acid rain and transported air pollutants.* New York: UNIPUB.

U.S. Environmental Protection Agency. 1982. *Air quality criteria for particulate matter and sulfur dioxide.* Research Triangle Park, N.C.: Office of Health and Environmental Assessment, EPA publication no. EPA/600/8-82/029. Available from NTIS, Springfield, Va., PBS4-156801/REB.

U.S. Environmental Protection Agency. Office of Air and Radiation. 1987. *EPA indoor air quality implementation plan.* Washington, D.C.: Government Printing Office. EPA publication no. EPA/600/8-87/031.

U.S. Environmental Protection Agency. Office of Health and Environmental Assessment. 1989. *Acid aerosols issue paper.* Washington, D.C.: Government Printing Office. EPA publication no. EPA/600/8-88/0005a.

U.S. Environmental Protection Agency. 1989. *National air quality and emission trends report, 1987.* Research Triangle Park, N.C.: Office of Air Quality Planning and Standards, Monitoring and Reports Branch. EPA publication no. EPA/450/4-89/001.

Walker, H. M. 1985. Ten year ozone trends in California and Texas. *J Air Pollut. Control Assoc.* 35:903–12.

Wilson, R., et al. 1980. *Health effects of fossil fuels.* Cambridge, Mass.: Ballinger Press.

World Health Organization. 1978. *Air quality in selected urban areas 1975–76.* Geneva: WHO Offset publication no. 41.

World Health Organization. EHE-EFP/85-5 *Urban air pollution in the People's Republic of*

*China, 1981–84.* (Not a formal publication, prepared to assist with implementation of WHO/UNEP Global Air Monitoring Project.)

Yaglou, C. P.; Riley, E. C.; and Coggins, D. I. 1936. Ventilation requirements. *ASHRAE Trans.* 42:133–62.

Yaglou, C. P., and Witheridge, W. N. 1937. Ventilation requirements: Part 2. *ASHRAE Trans.* 43:423–36.

# I. SOURCES, CONCENTRATIONS, AND EXPOSURE

# 2

# SOURCES AND CONCENTRATIONS OF INDOOR AIR POLLUTION

John D. Spengler, Ph.D., M.S.

Indoor air pollution arises from indoor and outdoor sources. This chapter describes indoor sources of air pollution. Information on outdoor sources can be obtained from standard texts such as Lippmann and Schlesinger (1979) and Stern et al. (1984). Indoor pollutants can be categorized by type of source, such as combustion, and by pollutant group, such as volatile organic compounds (VOCs) and fibers. Sources can be characterized by the pollutants emitted, by the source locations, and by the rate and pattern of emissions. In the context of mass-balance models, we consider the roles of source strength, volume of distribution, dilution, and removal in determining indoor concentrations (NRC 1981a). These models do not consider, however, patterns of source use and maintenance, which may be strong determinants of exposure. For some pollutants, the presence of a potential source does not necessarily indicate exposure. For example, the presence of fibrous asbestos-containing material in a building may not result in exposure to asbestos except under circumstances in which the material is disturbed or inadequately maintained.

Pollutant species are typically described under the broad source headings of combustion, evaporation, abrasion, biologic, and radon. Table 2.1 lists the major indoor sources and contaminants. Some sources are potential and contribute to indoor air pollution only when used or operated in an improper or unplanned fashion (e.g., asbestos).

Emission rates for indoor sources are reported in a variety of units. Physical mass-balance emission rates in models typically require units of mass per time, such as micrograms per second or grams per hour. Combustion sources that consume fuel can be characterized by mass released per unit of energy. If the fuel consumption rate and the energy per unit are known, fuel emissions can be reexpressed as mass per time. The emission rates for most conventional combustion

Table 2.1  Sources of Common Indoor Contaminants

| Contaminant | Source |
|---|---|
| **Asbestos** | |
| Chrysotile | Some wall and ceiling insulation installed between 1930 and |
| Crocidolite | 1950 |
| Amosite | Old insulation on heating pipes and equipment |
| Tremolite | Old wood stove door gaskets |
| | Some vinyl floor tiles |
| | Drywall joint-finishing material and textured paint purchased before 1977 |
| | Cement-asbestos millboard and exterior wall shingles |
| | Some sprayed and troweled ceiling finishing plaster installed between 1945 and 1973 |
| | Sprayed onto some structural steel beams as fire retardant |
| **Combustion By-products** | |
| Carbon monoxide | Gas range |
| Nitrogen dioxide | Wood and coal stoves |
| Sulfur dioxide | Gas and propane engines |
| Particulate soot | Fireplaces |
| Nitrogenated compounds | Backdrafting of exhaust flues |
| | Candles and incense |
| **Tobacco Smoke** | |
| Carbon monoxide | Cigarettes |
| Nitrogen dioxide | Pipes |
| Carbon dioxide | Cigars |
| Hydrogen cyanide | |
| Nitrosamines | |
| Aromatic hydrocarbons | |
| Benzo[a]pyrene | |
| Particles | |
| Benzene | |
| Formaldehyde | |
| Nicotine | |
| **Formaldehyde** | Some particle board, plywood, pressed-board, paneling |
| | Some carpeting and carpet backing |
| | Some furniture and dyed materials |
| | Urea-formaldehyde insulating foam |
| | Some household cleaners and deodorizers |
| | Combustion (gas, tobacco, wood) |
| | Some glues and resins |
| | Tobacco smoke |
| | Cosmetics |
| | Permanent-press textiles |
| **Biologic organisms** | |
| Fungal spores | Mold, mildew, and other fungi |
| Bacteria | Humidifiers with stagnant water |
| Virus | Water-damaged surfaces and materials |
| Pollens | Condensing coils and drip pans in HVAC systems |
| Arthropods | Drainage pans in refrigerators |
| Protozoa | Some thermophilics on dirty heating coils |
| | Animals |
| | Rodents |
| | Insects |
| | Humans |

*(continued)*

Table 2.1  (*Continued*)

| Contaminant | Source |
|---|---|
| Radon | |
| Radon gas and radon progeny | Radon gas emanating from soil, rocks, and water that diffuses through cracks and holes in the foundation and floor |
| | Radon in well water |
| | Radon in natural gas used near the source wells |
| | Some building materials such as granite |
| Volatile organic compounds | |
| Alkanes | Solvents and cleaning compounds |
| Aromatic hydrocarbons | Paints |
| Esters | Glues and resins |
| Alcohols | Spray propellants |
| Aldehydes | Fabric softeners and deodorizers |
| Ketones | Combustion |
| | Dry-cleaning fluids |
| | Some fabrics and furnishings |
| | Stored gasoline |
| | Outgasing from water |
| | Some building materials |
| | Waxes and polishing compounds |
| | Pens and markers |
| | Binders and plasticizers |

sources have been characterized in laboratory settings (Moschandreas 1983). For some sources, *in situ* measurements have been reported, and real-life emissions have been shown to vary considerably from the laboratory conditions.

This chapter does not provide detailed information on emission rates; emission rate data are published in several documents and reports, including the Environmental Protection Agency's *Preliminary Indoor Air Pollution Information Assessment Appendix*, published in June 1987 (EPA/600/8–87/014). This EPA document reports emission rates for combustion appliances and also summarizes emission rates of formaldehyde and other organic vapors from building materials. Emissions from cigarettes have been reported in considerable detail in recent reports (National Research Council [NRC] 1986; U.S. Department of Health and Human Services [U.S. DHHS] 1986).

Describing "steady-state" or even transient emission rates may not provide sufficient information. For the purpose of modeling, sources may be considered as having constant emission rates; but in actual use, emission rates vary. Combustion sources often emit more during start-up than during continued use, and fuel characteristics and fueling rates can cause emissions to vary. Cooking and smoking may take place both periodically and sporadically. Nevertheless, the routine contributions of these sources to indoor pollution can be estimated. For example, the potential for vented appliances to backdraft can be calculated from such factors as chimney height, emission buoyancy, and wind speed over the stack. However, the backdrafting of a water heater and the associated quantity of emissions released into the interior of the building cannot be readily predicted.

Some contaminants are outgased from materials. Although the overall emission rate depends upon the amount of material used, emission rates are usually not constant. For example, the release rate of formaldehyde from urea-formaldehyde foam insulation (UFFI) depends upon partial pressures of the gas, humidity, temperature, and the air exchange rate. Similarly, the leakage of soil gases such as radon into the basement of a home varies not only with the concentration beneath the slab, but with the fluctuation of air pressures in the basement.

Asbestos fibers are released into indoor air episodically and not at a constant rate. Fibers can become airborne when the surface of asbestos-containing materials is mechanically disrupted, but fibers can also be released through other mechanisms. Nicholson et al. (1978) measured an increased asbestos concentration in a school after a heavy rainstorm. The increase was attributed to asbestos washed from asbestos cement walkways and asbestos cement roof panels. Danish investigations have shown that generation of man-made mineral fibers from ceiling tiles depends upon the binders and other factors (Danish Building Research Institute 1987). Apparently, water-based resins absorb moisture and weaken the bond, releasing fibers more readily than epoxy-type binders.

At present, it is nearly impossible to characterize the source rate for biologic materials. Spores can be released periodically or only with an appropriate environmental stimulus (by heat or moisture, for example). Other biologically important material, such as house dust mites or the nonviable, but allergenic, material from fungal organisms, can be present but not airborne. Vacuuming, shaking blankets, or even a child's playing on a carpet can cause these materials to become airborne and result in antigen exposure. Unless samples are taken when the biologic material is actively introduced into the air, antigenic material may not be detected. Such biologic exposures illustrate the potential influence of human activities on source strength; however, it is impossible to predict the source strength in terms of mass of antigenic material released per unit of time for these activities.

## CONTAMINANTS BY SOURCE

### COMBUSTION

Combustion sources emit inorganic gases ($H_2O$, $NO$, $NO_2$, $CO$, $CO_2$) and particles. In addition, depending on fuel type and pyrolysis conditions, combustion sources can also emit hydrocarbon gases, vapors, and organic particles. Most liquid and solid fuels have impurities or additives. As the fuels burn, metals, mercaptans, sulfur oxides, and particles can be emitted. The particles may be partially burned carbon soot or minerals and are readily visible when released from oil-, wood-, or kerosene-fueled appliances. Many of the particles produced are large and settle out, contributing to soiling. However, even gas appliances, if operated below stoichiometric conditions, will emit particles in the submicron size range. Burning tobacco generates particles in the 0.1- to 1-$\mu$m range.

Because some combustion sources burn at temperatures high enough ($>900°C$)

to produce atomic nitrogen, these sources can produce nitrogenated species in the effluent. Traynor et al. (1983a, 1983b) have reported formation of nitrated polycyclic aromatic hydrocarbons from both well-tuned and maladjusted kerosene space heaters but at rates 10,000 to 100,000 times lower than the total particulate emission rates.

*Gas Combustion*    Unvented gas combustion is a ubiquitous source of $NO_2$ and CO in residences. Many studies indicate that gas ranges can increase indoor $NO_2$ concentrations above ambient levels. The $NO_2$ levels in homes with gas ranges are nearly always higher than the levels inside homes with electric ranges in the same community (Wade, Cote, and Yocom 1975; Spengler et al. 1979, 1983; Yocom et al. 1982; Moschandreas 1983; Marbury et al. 1988). Figure 2.1 displays week-long $NO_2$ averaged concentrations collected over a year-long study in Portage, Wisconsin. The ambient levels were between 15 and 20 $\mu g/m^3$. For electric cooking homes, the average indoor concentrations were less than ambient levels; in the gas cooking homes, indoor concentrations always exceeded ambient levels. Kitchen values were twice the bedroom concentrations. A distinct seasonal pattern was present, with higher concentrations in the fall and winter seasons.

In a more recent study, more than five hundred homes in the Los Angeles area were monitored for $NO_2$ three times during a year (Baker et al. 1987; Colome et al. 1987). In Los Angeles, the ambient levels of $NO_2$ were more than five times higher than in Portage. Although gas cooking sources were important contributors to indoor $NO_2$ air pollution, the ambient air had a major influence. A similar large-scale study of five hundred residential units was conducted in Boston (Ryan et al. 1988). Data from this study show the importance of gas pilot lights, which consume about one-third of the gas burned by a cooking stove and contribute about 12 ppb to the indoor $NO_2$ concentrations.

Most of the studies of indoor $NO_2$ report the time-averaged concentration over days to weeks. However, under most circumstances, range use usually lasts minutes, and most meals are prepared in less than one hour. Harlos (1988) equipped subjects with personal continuous $NO_2$ monitors and measured their exposures to $NO_2$ during the preparation of fifty meals (Figure 2.2). The short-term concentrations of one minute or less were independent of the longer averaging times and reflect the exposures received by a person working near the range or opening the oven door. Personal exposures for averaging times of three minutes and longer correlated with readings of a fixed-location monitor in the kitchen. This correlation indicates that mixing and dilution factors are more important than the individual's behavior in determining concentrations for longer averaging times.

Surveys of indoor $NO_2$ concentrations document considerable variation among homes, reflecting differences in source use, emission rates, mixing of the air, house volume, and air exchange rates. Most homes, even with unvented combustion sources, do not exceed the national ambient air quality standard for $NO_2$. Types of sources and home volume have been shown to underlie elevated con-

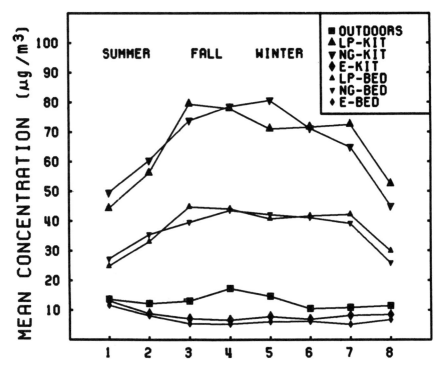

Figure 2.1. Seasonal variation (July 1980–June 1981) $NO_2$ concentrations ($\mu g/m^3$) in indoor locations and outdoors in Portage, Wisconsin. Kitchen, bedroom, and outdoors in homes with liquid propane (LP), natural gas (NG), and electricity (E) as cooking fuels. *Source:* Spengler et al. (1983), reprinted with permission.

centrations in some homes. Wall and floor furnaces were associated with increased concentrations in the Los Angeles study. In the Boston study, public housing units tended to have higher concentrations.

The studies by Goldstein et al. (1987) of $NO_2$ and CO in Harlem, New York, housing showed that excessive stove use and small-volume living units contributed to elevated concentrations. Parkhurst et al. (1988) reported a winter survey of $NO_2$ in public housing in Chattanooga, Tennessee. In this urban environment, housing units with gas appliances had multiweek averages exceeding 50 ppb. More than 10 percent of the housing units exceeded 200 ppb over the four weeks. The analysis by Parkhurst and co-workers indicates that units with smaller, vented space heaters located central to the apartment had higher indoor $NO_2$ levels. This association and the residents' own reports suggest that the residents were heating their kitchens with the gas range.

Carbon monoxide emissions from gas stoves are typically ten times the emission rate of $NO_2$. Yet, under typical conditions, concentrations do not exceed 10 ppm

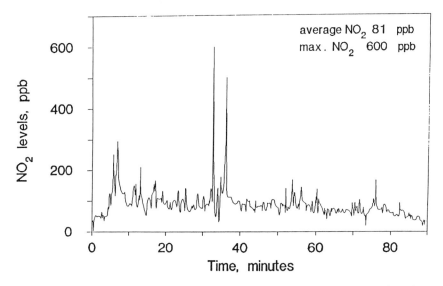

Figure 2.2. Real-time personal exposure to $NO_2$ concentrations (ppb) during meal preparation using a gas-fueled cooking range. *Source:* Harlos (1988), reprinted with permission.

over the cooking period. Nevertheless, the extreme conditions that result in elevated $NO_2$ concentrations also cause higher CO levels. Concentrations of 25–50 ppm have been measured in kitchens in New York City (Sterling and Kobayashi 1981). Gas ranges represent a potentially greater source of exposure than unvented space heaters. It is estimated that 45 percent of American homes, about 50 million housing units, use natural gas (U.S. Department of Energy 1987). Most of these units are in urbanized areas where ambient $NO_2$ and CO levels are elevated by stationary and mobile source emissions.

*Space Heaters*   In contrast, only 11 percent of the U.S. population is potentially exposed to gas or kerosene space heater emissions, which include particles, CO, and $NO_2$ and $SO_2$ if sulfur-containing fuel is burned. Leaderer et al. (1984) conducted a survey of indoor air quality in a small number of Connecticut homes. The $SO_2$ levels were less than 2 $\mu g/m^3$ inside homes without kerosene space heaters but were 60–150 $\mu g/m^3$ inside homes using this fuel. Apparently, in Connecticut at the time, commercial kerosene had a measurable amount of sulfur.

Kerosene space heaters and gas ranges emit particulate matter (Girman et al. 1982; Traynor et al. 1983a, 1983b). Bioassays have shown that kerosene heaters produce a carbonaceous particle that is highly mutagenic (Traynor et al. 1986). Most of the mutagenicity is attributed to the nitrated polycyclic aromatic hydrocarbons emitted. Particulate matter emitted from gas stoves was not found to be mutagenic (Sexton et al. 1986).

*Wood Burning*  In some regions of the country, wood stoves are an important source of primary heat in the home; about 6 percent of homes have wood stoves, and 19 percent have fireplaces. Emissions from wood stoves and fireplaces are vented to the outdoors. However, during start-up and stoking, and if the system is not airtight, emissions can contaminate the indoor air. Under such instances, transient particle levels may exceed a few hundred $\mu g/m^3$ (Hawthorne et al. 1988). But, on the average, only a few $\mu g/m^3$ of additional indoor particulate matter can be attributed to the presence of a home wood-burning or coal-burning stove (Sexton, Spengler, and Treitman 1984; Tennessee Valley Authority 1985).

Several investigators have indicated that wood burning produces highly mutagenic emissions. However, indoor air samples in homes with airtight wood stoves showed no mutagenic activity. In contrast, mutagenicity increased significantly with wood burning in open fireplaces and with tobacco smoking (Alfeim and Ramdahl 1984). Reports from the Environmental Protection Agency's integrated air cancer study indicated that the fraction of ambient particulate matter which is wood smoke is mutagenic (Lewtas, Claxton, and Mumford 1987). Wood combustion emissions that leak into the home may be a potential source of mutagenic material.

*Other Combustion Sources*  Significant exposure to combustion products may occur in numerous additional settings. Internal combustion engines running on gasoline or propane are used indoors. Spengler, Stone, and Lilley (1978) showed that CO in ice skating rinks might exceed 50 ppm for several hours due to exhaust emissions from resurfacing machines. Newspapers have published accounts of CO poisoning associated with hockey rinks.

Offices, hotels, hospitals, schools, shopping centers, and department stores often have attached or sublevel garages. Buildings with attached garages and offices connected to warehouses that use gasoline or propane forklifts can have elevated concentrations of combustion-related emissions. Often, sealed high-rise buildings have internal air pressures that are slightly positive on the upper floors but negative on the lower floors with respect to outside atmospheric pressure. Garage or roadside emissions can be entrained into these buildings. Cortese (1976), Ott and Flachsbart (1982), Akland et al. (1985), Flachsbart and Brown (1985a, 1985b), and Flachsbart and Ott (1986) have reported on CO in buildings in Washington, D.C., San Francisco, Honolulu, and Boston. Typically, indoor CO concentrations are lower than roadside ambient concentrations except when automobile emissions are entrained into the building. Under these conditions, the eight-hour (9 ppm) and one-hour (35 ppm) federal outdoor air quality standards can be exceeded indoors.

In more developed countries, nearly everyone spends time in automobiles or buses and is exposed to vehicle exhaust. Emissions can enter the passenger section of the vehicle from holes in the fire wall behind the engine, from faulty exhaust systems beneath the floor, from reentrainment in the negative pressure wake draft behind the car, or through windows and ventilation systems. Levels of CO exceeding 50 ppm may be produced. Cortese and Spengler (1976) estimated that 3–5 percent of all vehicles might produce such conditions. Cracks in the heating manifold have also caused high CO levels in the cockpits of small private airplanes. Even without faulty systems or entrained emission trapped in the wake of a vehicle, higher exposure will be experienced during vehicle transit. Spengler, Billick, and Ryan (1984) summarized exposures to lead particles in vehicles. Several studies have shown levels in vehicles three to ten times higher than concentrations measured at fixed locations in the urban environment.

Harlos (1988) conducted personal $NO_2$ monitoring in Boston. $NO_2$ concentrations varied depending on the mode of transportation (walking, bicycle, or automobile), time of day, and route. But in general, in-transit concentrations were 20–100 percent higher than concentrations measured at fixed locations in the city. Similar results were recently reported from a commuter exposure study conducted in Los Angeles (Shikiya et al. 1989). This study showed that other factors, such as time on the freeways and window and ventilation settings, influenced concentrations experienced by the driver.

Several investigators have shown that in-vehicle concentrations of CO are higher than those monitored at fixed urban locations (Cortese and Spengler 1976; Ott and Willits 1981; Ziskind et al. 1981; Akland et al. 1985; Flachsbart and Brown 1985b). Personal driving habits also can influence exposure. At stoplights (or in heavy traffic), CO concentrations can exceed 100 ppm if a driver brings the car close to the vehicle in front. Operating ventilation on *fresh air* intake setting instead of *recirculation* draws exhaust into the car.

*Tobacco Combustion*   The burning of tobacco products is a ubiquitous source of a great number of indoor contaminants. Tobacco burning produces a complex mixture of gases, vapors, and particulate matter. More than 4,500 compounds have been identified from burning tobacco, and 50 of these are known or suspected carcinogens (U.S. DHHS 1986). Tobacco smoke can be categorized as mainstream, sidestream, and environmental tobacco smoke. Mainstream (MS) emissions have been well characterized. These are the gases, vapors, and particles sucked from the "mouth end" of a cigarette. Under MS conditions, the burning cone of the tobacco may reach temperatures of 900°C. At this temperature, $N_2$ in the air dissociates to atomic nitrogen. In the cooling gas, atomic nitrogen reacts to form NO, $NO_2$, hydrogen cyanide (HCN), and highly carcinogenic *N*-nitrosamines (Hoffman and Brunneman 1983; U.S. DHHS 1986). Numerous other compounds are also found.

Sidestream smoke (SS) refers to the emissions from the smoldering cigarette; the cone temperature may drop as low as 400°C as the cigarette smolders. In the laboratory, these emissions are captured in close proximity to the cigarette. Approximately half of the tobacco is consumed during smoldering and the remainder during active puffing. Because the pyrolysis conditions are quite different during active puffing and smoldering, the components of MS and SS tobacco smoke differ. Klus and Kuhn (1982) characterized MS and SS smoke; the results are

Table 2.2  Distribution of Constituents in Fresh, Undiluted Mainstream Smoke and Diluted Sidestream Smoke from Nonfilter Cigarettes[a]

| Constituent | Amount in Mainstream Smoke | Range in Sidestream/ Mainstream Smoke |
|---|---|---|
| Vapor phase[b] | | |
| Carbon monoxide | 10–23 mg | 2.5–4.7 |
| Carbon dioxide | 20–40 mg | 8–11 |
| Carbonyl sulfide | 18–42 μg | 0.03–0.13 |
| Benzene[c] | 12–48 μg | 5–10 |
| Toluene | 100–200 μg | 5.6–8.3 |
| Formaldehyde | 70–100 μg | 0.1–≈50 |
| Acrolein | 60–100 μg | 8–15 |
| Acetone | 100–250 μg | 2–5 |
| Pyridine | 16–40 μg | 6.5–20 |
| 3-Methylpyridine | 12–36 μg | 3–13 |
| 3-vinylpyridine | 11–30 μg | 20–40 |
| Hydrogen cyanide | 400–500 μg | 0.1–0.25 |
| Hydrazine[d] | 32 ng | 3 |
| Ammonia | 50–130 μg | 40–170 |
| Methylamine | 11.5–28.7 μg | 4.2–6.4 |
| Dimethylamine | 7.8–10 μg | 3.7–5.1 |
| Nitrogen oxides | 100–600 μg | 4–10 |
| N-Nitrosodimethylamine[e] | 10–40 ng | 20–100 |
| N-Nitrosodiethylamine[e] | Nondetectable–25 ng | <40 |
| N-Nitrosopyrrolidine[e] | 6–30 ng | 6–30 |
| Formic acid | 210–490 μg | 1.4–1.6 |
| Acetic acid | 330–810 μg | 1.9–3.6 |
| Methyl chloride | 150–600 μg | 1.7–3.3 |
| Particulate Phase[b] | | |
| Particulate matter[c] | 15–40 mg | 1.3–1.9 |
| Nicotine | 1–2.5 mg | 2.6–3.3 |
| Anatabine | 2–20 μg | <0.1–0.5 |
| Phenol | 60–140 μg | 1.6–3.0 |
| Catechol | 100–360 μg | 0.6–0.9 |
| Hydroquinone | 110–300 μg | 0.7–0.9 |
| Aniline | 360 ng | 30 |
| 2-Toluidine | 160 ng | 19 |
| 2-Naphthylamine[c] | 1.7 ng | 30 |
| 4-Aminobiphenyl[c] | 4.6 ng | 31 |
| Benz[a]anthracene[e] | 20–70 ng | 2–4 |
| Benzo[a]pyrene[d] | 20–40 ng | 2.5–3.5 |
| Cholesterol | 22 μg | 0.9 |
| γ-Butyrolactone[e] | 10–22 μg | 3.6–5.0 |
| Quinoline | 0.5–2 μG | 8–11 |
| Harman[f] | 1.7–3.1 μg | 0.7–1.7 |
| N'-Nitrosonornicotine[e] | 200–3,000 ng | 0.5–3 |
| NNK[g] | 100–1,000 ng | 1–4 |
| N-Nitrosodiethanolamine[e] | 20–70 ng | 1.2 |
| Cadmium | 100 ng | 7.2 |
| Nickel[d] | 20–80 ng | 13–30 |
| Zinc | 60 ng | 6.7 |
| Polonium-210[c] | 0.04–0.1 pCi | 1.0–4.0 |
| Benzoic acid | 14–28 μg | 0.67–0.95 |
| Lactic acid | 64–174 μg | 0.5–0.7 |

(*continued*)

Table 2.2    (*Continued*)

| Constituent | Amount in Mainstream Smoke | Range in Sidestream/ Mainstream Smoke |
|---|---|---|
| Glycolic acid | 37–126 μg | 0.6–0.95 |
| Succinic acid | 110–140 μg | 0.43–0.62 |

[a]Diluted SS is collected with airflow of 25 ml/s, which is passed over the burning cone. Data from Elliot and Rowe (1975); Schmeltz et al. (1979); Hoffmann and Brunnemann (1983), Klus and Kuhn (1982), Sakuma et al. (1983, 1984a, 1984b), Hiller et al. (1982).
[b]Separation into vapor and particulate phases reflects conditions prevailing in mainstream smoke and does not necessarily imply same separation in sidestream smoke.
[c]Human carcinogen (U.S. DHHS 1986).
[d]Suspected human carcinogen (U.S. DHHS 1986).
[e]Animal carcinogen (Vainio, Hemminki, and Wilbourn 1985).
[f]1-Methyl-9H-pyrido(3,4-β)-indole.
[g]NNK = 4-(N-methyl-N-nitrosamino)-1-(3-pyridyl)-1-butanone.

summarized as a ratio of SS to MS emissions in Table 2.2. Many of these components have ratios greater than 1, indicating enrichment in the SS phase.

Environmental tobacco smoke (ETS) is the combination of exhaled MS and SS. The majority of ETS is made up of SS, which undergoes modification with dilution and aging after formation. Components with high vapor pressures may volatilize from particles to vapor phase. For example, nicotine is emitted in the SS particle phase and then evaporates to the vapor phase as it is diluted. The particles may accrete water, form aggregates, and change both in number count and diameter.

ETS cannot be measured directly in its entirety. Concentrations of individual ETS components have been reported: CO, nicotine, nitrogen oxides, aromatic hydrocarbons, acrolein, acetone, benzene, nitrous compounds, benzo[a]pyrene, and respirable suspended particles (RSP). These components have been measured in a variety of locations including homes, offices, restaurants, bars, clubs, arenas, trains, and airplanes, among others (see NRC 1986 and U.S. DHHS 1986 for reviews).

The concentrations of ETS constituents vary among indoor locations and over time. The number of smokers and the pattern of smoking determine the source strength for generation of ETS. An average smoker may smoke two cigarettes per hour over the day. But in some situations, such as in an airplane, smokers tend to light up at predictable times and produce high peak concentrations. In buildings with heating, ventilating, and air conditioning systems, the concentrations of ETS components are influenced by the ventilation rate, mixing, and directional flow of air currents. In homes, the volume of the room and the air exchange rate are determinants of ETS concentration.

Thus, the concentrations of ETS components to which nonsmokers are exposed depends on the degree of dilution of the smoke. As the intact plume of a smoldering cigarette passes by the nose or eyes, acute irritation can be experienced. The concentrations of formaldehyde and acrolein can still be several ppm a few feet from the burning cone of tobacco if the plume has not been mixed by air turbulence (Ayer and Yeager 1982).

More typically, however, ETS exposure occurs after SS and exhaled MS have been diluted several thousand times. Under these conditions, the concentrations experienced depend mostly on ventilation rates, smoking frequency, and room volume. In smoky bars, waiting areas, restaurants, automobiles, airplanes, or even in the home, short-term concentrations of ETS can be quite high. ETS particulate matter can range from 100 to more than 1,000 $\mu g/m^3$. Under these conditions, nicotine in closed environments can range from a few $\mu g/m^3$ to more than 100 $\mu g/m^3$. Nicotine concentrations up to 1,000 $\mu g/m^3$ have been reported (U.S. DHHS 1986, 155).

For some health end points, such as cancer and susceptibility to respiratory infection, a longer averaging time for assessing ETS impact on indoor environments may be most relevant. Comparatively few studies have sampled for ETS over days and months in an attempt to characterize long-term conditions. However, a rather consistent pattern emerges from the limited data available. Respirable particle levels in homes are associated with the number of cigarettes smoked (Spengler et al. 1981). On average, about 1 $\mu g/m^3$ of respirable-size particles is added to the long-term indoor concentrations for each cigarette smoked per day (Dockery and Spengler 1981). Figure 2.3 displays the results of repeated monitoring in 80 homes in six cities. On average, a home with one smoker had about 20 $\mu g/m^3$ greater concentration of RSP than one without smokers. Personal monitoring of nonsmokers confirms the importance of ETS exposure in determining personal exposures to particulates (Figure 2.4) (Spengler et al. 1985).

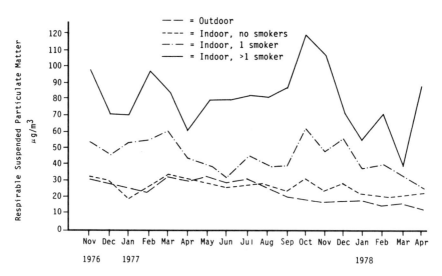

Figure 2.3. Monthly mean mass respirable particulate concentrations ($\mu g/m^3$) in homes with smokers and without smokers and in the outdoors across six cities. *Source:* Reprinted with permission from *Atmospheric Environment* 15, Spengler JD et al., Long-term measurements of respirable sulfates and particles inside and outside homes, Copyright 1981, Pergamon Press PLC.

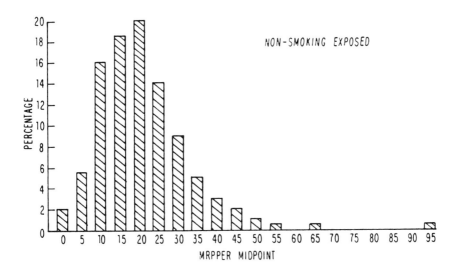

PERCENTAGE DISTRIBUTION OF PERSONAL DISTRIBUTION
PERCENTAGE BAR CHART

NON-SMOKING EXPOSED

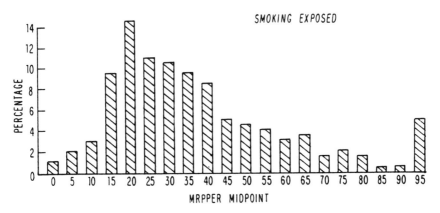

SMOKING EXPOSED

Figure 2.4. Percentage distribution of personal exposures to respirable particles with and without exposures to environmental (passive) tobacco smoke. *Source:* Spengler and Tosteson (1981), reprinted with permission.

Increases in levels of other ETS components have also been documented in association with cigarette smoking. Nitrogen dioxide is increased by a few $\mu g/m^3$ in homes with smokers. Studies on volatile organic vapors conducted in the United States and Germany indicated that benzene is 1–2 ppb higher in homes with smokers. Wallace et al. (1987) reported an average of 4 ppb benzene in homes of nonsmokers and 6 ppb in homes with smokers.

*General Sources* Modern furnishings, construction materials, and consumer products contaminate indoor air with numerous vapor-phase organic compounds (Table 2.3). In a recent Environmental Protection Agency study of air quality in ten public access buildings more than five hundred VOCs were identified (Sheldon et al. 1988); this study and others (Miksch, Hollowell, and Schmidt 1982; Molhave 1982; Özkaynak 1987; Wallace 1987) have described emission rates of VOCs from hundreds of materials and products, as mass of VOC per mass of material or as emission rate per unit.

Although VOC emission rates from materials and other sources may be used to predict indoor concentration, this approach is limited because emission rates may decrease as materials age. In one study, concentrations of VOCs from construction materials decreased with half-lives of two to twenty weeks after completion of the building (Sheldon et al. 1988). The concentrations of many VOCs decrease after a new building is occupied (Table 2.4), but concentrations of VOCs produced by furnishings, equipment, and occupant use can increase over time. Emission rates may also fluctuate with temperature and humidity (Girman et al. 1987).

Volatile and semivolatile organic compounds overlap in characteristics to some extent. The VOCs are compounds that exist as vapors over the normal range of air

Table 2.3   Sources of Volatile Organic Compounds in Indoor Air

| General Category | Examples | Important Emissions |
|---|---|---|
| Construction materials | Foam insulation, carpet glue, paint | Methyl chloroform, formaldehyde, styrene, xylene, tetrachloroethylene, ethylbenzene, benzene, 1,1,1-trichloroethane |
| Structural components | Particle board, vinyl tile, sheetrock | $n$-Decane, xylene, formaldehyde, acetone, hexanal, benzyl chloride, benzal chloride |
| Furnishings | Foam, textured carpet, drapery and upholstery fabric | Methyl chloroform, formaldehyde, tetrachloroethylene, $n$-undecane, benzene, 1,1,1-trichloroethane |
| Cleansers and solvents | Liquid detergent, chlorine bleach, scouring powder, furniture wax | $n$-Dodecane, $n$-undecane, xylene, $n$-decane, chloroform, benzene, 1,1,1-trichloroethane |
| Personal care products | Eyeliner pencil, deodorant, skin lotion | Methylchloroform, styrene, tetrachloroethylene, trichloroethylene, benzene, lisopene |
| Insecticides/pesticides | Rodenticide (solid) | $n$-Decane |
|  | Insecticide (solid) | Xylene |
|  | Insecticide (spray) | 1,1,1-Trichloroethane |
| Electrical equipment | Home computer, cassette tape recorder, VCRs, video cameras, videotapes | Ethyl benzene, chloroform |
| Combustion | Wood, kerosene | Acrolein, formaldehyde, 1-nitropyrene, 1-nitronaphthalene |

Table 2.4  Volatile Organic Compounds in a New Office Building

| Chemical | Concentration (μg/m³) | | | |
|---|---|---|---|---|
| | Indoors[a] | | | Outdoors[b] |
| | July | September | December | All Trips |
| Aliphatics | | | | |
| Decane | 380 | 38 | 4 | 2 |
| Undecane | 170 | 48 | 13 | 1 |
| Dodecane | 47 | 19 | 5 | 0.2 |
| Aromatics | | | | |
| m + p-Xylene | 140 | 19 | 9 | 2 |
| o-Xylene | 74 | 8 | 4 | 1 |
| Ethylbenzene | 84 | 6 | 5 | 1 |
| Benzene | 5 | 7 | 7 | 3 |
| Sytrene | 8 | 7 | 4 | 1 |
| Halocarbons | | | | |
| 1,1,1-Trichloroethane | 380 | 100 | 49 | 6 |
| Tetrachloroethylene | 7 | 2 | 3 | 1 |
| Trichloroethylene | 1 | 38 | 27 | 0.3 |
| Carbon tetrachloride | 1 | 1 | 1 | 1 |
| Chloroform | 1 | 2 | 18 | 6 |
| p-Dichlorobenzene | 1 | 1 | 1 | ND[c] |
| Total of 14 organics | 1,299 | 296 | 150 | 25.5 |

*Source*: Adopted from Sheldon et al. (1988).
[a]Mean of six 12-hour averages at five indoor locations.
[b]Mean of eighteen 12-hour averages at one outdoor location.
[c]ND, not determined.

temperatures and pressures. Semivolatiles are compounds that exist as liquids or solids but also evaporate. Termiticides such as chlordane and heptachlor are injected into the ground as liquids but are effective against termites because of emanating vapors. Many semivolatile insecticides and pesticides behave in a similar fashion. Some higher molecular weight organic molecules are in the form of particulate matter in air.

Benzo[a]pyrene is one of the most widely known polycyclic aromatic hydrocarbons. These compounds, formed by the combustion of coal, oil, kerosene, gasoline, wood, and tobacco, may condense as particles. Such organic particles and some inorganic particles can absorb gases and vapors and undergo chemical transformation. For example, dioxins may be formed in the cooling combustion gases of municipal waste incinerators.

Because many organic compounds that evaporate at ambient temperatures undergo adsorption and/or chemical reactions, sampling and identification are challenging, and no single sampling method is suitable for all organic compounds (see Chapters 4 and 11).

*Formaldehyde*  Formaldehyde (HCHO) is one of the most ubiquitous organic vapors indoors (Table 2.5). Long before the EPA's VOC total exposure assessment methodology (TEAM) studies (see Chapter 10) documented the indoor presence of

Table 2.5  Examples of Formaldehyde (Aldehyde) Uses and Potential Indoor Sources

| Source Categories | Examples |
| --- | --- |
| Paper products | Grocery bags, waxed paper, facial tissues, paper towels, disposable sanitary products |
| Stiffeners, wrinkle resistors, and water repellants | Floor coverings (rugs, linoleum, varnishes, plastics), carpet backings, adhesive binders, fire retardants, permanent-press clothes |
| Insulation | Urea-formaldehyde foam insulation |
| Combustion devices | Natural gas, kerosene, tobacco |
| Pressed-wood products | Plywood, particle board, decorative paneling |
| Other | Cosmetics, deodorants, shampoos, fabric dyes, inks, disinfectants |

*Source*: Sterling (1985).

organic compounds, HCHO had been recognized as a pungent water soluble gas that causes irritation of the eyes and mucous membranes (NRC 1981b). It is now considered a potential cause of other symptom complaints and some diseases (see Chapter 11). Sources and concentrations of formaldehyde are briefly presented in this chapter.

Formaldehyde is a widely used chemical that can be found in hundreds of products. Formaldehyde is added as a preservative to medicines, cosmetics, toiletries, and some food containers. The largest single use of formaldehyde is in the production of urea- and phenol-formaldehyde resins, which are used to bond laminated wood products and to bind wood chips in particle board. These wood products are used as shelving, counters, bookcases, cabinets, floors, and wall covers common to many homes and offices.

Formaldehyde has been used as a carrier solvent in the dyeing of textiles and paper products and is particularly effective on synthetic fibers. For this reason, most customers visiting fabric or carpeting stores can smell formaldehyde, and contact lens wearers often report acute eye irritation.

Formaldehyde is also released during combustion. Gasoline and, more important, diesel engine emissions, react to form formaldehyde and other aldehydes. Gas stoves and cigarettes are minor indoor sources. Although the HCHO concentrations measured in the intact plume of a cigarette can be as high as 40 ppm, high enough to cause intense eye irritation, dilution of tobacco smoke by room air produces much lower levels. For example, it required intense smoking of seventy cigarettes within thirty minutes to increase the HCHO concentration in an average size room from 0.01 to 0.27 ppm (Gammage and Gupta 1984).

In the mid-1970s, urea-formaldehyde foam insulation became a popular insulation material. To make UFFI, urea-formaldehyde partially polymerized resin is mixed with an acidic hardening agent. The mixed liquid is sprayed into attic and wall cavities by injecting compressed air. Small bubbles form as the resin hardens into a foam. The foam prevents convective air movement within the cavity while the billions of air bubbles form an insulating barrier.

Formaldehyde is emitted from UFFI in an initial burst and then continuously at a lower level (Allan, Dutkiewicz, and Gilmartin 1980). The initial release is unavoidable because of a slight excess of free formaldehyde in the resin. In the past, some installers either used inappropriate formulations of UFFI or installed the UFFI at an inappropriate ambient temperature, thereby increasing the initial release. Allan and colleagues (1980) described a second contribution to the initial fast release of formaldehyde from UFFI. The UFFI reaction forms methylene and diethylene ester bridges; if these links are not formed, a methylol ending group ($CH_2OH$) is left. These weaker bonds can break and release formaldehyde. In homes with UFFI, the HCHO concentration decays with a half-life of about two years (Dally et al. 1981a). However, because UFFI continues to degrade slowly, HCHO will be released chronically.

In the United States, about 500,000 homes had UFFI installed between 1970 and the early 1980s. In 1982, the Consumer Product Safety Commission (CPSC) banned the sale of UFFI. Even though the U.S. Fifth Circuit Court of Appeals reversed this decision, the controversy over UFFI effectively eliminated its use. In Canada, UFFI was installed in almost 100,000 homes as part of an active program of energy conservation. Extensive formaldehyde monitoring has been conducted in homes insulated with UFFI (Table 2.6). The CPSC reports that the average

Table 2.6  Selected Examples of Observed Formaldehyde Concentrations

| | Concentration (ppm) | |
|---|---|---|
| Sampling Site | Range | Mean |
| 28 Residences[a] | | |
| UFFI | 0.02–0.13 | 0.07 |
| Control | 0.03–0.07 | |
| 78 Structures[b] | | |
| Apartments | | 0.08 |
| UFFI and non-UFFI | 0.03–0.20 | 0.05 |
| Public buildings | | 0.04 |
| 3 Residences[c] | | |
| UFFI | 0.11–0.16 | |
| Non-UFFI | 0.06–0.08 | |
| Energy-efficient non-UFFI | 0.13–0.17 | |
| 164 Mobile homes[d] | <0.02–0.78 | 0.15 |
| 65 Mobile homes[e] | <0.01–3.68 | 0.47[f] |
| 65 Mobile homes[g] | <0.10–0.80 | 0.16[f] |

*Source*: Sterling (1985).
[a]Godish (1981).
[b]TerKonda and Liaw (1983).
[c]Gammage et al. (1983).
[d]Stock et al. (1984).
[e]Dally et al. (1981a, 1981b).
[f]Median.
[g]Hanrahan et al. (1984).

HCHO concentrations in homes insulated with UFFI were 0.12 ppm in contrast to 0.03 ppm in homes not insulated with UFFI (CPSC 1982; Gupta, Ulsamer, and Preuss, 1982).

Indoor HCHO concentrations do not reach a steady state. Not only can emission rates fluctuate with temperature and humidity, but the absorption rate can also vary. HCHO concentrations in one home in which UFFI was installed three years earlier were tracked over a year. In the winter, the HCHO concentration was about 0.05 ppm; as the outdoor temperature rose to 25°C in the summer, the concentration more than tripled (Schutte et al. 1981). Changes in ventilation (air exchange) and occupant activities also influence concentrations. Figure 2.5 shows diurnal HCHO concentrations in two Oak Ridge, Tennessee, homes (Gammage et al. 1982). Concentrations in the UFFI-containing home fluctuated from 0.1 to nearly 0.18 ppm.

Products formulated with phenol- or urea-formaldehyde resins or treated with formaldehyde to make them crease resistant or to adhere pigments can be found in almost all homes and modern office buildings. Besides the products listed in Table

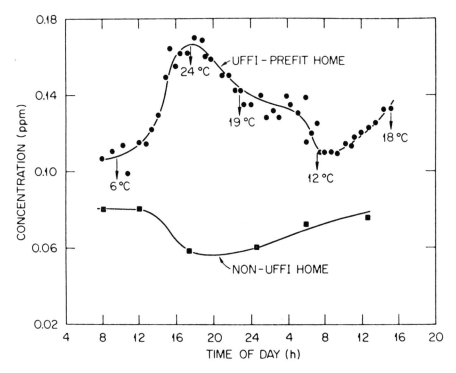

Figure 2.5. Diurnal fluctuations in formaldehyde levels (ppm) inside a three-year-old UFFI-prefit house and a ten-year-old non-UFFI house in Oak Ridge, Tennessee. *Source:* Reprinted with permission from Gammage RB and Gupta KC, Formaldehyde. In *Indoor Air Quality,* ed. Walsh PJ, Dudney CS, Copenhaver ED. Copyright 1984, CRC Press, Inc., Boca Raton, Fla.

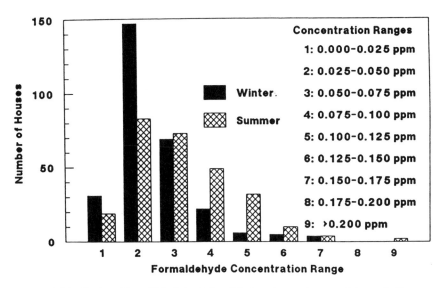

Figure 2.6. Distribution of formaldehyde levels (ppm) during winter and summer in homes in Kingston and Harriman, Tennessee. *Source:* Hawthorne et al. (1988), reprinted with permission.

2.5, formaldehyde can be in wall paper, especially the prepasted kind, floor covering, and in the binder used in fiberglass insulation. Sources in offices include partitions, pressed-board desks, wall paneling, and fiberglass-lined ventilation ducts. Even without UFFI, homes and office buildings can have HCHO concentrations of 0.2 ppm or more. Mobile homes, which have small volumes, low air exchange rates, and extensive particle board, may have concentrations of 1 ppm or greater. Hollowell et al. (1980) reported that just adding furniture to an unoccupied house increased HCHO concentrations from 0.07 to 0.19 ppm. Figure 2.6 summarizes week-long winter and summer monitoring in over three hundred homes in eastern Tennessee (Hawthorne et al. 1988), and Table 2.6 summarizes several studies of indoor HCHO concentrations.

ASBESTOS

Asbestos refers to several fibrous inorganic materials characterized by chemical formulation and crystalline structure. Chrysotile asbestos, a serpentine mineral, has been most widely used commercially. The other types of asbestos are amphibole minerals with straight fibers, in contrast to the undulating chrysotile fibers. Of the amphiboles, crocidolite and amosite have been most extensively mined, but most asbestos used in the United States has been chrysotile; both tremolite and cummington-grunerite, also amphiboles, may contaminate other minerals.

The health effects of exposure to asbestos have been amply documented by epidemiologic studies of workers exposed to high concentrations. Asbestos exposure is associated with asbestosis (fibrosis of the lung), pleural effusion and pleural plaques (fluid in the space around the lung and scarring of the pleura, respectively), mesothelioma (cancer of the pleural sac lining the lung or of the peritoneal sac lining the abdomen), cancer of the lung, cancer of the larynx, and, possibly, cancers of the gastrointestinal tract (CPSC 1983; NRC 1984; Ontario Royal Commission 1984; U.S. EPA 1984; British Health and Safety Commission 1985; Omenn et al. 1986). The epidemiologic studies suggest greater carcinogenicity for the amphiboles, particularly in relation to mesothelioma. The confirmed occupational hazards of asbestos have raised concern that nonoccupational exposure to asbestos may also have adverse consequences.

To date, our understanding of the health risks of indoor asbestos is derived largely from risk assessment, using risk projection models based on occupationally exposed workers. To estimate risks of lung cancer and mesothelioma, these models extrapolate from relatively high workplace exposures to the much lower levels generally encountered indoors. Because the models do not incorporate a threshold exposure that must be exceeded for cancer to develop, some risk is projected for any level of exposure. Diverse models have been developed (recent reviews include Mossman et al. [1990] and Spengler et al. [1989]).

Because of its high tensile strength and thermal properties, asbestos has been used extensively in building materials since the beginning of this century (Table 2.7). The broad use categories are thermal and acoustical insulation, fire protection, and the reinforcement of building products. In addition to its use in acoustical ceiling tiles and vinyl floor tiles, asbestos has been used in paints and wall and ceiling plaster. Until banned in the late 1970s, asbestos materials were used to coat pipes, boilers, and steel structural beams. The use of asbestos in the United States has decreased since 1973, coincident with the banning of certain applications by the EPA (Figure 2.7). However, asbestos-containing materials are still present in many homes, offices, and schools.

Based on surveys, the EPA has estimated that 20 percent of the nation's buildings, about 733,000 not including schools and residential buildings with fewer than ten units, contain some asbestos materials (U.S. EPA 1988a, 1988b). Sixteen percent have thermal insulation containing asbestos. Separate surveys of the city of New York suggest that 67 percent (158,000) of the buildings contain asbestos (Price 1988, U.S. EPA 1988a, 1988b). Concern about the potential health effects of exposure has led to the removal of asbestos-containing materials from private and public buildings. However, asbestos removal is expensive, and the costs are rising. For example, the General Services Administration estimated a cost of over $50 billion to remove asbestos from federal buildings alone (U.S. EPA 1988a). Under Section 6 of the Toxic Substances Control Act, the EPA has banned manufacturing, importing, and processing of most asbestos products. This phased ban will start in 1990 and continue through 1997.

Several issues have arisen regarding the measurement and exposure of asbestos in buildings. A rapidly enlarging data base on airborne asbestos concentrations in buildings demonstrates extremely low average values under normal building use

Table 2.7   Summary of Asbestos-Containing Building Products

| Product | Dates Used | Average Percent Asbestos |
|---|---|---|
| Floor tile and sheet | 1950–present | 20 |
| Asphaltic coatings and sealants | 1900–present | 10 |
| Cement pipe and sheet | 1930–present | 30 |
| Roofing felt | 1910–present | 15 |
| Corrugated paper pipe wrap | 1910–present | 80 |
| Sprayed insulation | 1935–78 | 50 |
| Troweled insulation | 1935–75 | 70 |
| Preformed pipe wrap | 1926–75 | 50 |
| Insulation board | Unknown | 30 |
| Boiler insulation | 1930–78 | 10 |
| Other uses | 1900–present | <50 |

*Source*: Oppenheim-McMullen, J. and Turner, B. *Progressive Builder* (1986).

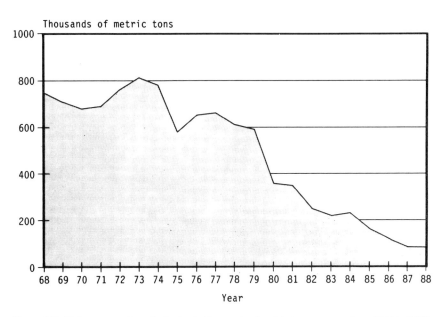

Figure 2.7. U.S. consumption of asbestos in thousands of metric tons per year from 1968 to 1988. *Source:* Bureau of Mines, and Zurer, P. *Chemical & Engineering News,* March 4, 1985, *63*(9), p. 29. Published 1985 by the American Chemical Society.

conditions. Early measurements of airborne asbestos levels made by transmission electron microscopy (U.S. EPA 1975, 1980, 1983; Nicholson et al. 1978) were obtained using the indirect filter preparation method. Measurements by indirect transmission electron microscopy are likely to overestimate the number of respirable asbestos fibers. These measurements were reported in mass units (nanograms per cubic meter of air). A concentration in mass units, however, does not predict potential health risk as directly as concentration measured in fibers per cubic centimeter of air ($f/cm^3$). More recent data, obtained using transmission electron microscopy and the direct filter preparation method, are reported as $f/cm^3$ and indicate lower average exposure levels than were implied by the earlier measurements obtained with the indirect method.

The EPA's recent report to Congress concerning asbestos in public and commercial buildings (U.S. EPA 1988a) provides a summary of direct transmission electron microscopy data for forty-one schools and ninety-four buildings other than schools. The average airborne asbestos concentration in nonschool buildings was $0.006\ f/cm^3$; the average for the school buildings was $0.03\ f/cm^3$. Since these data were compiled from different air monitoring studies with varying documentation, the averages should be interpreted as representing concentrations for all asbestiform matter visible with transmission electron microscopy (i.e., fibers both longer and shorter than 5 $\mu$m, and other asbestoslike materials that may not be considered respirable).

More fully documented data are available for the 43 nonschool buildings with asbestos-containing material studied by the EPA and for seventy-three schools about to undergo asbestos removal studied by asbestos product manufacturers (Price 1988; U.S. EPA 1988b). In the study by the EPA, the average airborne asbestos concentration, counting all fibrous particles, was $0.0007\ f/cm^3$. Of the 387 samples collected, including forty-eight outdoor samples and samples in six buildings with no friable asbestos-containing material, 83 percent yielded no measurable asbestos fiber counts. Restricting the asbestos count to only those fibers 5 $\mu$m in length or longer resulted in an average concentration level approximately eight times lower, $0.00008\ f/cm^3$. In the seventy-three school buildings, the average airborne concentration, counting all asbestos structures, was $0.01773$ $f/cm^3$. Restricted to fibers 5 $\mu$m or longer, the average concentration was $0.00022$ $f/cm^3$. The average of the outdoor measurements in these studies was comparable to the measured indoor level. These indoor concentrations are many orders of magnitude less than were measured in the asbestos-contaminated workplaces that have been associated with disease (e.g., $>1\ f/cm^3$).

Occupant risk is determined by exposures to airborne fibers rather than the presence of asbestos-containing materials in the building. At present, information is lacking on the relationship between the presence of asbestos-containing material and indoor concentrations of airborne asbestos fibers. This relationship cannot be evaluated readily because of the episodic fashion in which much of the asbestos is released into indoor air.

Personal exposures to asbestos are determined by the fiber concentrations in the immediate vicinity of a person. Fixed location monitoring within a structure only provides an estimate of what exposures might be for occupants of that building. For example, the exposure in the breathing zone of a facility maintenance employee during replacement of ceiling panels could be quite different from concentrations monitored at another location. Building occupants have substantially different likelihoods of exposure depending on their activities. The low fiber counts documented in building surveys imply minimal health risks for most persons working in buildings with asbestos-containing materials. However, exposures of persons involved with building maintenance and alteration may be substantially higher than the concentrations measured during surveys.

After asbestos has been removed from a building or an area, monitoring is required before reoccupancy. This EPA requirement states that indoor fiber concentrations cannot exceed outdoor levels. However, settled fibers might be resuspended at a later point. Aggressive sampling in postabatement areas has shown fiber levels increased three- to sixfold (Karaffa et al. 1987). Burdett et al. (1988) found fiber levels increased ten to one hundred times after incomplete dry removal. Further, the comparison with ambient fiber concentrations as the criterion for reoccupancy does not address the change in exposures to occupants before and after removal. It is the net change in estimated lifetime exposures before and after asbestos removal which will determine the efficacy of the mitigation strategy.

## RADON

Radon-222, a noble gas, is produced in the decay of naturally occurring uranium–238. It decays with a half-life of 3.8 days into a series of short-lived progeny: polonium–218, lead–214, bismuth–214, and polonium–214, all with half-lives less than thirty minutes (Evans 1969). Polonium–218 and polonium–214 release $\alpha$-particles during decay; these $\alpha$-emissions are presumed to produce lung cancer by damaging cells of the tracheobronchial epithelium. The health effects of radon are covered in Chapter 16; Chapter 4 discusses measurement techniques.

The principal source of radon in buildings is naturally occurring gas in the soil. The soil gas penetrates through sump pump wells, drains, cracks, utility access holes, and the foundation into the air in homes. The driving pressure for entry of soil gas comes from the pressure gradient established by a home across the soil; the gradient varies with atmospheric pressure, wind flow over a structure, and/or buoyancy of air within the structure. According to Nero and Nazaroff (1984), soil gas typically contains enough radon so that only 0.1 percent of air infiltrating a home would have to be drawn from the soil to produce potentially significant contamination. Generally, building materials and potable water do not contribute significantly to concentrations of radon indoors. However, potable water drawn from wells in areas in which soils and rocks are enriched in radium may be an important source of radon. Natural gas may also contribute radon if transport and storage times are brief.

Nero (1985) summarized the results of radon entry studies conducted in five countries. Figure 2.8 shows the distribution of radon entry rates; the median entry rate for U.S. single-family homes is about 0.5 pCi/liter/h (about 15–20 Bq/m³/h). As Nero indicated, this rate is much higher than the estimated rate of emissions from concrete, only 0.07 pCi/liter/h (Ingersoll 1983).

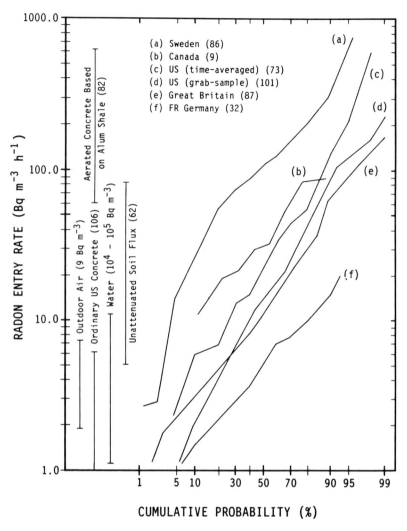

Figure 2.8. Cumulative frequency distribution of radon entry rate determined in dwellings in several countries as the product of simultaneously measured ventilation rate and radon concentration. *Source:* From *Indoor Air and Human Health,* edited by Richard B. Gammage and Stephen V. Kaye. Copyright 1985, Lewis Publishers, Inc., Chelsea, Mich. Used with permission.

On a short-term basis, radon concentrations vary with the ventilation rate of the structure. For example, Figure 2.9 shows radon measurements made in an elementary school over six days. During the week, the perimeter unit ventilators were operating during the day. Radon levels quickly dropped to below 4 pCi/liter with the units operating. When the univents were turned off, levels rose to 20–30 pCi/liter. Over the weekend, without mechanical ventilation, the air exchange rate

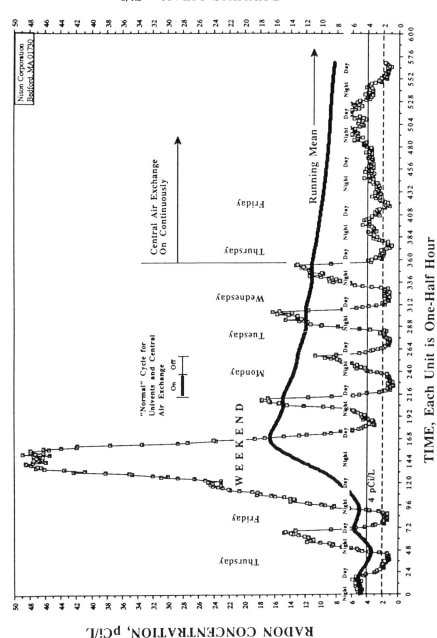

Figure 2.9. Half-hour and running mean indoor radon concentration (pCi/liter) in a school room over twelve days. Variation in concentrations over first week demonstrates the influence of ventilation. *Source:* Grodzins (1990), reprinted with permission.

57

must be assumed to have dropped sharply. Levels of radon increased to nearly 100 pCi/liter from Friday evening to Sunday morning.

The indoor concentration of radon at any particular time is determined in a complex fashion by the interplay of several dynamic factors including meteorology, soil characteristics, and building use and operations. Therefore, it is not unexpected that radon concentrations vary over several orders of magnitude among homes (0.05 to greater than 100 pCi/liter) and over an order of magnitude for a particular home. Because of variations in entry rates and air exchange rates, homes may have short-term fluctuations in radon concentrations as large as those documented in the public school (Figure 2.9).

Smoothing these diurnal patterns by monitoring radon with integrating samplers reveals temporal variations on the seasonal scale. Researchers at Oak Ridge National Laboratories participated in an indoor air quality study in Kingston and Harriman, Tennessee (Hawthorne et al. 1988). Radon monitoring was conducted in 248 homes over six winter months and in 287 homes during a five-month summer phase. Figure 2.10 presents the distribution of winter and summer concentrations. In this study, the downstairs radon concentrations were higher, by about a factor of two, than the upstairs concentrations. Other studies have shown a similar spatial gradient.

MICROBIOLOGIC CONTAMINANTS

Microbiologic contaminants have a wide variety of forms. Pollens from trees, grasses, and other plants are familiar to most people through their associations with allergens and the clinical syndromes of allergy. Microbiologic contaminants of indoor air also include microbial cells such as viruses and bacteria in addition to fungal spores, protozoans, algae, animal dander and excreta, and insect excreta and fragments. A broad definition of microbiologic contaminants would also include the volatile metabolites of living and decaying organisms. The contaminants may be viable organisms that multiply in an infected host or they may live in dust, soil, water, oil, organic films, food, vegetative debris, or wherever the microclimate provides the correct temperature, humidity, and nutrients for growth. Bathroom walls and window casements as well as damp basements are typical locations in which water condenses. Dust can accumulate on heat exchanger coils of heating and cooling systems and refrigerators as well as in the duct lining of these mechanical devices. During the summer cooling season, moisture condenses on cooling coils and encourages the proliferation of microflora. Similarly, the drainage pans under the condensing coils in building heating, ventilating, and air-conditioning (HVAC) systems often provide favorable conditions for microbial growth. Table 2.8 summarizes the potential occurrence of microbiologic contamination at various locations in HVAC systems. Table 2.9 lists some of the aeroallergens and aeropathogens commonly found indoors.

Microbiologic contamination has also been found in a variety of other locations. For example, the use of cool mist humidifiers in the home can result in microbiologic contamination. Ultrasonic humidifiers can also disseminate bacteria if tap

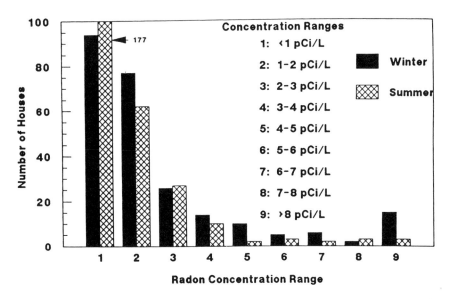

Figure 2.10. Distribution of indoor radon levels (pCi/liter) during winter and summer in homes in Kingston and Harriman, Tennessee. *Source:* Hawthorne et al. (1988), reprinted with permission.

water is used and becomes contaminated. Humidification by steam in a central air handling system usually does not present a problem since biocides are added to most steam supplies. However, the addition of moisture to dust-contaminated ducts can lead to biologic contamination.

In general, moisture control of buildings is very important in preventing conditions that lead to fungal or bacterial growth. At relative humidities above 70 percent, fabrics, leather, and wood materials can absorb sufficient water to support fungal growth. Even when air humidities are lower, surfaces may be colder than air temperature or water damaged and hence have higher local relative humidities. Other biologic agents are less dependent on moisture conditions. Animal dander, dust mites, and insect parts can become aerosolized when shaking out bedding or vacuuming rugs. Children playing on carpets or with stuffed animals can be exposed to potentially allergenic antigens. Birds nesting near or in air intake vents can also be a source of exposure.

Chapters 13 and 14 discuss in detail the health consequences of indoor biologic contamination. Many of the airborne allergenic and infectious materials are commonly found in the outdoor and indoor environment. For a building to become contaminated, there needs to be a reservoir in which the organism can colonize and in which there are conditions favorable for its amplification. However, even these are not sufficient if a potential host does not come in close contact with the organism. Contact is facilitated by dissemination of the organism or agents through a ventilation system, air conditioner, or humidifier or by mechanical

Table 2.8  Probabilities of Occurrence of Microbial Contamination at Various Locations in HVAC Systems

| HVAC Process or Location | System Time | | | | | | |
| --- | --- | --- | --- | --- | --- | --- | --- |
| | Central Forced Air | | | | Local or Distributed | | |
| | Conventional Heating and Refrigeration | Heat Pump | Evaporative Cooler | Heat Recovery | Window/Wall Air Conditioners | Evaporative Cooler | Heat Recovery |
| Outdoor air intake | Moderate | Moderate | High | Moderate | Moderate | High | Moderate |
| Duct lining | Moderate | Moderate | High | Moderate | Moderate | High | Moderate |
| Air cleaners | Low to moderate | Low to moderate | Low | Low to moderate | Low to moderate | Low | Low to moderate |
| Humidifier | High | High | | | | | |
| Condensate pans/drain liner | High | High | Very high | Moderate | High | Very high | Moderate |
| Return/exhaust air | Moderate to high | Moderate to high | | Moderate to high | Low to moderate | | Low to moderate |

Source: Woods (1989).

Table 2.9 Aeroallergens and
Aeropathogens Found Indoors[a]

Bacteria
  *Staphylococcus aureus*
  *Streptococcus faecalis*
  *Escherichia coli*
  *Salmonella typhosa*
  *Salmonella choleraesuis*
  *Pseudomonas aeruginosa*
  *Mycobacterium smegmatis*
  *Mycobacterium tuberculosis*
  *Streptococcus mutans*
  *Klebsiella pneumoniae*
  *Enterobacter agglomerans*
  *Staphylococcus epidermidis*
  *Acinetobacter calcoaceticus*
  *Legionella*
Yeasts
  *Saccharomyces cerevisae*
  *Candida albicans*
Fungi
  *Aspergillus niger*
  *Aspergillus flavus*
  *Aspergillus terreus*
  *Chaetomium globosum*
  *Penicillium funiculosum*
  *Trichophyton interdigitale*
  *Aureobasidium pullulans*
Amoeba
Arthropods
  Mites
  Cockroach
Dander
  Cat
  Dog
  Hamster

[a]This table represents only a small number of the total microorganisms that may be present in the indoor environments.

disruption. However, it is not limited to these mechanisms alone; the release of spores by some fungal organisms is regulated by biologic mechanisms.

## SUMMARY

Concentrations indoors vary not only with the strength of the pollution sources, but with the volume of the polluted space, the rate of air exchange between indoor and outdoor air, and other factors that affect removal. Health risks from indoor pollution depend not only on indoor concentrations, but on patterns of human activity and source use, which, along with indoor concentrations, determine personal exposures (see Chapter 5). For some health effects, short-term patterns of source emissions may be relevant whereas long-term patterns may be more pertinent for others. Thus, to assess and control the health effects of indoor air pollution, the contributions of indoor sources to personal exposures must be characterized. However, sources of indoor air pollution are myriad and may vary with age, race, and ethnicity of a home's occupants and with climate and geology. For example, inner city residents may have much greater exposure to cockroach antigen than persons residing in the suburbs.

## REFERENCES

Akland, G. G., et al. 1985. Measuring human exposure to carbon monoxide in Washington, D.C., and Denver, Colo., during the winter of 1982–1983. *Environ. Sci. Technol.* 19:911–18.

Alfeim, I., and Ramdahl, T. 1984. Contribution of wood combustion to indoor air pollution as measured by mutagenicity in *Salmonella* and polycyclic aromatic hydrocarbon concentration. *Environ. Mutagen* 6:121–30.

Allan, G. G.; Dutkiewicz, J.; and Gilmartin, E. J. 1980. Long-term stability of urea-formaldehyde foam insulation. *Environ. Sci. Technol.* 14:1237.

Ayer, H. E., and Yeager, D. W. 1982. Irritants in cigarette smoke plumes. *Am. J. Public Health* 72:1283–85.

Baker, P. E., et al. 1987. An overview of the residential indoor air quality characterization study of nitrogen dioxide. In *Indoor air '87: Proceedings of the fourth international conference on indoor air quality and climate.* Ed. B. Seifert et al., Vol. 1, 395–99. Berlin: Institute for Water, Soil, and Air Hygiene.

British Health and Safety Commission. 1985. Health and Safety Executive, *Asbestos: Effects on health of exposure to asbestos,* Guidance note EH35. London: H. M. Stationery Office.

Burdett, G. J., et al. 1988. Airborne asbestos fiber levels in buildings and their impact on risk management. Paper presented at the symposium on health effects of exposure to asbestos in buildings, 14–16 December, Harvard University.

Colome, S. D., et al. 1987. Analysis of factors associated with indoor residential nitrogen dioxide: Multivariate regression results. In *Indoor air '87: Proceedings of the fourth international conference on indoor air quality and climate.* Ed. B. Seifert et al., Vol. 1, 405–7. Berlin: Institute for Water, Soil, and Air Hygiene.

Cortese, A. D. 1976. Ability of fixed monitoring stations to represent personal carbon monoxide exposure. Ph.D. diss., Harvard University School of Public Health, Boston.

Cortese, A. D., and Spengler, J. D. 1976. Ability of fixed monitoring stations to represent personal carbon monoxide exposure. *J. Air. Pollut. Control Assoc.* 26:1144–50.

Dally, K. A., et al. 1981a. A follow-up study of indoor air quality in Wisconsin homes. Paper presented at the international symposium on indoor air pollution, health and energy conservation. 13–16 October, Amherst, Mass.

Dally, K. A., et al. 1981b. Formaldehyde exposure in nonoccupational environments. *Arch. Environ. Health* 36:277–84.

Danish Building Research Institute. 1987. Report on man-made mineral fibers in the indoor air. (In Danish.)

Dockery, D. W., and Spengler, J. D. 1981. Indoor-outdoor relationships of respirable sulfates and particles. *Atmos. Environ.* 15:335–43.

Elliott, L. P., and Rowe, D. R. 1975. Air quality during public gatherings. *J. Air Pollut. Control Assoc.* 25:635–36.

Evans, R. D. 1969. Engineers' guide to the elementary behavior of radon daughters. *Health Phys.* 17:229–52.

Flachsbart, P. G., and Brown, D. E. 1985a. Merchant exposure to CO from motor vehicle exhaust at Honolulu's Ala Moana shopping center. Paper 85-85.3, presented at the seventy-eighth annual meeting of the Air Pollution Control Association, 16–25 June, Pittsburgh, Pa.

Flachsbart, P. G., and Brown, D. E. 1985b. Surveys of personal exposure to vehicle exhaust in Honolulu microenvironments. *Final report under cooperative agreement CR-808541-01-3.* Research Triangle Park, N.C.: U.S. Environmental Protection Agency.

Flachsbart, P. G., and Ott, W. R. 1986. A rapid method for surveying CO concentrations in high-rise buildings. *Environ. Int.* 12:255–64.

Gammage, R. B., and Gupta, K. C. 1984. Formaldehyde. In *Indoor air quality.* Ed. P. J. Walsh, C. S. Dudney, and E. D. Copenhaver, 109–42. Boca Raton, Fla.: CRC Press.

Gammage, R. B., et al. 1982. *Identification and measurement of air pollutants in homes.* U.S. Consumer Product Safety Commission, Oak Ridge National Laboratory, Publication no. CPSC-IAG/81/1403. Monthly Reports for September 1981 and March, May, June, July, August, and October 1982.

Gammage, R. B., et al. 1983. Temporal fluctuations of formaldehyde levels inside residences. *Proceedings of the Air Pollution Control Association specialty conference: Measurement and monitoring of non-criteria (toxic) contaminants in air,* 22–24 March, Chicago.

Girman, J. R., et al. 1982. Pollutant emission rates from indoor appliances and sidestream cigarette smoke. *Environ. Int.* 8:213–21.

Girman, J. R., et al. 1987. Bake-out of an office building. In *Indoor air '87: Proceedings of the fourth international conference on indoor air quality and climate.* Ed. B. Seifert et al., Vol. 1, 22–26. Berlin: Institute for Water, Soil, and Air Hygiene.

Godish, T. 1981. Formaldehyde and building related illness. *J. Environ. Health* 44:116–21.

Goldstein, I. F., et al. 1987. Acute exposure to nitrogen dioxide and pulmonary function. In *Indoor air '87: Proceedings of the fourth international conference on indoor air quality and climate.* Ed. B. Seifert et al., Vol. 1, 293–97. Berlin: Institute for Water, Soil, and Air Hygiene.

Grodzins, L. 1990. Radon in schools in Massachusetts: A report on testing and mitigation of eighty school systems. *U.S. EPA 1990 international symposium on radon and radon reduction technology.* 19–23 February, Atlanta, Ga.

Gupta, K. C.; Ulsamer, A. G.; and Preuss, P. W. 1982. Formaldehyde in indoor air: Sources and toxicity. *Environ. Int.* 8:349–58.

Hanrahan, L., et al. 1984. Formaldehyde vapor in mobile homes: A cross-sectional survey of concentrations and irritant effects. *Am. J. Public Health* 74:1026–27.

Harlos, D. P. 1988. Acute exposure to nitrogen dioxide during cooking or commuting. Ph.D. diss. Harvard School of Public Health, Boston.

Hawthorne, A. R., et al. 1988. *Indoor air quality in 300 homes in Kingston/Harriman, Tennessee.* Oak Ridge, Tenn.: Oak Ridge National Laboratory, Publication no. ORNL/6401.

Hiller, F. C., et al. 1982. Deposition of sidestream cigarette smoke in the human respiratory tract. *Am. Rev. Respir. Dis.* 125:406–8.

Hoffman, D., and Brunneman, K. D. 1983. Endogenous formation of $N$-nitrosopoline in cigarette smokers. *Cancer Res.* 43:69–83.

Hollowell, C. D., et al. 1980. *Building ventilation and indoor air quality.* LBL Report no. 10391. Berkeley, Calif.: Lawrence Berkeley Laboratory.

Ingersoll, J. G. 1983. A survey of radionuclide contents and radon emanation rates in materials used in the United States. *Health Phys.* 45:363–68.

Karaffa, M. A., et al. 1987. Preliminary evaluation of potential asbestos exposure during carpet vacuuming in buildings containing friable asbestos material. Cincinnati, Ohio: U.S. Environmental Protection Agency, unpublished draft report.

Klus, H., and Kuhn, H. 1982. Distribution of various tobacco smoke constituents in main and sidestream smoke: A review. *Bietr. Tabakforsch. Int.* 15:340–56.

Leaderer, B. P., et al. 1984. Residential exposure to $NO_2$, $SO_2$, and HCHO associated with unvented kerosene space heaters, gas appliances, and sidestream tobacco smoke. In B. Berglund, T. Lindvall, and J. Sundell, *Indoor air, Vol. 4: Chemical characterization and personal exposure,* 151–56. Stockholm: Swedish Council for Building Research, Publication no. NTIS/PB85-104214.

Lewtas, J.; Claxton, L. D.; and Mumford, J. L. 1987. Human exposure to mutagens from indoor combustion sources. In *Indoor air '87: Proceedings of the fourth international conference on indoor air quality and climate.* Ed. B. Seifert et al., 473–77. Berlin: Institute for Water, Soil, and Air Hygiene.

Lippmann, M., and Schlesinger, R. B. 1979. *Chemical contamination in the human environment.* New York: Oxford University Press.

Marbury, M. C. 1988. Indoor residential $NO_2$ concentrations in Albuquerque, New Mexico. *J. Air Pollut. Control Assoc.* 38:392–98.

Miksch, R. R.; Hollowell, C. D.; and Schmidt, H. E. 1982. Trace organic chemical contaminants in office spaces. *Environ. Int.* 8:129–37.

Molhave, L. 1982. Indoor air pollution due to organic gases and vapours of solvents in building materials. *Environ. Int.* 8:117–27.

Moschandreas, D. J. 1983. Emission factors of volatile organic compounds and other air constituents from unvented gas appliances. *Proceedings of the Air Pollution Control Association specialty conference: Measurement and monitoring of noncriteria (toxic) contaminants in air,* 22–24 March, Chicago. Publication no. SP-50.

Mossman, B. T., et al. 1990. Asbestos: Scientific developments and implications for public policy. *Science* 247:294–301.

National Research Council. 1981a. *Indoor pollutants.* Washington, D.C.: National Academy Press.

National Research Council. 1981b. *Formaldehyde and other aldehydes.* Washington, D.C.: National Academy Press.

National Research Council. 1984. *Asbestiform fibers: Nonoccupational health risks.* Washington, D.C.: National Academy Press,

National Research Council. 1986. *Environmental tobacco smoke: Measuring and assessing health effects.* Washington, D.C.: National Academy Press.

Nero, A. V. 1985. Indoor concentrations of radon-222 and its daughters: Sources, range, and environmental influences. In *Indoor air and human health.* Ed. R. B. Gammage and S. V. Kaye. Chelsea, Mich.: Lewis Publishers.

Nero, A. V., and Nazaroff, W. W. 1984. Characterizing the sources of radon indoors. *Radiation Protection Dosimetry* 7:23–39.

Nicholson, W. J., et al. 1978. Control of sprayed asbestos surfaces in school buildings: A feasibility study. *Report to the National Institute of Environmental Health Sciences.*

Omenn, G. S., et al., 1986. Contribution of environmental fibers to respiratory cancer. *Environ. Health Perspect.* 70:51–56.

Ontario Royal Commission. 1984. *Report of the Royal Commission on matters of health and safety arising from the use of asbestos in Ontario,* Vol. 1–3. Toronto, Canada: Ontario Ministry of the Attorney General.

Oppenheim-McMullen, J., and Turner, B. 1986. Facing the asbestos menace. *Progressive Builder,* September:21–22.

Ott, W., and Flachsbart, P. 1982. Measurement of carbon monoxide concentrations in indoor and outdoor locations using personal exposure monitors. *Environ. Int.* 8:295–304.

Ott, W. R., and Willits, N. H. 1981. CO exposures of occupants of motor vehicles: Modeling the dynamic response of the vehicle. *SIMS technical report no. 48.* Stanford, Calif.: Stanford University.

Özkaynak, H., et al. 1987. Sources of emission rates of organic chemical vapors in homes and buildings. In *Indoor air '87: Proceedings of the fourth international conference on indoor air quality and climate.* Ed. B. Seifert et al., Vol. 1, 3–7. Berlin: Institute for Water, Soil, and Air Hygiene.

Parkhurst, W. J., et al. 1988. Influence of indoor combustion sources on indoor air quality. *Environ. Prog.* 7:257–61.

Price, B. 1988. Assessing asbestos exposure potential in buildings. Paper presented at the symposium on health effects of exposure to asbestos in buildings, 14–16 December, Harvard University.

Ryan, P. P., et al. 1988. The Boston residential $NO_2$ characterization study, I: Preliminary evaluation of the survey methodology. *J. Air Pollut. Control Assoc.* 38:22–27.

Sakuma, H., et al. 1983. The distribution of cigarette smoke components between mainstream and sidestream smoke: 1. Acidic components. *Beiträge Tabakforsch.* 12:63–71.

Sakuma, H., et al. 1984a. The distribution of cigarette smoke components between mainstream and sidestream smoke: 2. Bases. *Beiträge Tabakforsch.* 12:199–209.

Sakuma, H., et al. 1984b. The distribution of cigarette smoke components between mainstream and sidestream smoke: 3. Middle and higher boiling components. *Beiträge Tabakforsch.* 12:251–58.

Schmeltz, I.; Wenger, A.; Hoffman, D.; and Tso, T. C. 1979. On the fate of nicotine during pyrolysis and in a burning cigarette. *Agric. Food Chem.* 27:602–8.

Schutte, W. C., et al. 1981. Problems associated with the use of urea-formaldehyde foam for residential insulation, II. Residential studies in Colorado and Wisconsin. Oak Ridge, Tenn.: Oak Ridge National Laboratory, Publication no. ORNL-SUB/7559/3.

Sexton, K.; Spengler, J. D.; and Treitman, R. D. 1984. Effects of residential wood combustion on indoor air quality: A case study in Waterbury, Vermont. *Atmos. Environ.* 18:1371–83.

Sexton, K., et al. 1986. Characterization of particle composition, organic vapor constituents, and mutagenicity of indoor air pollution emissions. *Environ. Int.* 12:351–62.

Sheldon, L. S., et al. 1988. *Indoor air quality in public buildings, Vol. 1: Project summary.* Washington, D.C.: U.S. Environmental Protection Agency. Publication no. EPA/600/S6-88/009a.

Shikiya, D. C., et al. 1989. *Vehicle air toxins characterization study in the south coast air basin.* El Monte, Calif.: South Coast Air Quality Management District.

Spengler, J. D., and Tosteson, T. D. 1981. Personal exposures to respirable particles.

Presented at Environmetrics '81, April, Society for Industrial and Applied Mathematics, Alexandria, Va.

Spengler, J. D.; Billick, I.; and Ryan, P. B. 1984. Modeling population exposures to airborne lead. In *Indoor Air: Proceedings of the third international conference on indoor air quality and climate.* Ed. B. Berglund, T. Lindvall, and J. Sundell, Vol. 4, 87–94. Stockholm, Sweden: Swedish Council for Building Research. Available from NTIS, Springfield, Va. PB85-104214.

Spengler, J. D.; Stone, K. B.; and Lilley, F. W. 1978. High carbon monoxide levels measured in enclosed skating rinks. *J. Air Pollut. Control Assoc.* 28:776–79.

Spengler, J. D., et al., 1979. Sulfur dioxide levels and nitrogen dioxide levels inside and outside homes and the implications on health effects research. *Environ. Sci. Technol.* 13:1276–80.

Spengler, J. D., et al. 1981. Long-term measurements of respirable sulfates and particles inside and outside homes. *Atmos. Environ.* 15:23–30.

Spengler, J. D., et al., 1983. Nitrogen dioxide inside and outside 137 homes and implications for ambient air quality standards and health effects research. *Environ. Sci. Technol.* 17:164–68.

Spengler, J. D., et al., 1985. Personal exposures to respirable particulates and implications for air pollution epidemiology. *Environ. Sci. Technol.* 19:700–707.

Spengler, J. D., et al., eds. 1989. *Proceedings of the symposium on health aspects of exposure to asbestos in buildings.* Cambridge, Mass.: Harvard University Energy and Environmental Policy Center.

Sterling, D. A. 1985. Volatile organic compounds in indoor air: An overview of sources, concentrations, and health effects. In *Indoor air and human health.* Ed. R. B. Gammage and S. V. Kaye, 387–402. Chelsea, Mich.: Lewis Publishers.

Sterling, T. D., and Kobayashi, D. 1981. Use of the gas ranges for cooking and heating in urban dwellings. *J. Air Pollut. Control Assoc.* 29:238–41.

Stern, A. C., et al. 1984. *Fundamentals of air pollution.* 2d ed. Orlando, Fla.: Academic Press.

Stock, T. H.; Sterling, D. A.; and Monsen, R. M. 1984. A survey of indoor air quality in Texas mobile homes. In *Indoor air: Proceedings of the third international conference on indoor air quality and climate.* Ed. B. Berglund, T. Lindvall, and J. Sundell, Vol. 4, 331–34. Stockholm, Sweden: Swedish Council for Building Research.

Tennessee Valley Authority. 1985. *Indoor air quality study, phase II.* Chattanooga, Tenn.: Tennessee Valley Authority, Division of Conservation and Energy Management.

TerKonda, P., and Liaw, S. 1983. Monitoring of indoor aldehydes. *Proceedings of the Air Pollution Control Association specialty conference: Measurement and monitoring of non-criteria (toxic) contaminants in air,* 22–24 March, Chicago.

Traynor, G. W., et al. 1983a. Pollutant emissions from portable kerosene-fired space heaters. *Environ. Sci. Technol.* 17:369–71.

Traynor, G. W., et al. 1983b. Indoor air pollution from portable kerosene-fired space heaters. Washington, D.C.: U.S. Department of Energy, Office of Energy Research, Office of Health and Environmental Research. Publication no. 20585NTIS DE83-009140.

Traynor, G. W., et al. 1986. Selected organic pollutant emissions from unvented kerosene heaters. Paper 86-52.5, presented at the seventy-ninth annual meeting of the Air Pollution Control Association, 22–27 June, Minneapolis, Minn. Pittsburgh, Pa.: Air Pollution Control Association.

U.S. Consumer Product Safety Commission. 1982. Part IV: Ban of urea-formaldehyde foam insulation, withdrawal of proposed information labeling rule, and denial of petition to issue a standard. *Fed. Reg.* 47:14366.

U.S. Consumer Product Safety Commission. 1983. *Report of the chronic hazard advisory panel on asbestos.* Washington, D.C.: U.S. Consumer Product Safety Commission Directorate for Health Sciences.

U.S. Department of Energy. 1987. *Indoor air quality environmental information handbook: Combustion sources.* Washington, D.C.: U.S. Department of Energy. Publication no. DOE-EV/10450-821.

U.S. Department of Health and Human Services. 1986. *The health consequences of involuntary smoking: A report of the surgeon general.* Washington, D.C.: U.S. Government Printing Office. DHHS Publication no. CDC/87/8398.

U.S. Environmental Protection Agency. 1975. *Asbestos contamination of the air in public buildings.* Research Triangle Park, N.C.: U.S. Environmental Protection Agency. Publication no. EPA/450/3-76/004.

U.S. Environmental Protection Agency. 1980. *Measurement of asbestos air pollution inside buildings sprayed with asbesetos.* Washington, D.C.: U.S. Environmental Protection Agency. Publication no. EPA/560/13-80/026.

U.S. Environmental Protection Agency. 1983. *Airborne asbestos levels in schools.* Washington, D.C.: U.S. Environmental Protection Agency. Publication no. EPA/560/5-81-006.

U.S. Environmental Protection Agency. 1984. *Asbestos in buildings: A national survey of asbestos-containing friable materials.* Washington, D.C.: U.S. Environmental Protection Agency, Office of Toxic Substances. Publication no. EPA/560/5-84/006.

U.S. Environmental Protection Agency. 1987. *Preliminary indoor air pollution information assessment appendix.* Washington, D.C.: U.S. Environmental Protection Agency. Publication no. EPA/600/8-87/014.

U.S. Environmental Protection Agency. 1988a. *Study of asbestos-containing materials in public buildings: A report to Congress.* Washington, D.C.: U.S. Environmental Protection Agency.

U.S. Environmental Protection Agency. 1988b. *Assessing asbestos exposure in public buildings.* Washington, D.C.: U.S. Environmental Protection Agency. Publication no. EPA/560/5-88/002.

Vainio, H.; Hemminki, K.; and Wilbourn, J. 1985. Data on the carcinogenicity of chemicals in the IARC Monographs Programme. *Carcinogenesis* 6:1653–65.

Wade, W. A., III; Cote, W. A.; and Yocum, J. E. 1975. A study of indoor air quality. *J. Air Pollut. Control Assoc.* 25:933–39.

Wallace, L. A., et al. 1987. Emissions of volatile organic compounds from building materials and consumer products. *Atmos. Environ.* 21:385–93.

Woods, J. 1989. *HVAC systems as sources or vectors of microbiological contaminants.* COSC/ALA Workshop on Biological Pollutants in the Home, 10–11 July, Alexandria, Va.

Yocom, J. E. 1982. Indoor-outdoor air quality relationships: A critical review. *J. Air Pollut. Control Assoc.* 32:904–20.

Ziskind, R. A., et al. 1981. Carbon monoxide intrusion into sustained-use vehicles. *Environ. Int.* 5:109–23.

Zurer, P. 1985. Asbestos: The fiber that is panicking America. *Chem. Eng. News* 63:28–41.

# 3

# BUILDING DYNAMICS AND INDOOR AIR QUALITY

David T. Harrje, M.S.

The question may be asked—Why are building characteristics important to the understanding of indoor air quality? The answer is that indoor air quality is determined by the way a building is constructed and the materials used, and by the way the building is operated (Fanger 1987; American Society of Heating, Refrigerating, and Air-Conditioning Engineers [ASHRAE] 1989). Building characteristics are a major influence on indoor air quality in even the smallest house and in the largest commercial building.

The minimum ventilation necessary to maintain reasonable indoor air quality is treated in ASHRAE *Standard 62, Ventilation for Acceptable Indoor Air Quality* (ASHRAE 1989). *Standard 62* points out the need for concern not only for occupant factors, but also for factors related to building materials and the mechanical systems. Fanger emphasizes this point in two recent papers (Fanger 1987); (Fanger et al. 1988) based on an investigation of twenty Danish buildings. Fanger found the polluting effect of mechanical systems to cause 38 percent of the building indoor air quality problem: material outgasing, 36 percent; people, 7 percent; and smoking, 19 percent. From these and other studies it is evident that in any building the approach to maintaining indoor air quality must be first to limit the source of pollution (source control) or to control the pollution with local exhaust from the area, and only if these measures fail should ventilation be used to dilute the pollutants to acceptable concentration levels. These principles apply to all buildings, and the building dynamics can interact directly with both the spread and the control of pollutants. Inside-outside pressure differences caused by temperature and wind effects, air systems operation, the use of equipment in the building, and the activities of the occupants also influence indoor air quality. This chapter reviews the critical factors that determine the presence or absence of problems in indoor air quality, with a focus on building features and dynamics and the movement of air into and within buildings.

## CHARACTERISTICS OF THE BUILDING AND ASSOCIATED AIRFLOWS

The building envelope, that part of the building which separates the inside environment from the vagaries of the weather outside, is an important determinant of air infiltration (ASHRAE 1985a; Harrje, Dutt, and Beyea 1979) which has been defined as inward air leakage through cracks and interstices and through ceilings, floors, and walls (ASHRAE 1989). Air infiltration supplies most of the required ventilation in dwellings and, even in more sophisticated buildings, a substantial amount of the outside air that reaches the building occupants (Harrje 1985; Grot and Persily 1986). The location of the openings in the building envelope directly affects how much air can enter and the timing of air entry (Blomsterberg and Harrje 1979a, 1979b; ASHRAE 1985a).

The contribution of leakage sites to air infiltration and energy consumption has prompted studies of how leakage is distributed in residential structures. In most of the homes surveyed, the windows and doors accounted for 20–25 percent of the leakage (Figure 3.1), with four to five times as much leakage occurring through other sites (Harrje and Born 1982; Reinhold and Sonderegger 1983). Many of the other leakage sites were in the lower portion of the house, where soil gas and other pollutants can easily enter. Air inversion layers near buildings (Geiger 1965) can cause pollutants to collect from the soil or from nearby vehicular traffic and can funnel the pollutants to the building air inlet.

The degree of structural tightness between floors directly influences vertical airflow in a building. This vertical airflow is stack driven; that is, temperature-related density differences provide pressure that causes vertical air movement, with warmer air rising and cooler air falling. If the floors are structurally well separated, these vertical air movements will be impeded (ASHRAE 1985a). Open staircases and other easy airflow paths facilitate a free exchange of air between floors. Mechanically driven air movement in a building may suppress or enhance these natural air flows (Elmroth and Levin 1983).

Natural vertical air movement can be maximized with openings at the top of the building to allow warm building air to exfiltrate during the heating season and with openings at the lowest building level for air infiltration. Window openings in a high-low pattern can also be used to ventilate the building, utilizing the stack effect. Window openings also involve cross-ventilation, which changes with wind direction and pressures caused by the wind. Opening windows to allow air to enter on the windward (higher pressure) side and exit on the leeward (lower pressure) side of the building can optimize airing of the interior space (Blomsterberg and Harrje 1979a, 1979b; Persily 1982). Unintentional building openings function in the same manner to produce ventilation, although in an uncontrolled and often undesirable fashion.

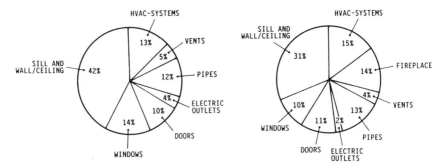

Figure 3.1. Typical air leakage distributions are shown for components in residential buildings. Eleven houses without fireplaces and nineteen houses with fireplaces were used as the data base. *Source: Reinhold and Sonderegger (1983), reprinted with permission.*

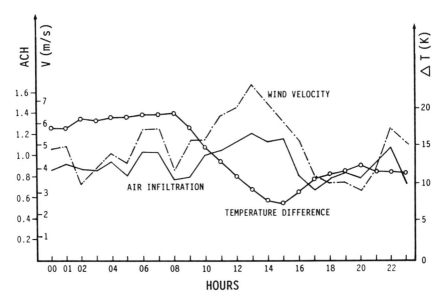

Figure 3.2. Air infiltration rates change rapidly due to stack, wind, and occupant effects. Ventilation levels may be excessive one minute and too low the next, as the wind changes direction or windows are closed. Minute-by-minute monitoring reveals the dynamic behavior.

Unfortunately, the effects due to wind and stack-induced pressures that cause air infiltration are not necessarily additive (Sinden 1978) and may actually oppose each other (Sinden 1978; Blomsterberg and Harrje 1979a, 1979b). Figure 3.2 illustrates how complex these combinations of effects may be as the variation of air infiltration is recorded over a period of time in a simple house.

A number of methods have been developed to identify sites of air infiltration and to describe the extent of the openings. These methods range from simple smoke tracers to indicate airflow to infrared scanning devices that rapidly determine details of the actual air leakage sites (Harrje, Dutt, and Beyea 1979; American Society for Testing Materials [ASTM] 1988c). Other methods such as fan pressurization (ASTM 1988b) and gas tracer techniques (ASTM 1988a) are used to determine the extent of the resultant air infiltration. These methods are used when air infiltration is likely to be a major factor in an indoor air quality problem and enable building diagnosticians to determine whether air exchange rates are acceptable, below standards, or excessive. The methods can also be used to find solutions to ventilation or infiltration problems.

## METHODS OF CHECKING FOR VENTILATION/AIR INFILTRATION

### FAN PRESSURIZATION

The simplest test for assessing the tightness of the building envelope is fan pressurization (Blomsterberg and Harrje 1979a, 1979b; Harrje and Born 1982; Persily 1982; Reinhold and Sonderegger 1983; ASTM 1988b). When applied to houses, this technique may use a blower door; that is, a flow-calibrated fan or blower is adjusted to fit an exterior doorway. Blower doors change the pressure difference between inside and outside by varying the airflow rate and flow direction. This procedure, detailed in ASTM *Standard Procedure E779–87*, provides a pressure versus flow profile for the house (Figure 3.3), indicating whether the house is too leaky, reasonably tight, or too tightly constructed. Too leaky implies unnecessary air infiltration, with energy waste and discomfort from drafts; too tight means that mechanical ventilation may be required to maintain air quality.

The fan pressurization/depressurization technique is not a precise measure of the amount of ventilation needed to achieve acceptable air quality but rather provides a gauge of the building envelope tightness. For an average house with 1,600 ft$^2$ of floor area, seven house volume air changes per hour at a pressure difference of 0.02 inches of water (50 Pascal) is calculated to be a desired goal. Using a rule of thumb translation to air changes per hour (ACH), under average outside heating season conditions, the 7 ACH is divided by twenty, giving 0.35 ACH as an average air infiltration rate (Kronvall 1980; Reinhold and Sonderegger 1983; Brunsell 1987). The value of 0.35 ACH is the prescribed air exchange rate for residential buildings in the latest draft version of ASHRAE *Standard 62–1989* (ASHRAE 1989). This version of ASHRAE *Standard 62* also states that smaller houses and a higher density of occupancy both require 15 cfm per person, minimum. In this case, for a 1,000 ft$^2$ home with four to five occupants, the blower door target becomes 10 ACH at 50 Pa, and the ventilation rate will equal 0.5 ACH under average conditions.

### TRACER GAS TECHNIQUES

Tracer gas techniques offer another approach to evaluation of air infiltration/ventilation rates (Harrje, Grot, and Grimsrud 1981). Standards have been established for tracer gas use; ASTM *Standard Practice E741–83* (ASTM 1988a)

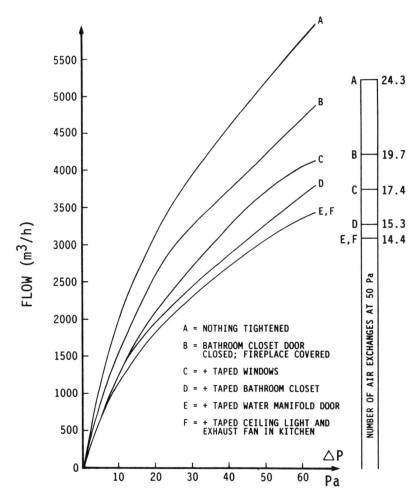

Figure 3.3. Fan pressurization produces flow profiles indicating the tightness of the structure. Evaluated at 50 Pa, curve A shows a very leaky structure. Even profile E,F predicts a 14.5 ACH. If we divide by twenty, a value of 0.73 ACH air infiltration seasonal rate is indicated, which is twice the required ventilation value.

discusses the different techniques, which include tracer gas dilution (decay of tracer concentration over time), constant injection of tracer into the spaces evaluated, and constant concentration of tracer gas maintained in each zone of the building (tracer gas sent to each zone is then directly proportional to the air infiltrating into the zone) (Harrje, Grot, and Grimsrud 1981).

*Tracer Gas Dilution*   The space to be evaluated is "seeded" with tracer gas by mixing the tracer in the space to a uniform concentration and then measuring the concentration of tracer gas over time. The rate of decay is directly related to the air exchange rate in the space being measured. An average air infiltration rate in the period of decay can be calculated from repeated measurements during the period.

The application of the dilution (or decay) technique can be simplified and made less costly by periodically capturing air samples in special bags or plastic bottles for later analysis rather than using on-site measuring equipment. This method has been used in relatively large field studies (Grot and Clark 1981; Harrje, Gadsby, and Linteris 1982). For example, in a study by Grot and Clark (1981), more than two hundred houses were measured using the bag sampling and tracer dilution technique. The purpose of the project was to evaluate the potential for weatherization of the homes of lower-income people. The tracer gas was dispersed with syringes so that each zone in the house could receive a roughly proportionate amount of tracer.

*Constant Injection of Tracer Gas*    In this method of evaluating air exchange rates, the tracer is injected at a constant rate, and the concentration is generally measured continuously (Harrje, Grot, and Grimsrud 1981; ASTM 1988a).

A simple passive version of the constant injection method uses perfluorocarbon tracers (Grot and Clark 1981; Dietz and Cote 1982; Dietz et al. 1986). The perfluorocarbon tracer technique uses capillary adsorption tube samplers (CATS), which are small glass tubes half the length of a cigarette and holding a charcoal-like material. The tracer gas is released at a controlled rate from even smaller containers. The tracer gas adsorbed in the CATS is recovered by heating the tube to 750–850°F and analyzing the gases with a gas chromatograph. By using the tracer diffusion rate and exposure time of the CATS, the tracer gas volume can be converted to an average concentration and the ventilation/air infiltration rate estimated. Using different tracers in various rooms allows interzone estimates of flow rates in addition to the primary measurements.

*Constant Concentration of Tracer Gas*    This third measurement method has gained considerable favor in the last few years (Harrje, Grot, and Grimsrud 1981; Harrje, Bohac, and Nagda 1985; Harrje et al. 1985; Liddament 1986; Bohac and Harrje 1987; Harrje, Bohac, and Fortmann 1987; ASTM 1988a). Although the measurement system requires the use of a computer, it can monitor ten (or even more) zones simultaneously. The rate of gas injection into each zone to maintain constant tracer gas concentration is used to calculate the air exchange rate.

The constant concentration measurement approach eliminates the influences of flow between zones and supplies individual air infiltration/ventilation values for each zone. By stopping tracer injection in one or more of the zones, information on interzone effects can also be obtained (Bohac and Harrje 1987). Another more commonly used approach is to employ multiple tracer gases so that individual tracers may reveal the interzone flows (I'Anson, Irwin, and Howarth 1982; Dietz, D'Ottavio, and Goodrich 1985).

Residential buildings, when studied using the techniques described above, show a log normal distribution of air infiltration (Figure 3.4) (Grot and Clark 1981). This distribution implies that many homes are much too leaky and require excessive heating and cooling to maintain comfort conditions. The homes with less than the one-third to one-half air change per hour are at risk for indoor air quality problems. Although Figure 3.4 places relatively few houses in that category, these data (Grot and Clark 1981) were taken in older homes of lower-income people. Data on newer housing indicate a greater proportion of homes in the "too tight" category and a lesser proportion in the "tail" of houses that are overventilated. To guide home builders in targeting the appropriate range of tightness, a proposed standard, SPC 119, has been written by an ASHRAE special committee. Titled "Air Leakage Performance for Detached Single-Family Residential Buildings," the proposed standard concentrates on weather influences in North America and provides guidelines for air infiltration and building tightness control to achieve a balance between energy needs and indoor air quality.

INSIDE-OUTSIDE TEMPERATURE DIFFERENCES: THE STACK EFFECT

The stack effect is an important but often overlooked factor that influences airflow in buildings. Nearby buildings or surrounding vegetation tend to shield the majority of buildings from much of the effect of the wind. In contrast, the stack effect reflects the inside-outside temperature difference, and from an air infiltration standpoint, it often becomes nature's dominant force (Blomsterberg and Harrje 1979a, 1979b; ASHRAE 1985a; Harrje 1985).

The stack effect increases air infiltration on the lowest floors of the building and maximizes air exfiltration at the highest floor level. This pressure-driven flow causes soil gases to enter buildings, producing a variety of pollutant problems including the entry of radon gas (Highland et al. 1985; Nazaroff et al. 1985; Harrje 1986; Harrje and Gadsby 1986; Harrje, Hubbard, and Sanchez 1987, 1988; Erickson 1988). The height at which interior and exterior pressures are equal is termed the *neutral pressure level* (NPL), that is, the height at which building envelope air leakage would have the least effect.

Even in a single-story building the influence of stack effect can be evident (ASHRAE 1985a; Harrje 1986; Harrje and Gadsby 1986). In multistory buildings, the effect can become much more pronounced as the number of floors increases unless the floors are isolated from each other. Even if the floors communicate, however, the vertical flow may not provide effective mixing of the air on each floor (Jun and Sheng 1987), and air moving up staircases may prove ineffective in removing pollutants from the floors it passes. Because of the stack effect, upper floors may receive little air directly from the outside and instead get "used air" from the lower floors.

The stack effect is usually conceptualized as most prominent during the heating season when the air within a building becomes increasingly more buoyant as the

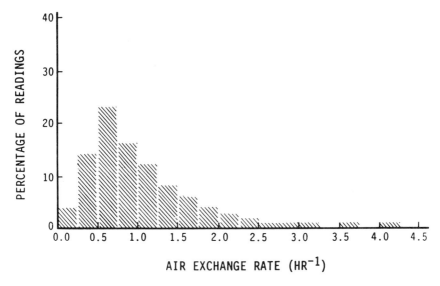

Figure 3.4. The typical histogram of measured air infiltration versus percent of readings follows a log normal distribution. The data shown are for 14 cities, 266 houses, and 1,048 readings with an average air infiltration of 1.12 ACH. Many of the houses exceed the 0.35–0.50 ACH goal, indicating energy waste, but there are also a number of houses with marginal air exchange rates, pointing to possible indoor air quality problems. *Source:* Grot and Clark (1981), reprinted with permission.

outside temperature drops. During the cooling season, reversal of the stack effect, with air entering upper stories and flowing to the lower stories and basement, might be anticipated. However, the temperature difference across a building in the cooling season is not so great as in the heating seasons in most areas of the United States. Furthermore, extremely high attic temperatures, 120°F or more, produce upward flow from the attic to outdoors in the summer. To make up for that flow, air may be drawn from the living space and thereby counteract the downward flow from the reversed stack effect. Because of such counteracting flows, the consequences of the stack effect cannot be readily predicted during the cooling season. Summer weather conditions have been shown repeatedly to produce the least air infiltration and to lead to major indoor air quality problems in houses (Harrje, Bohac, and Nagda 1985; Harrje, Bohac, and Fortmann 1987) when open windows are not used for cooling.

The stack effect and other pressure-driven flows cause soil gases to enter buildings (Nazaroff et al. 1985; Harrje 1986; Harrje and Gadsby 1986; Harrje, Hubbard, and Sanchez 1987, 1988). Although the problem of radon gas has received the most publicity, other undesirable pollutants emanate from in and around the building foundation or are constituents of soil gases. The pollutants of concern include pesticides, especially termicides, and constituents in ground water (Highland et al. 1985; Harrje 1986). The movement of soil gas has not yet been well characterized (Nazaroff et al. 1985; Harrje, Hubbard, and Sanchez 1987, 1988). The quantity of soil gas measured experimentally indicates that the gas may travel many feet through the soil.

Prevailing wind conditions also produce pressure-driven flows (Blomsterberg and Harrje 1979a, 1979b; ASHRAE 1985a). Wind effects can be very complex and have both static and dynamic features. For the unprotected building, wind can be the dominant effect, and if wind speeds are high, for example, greater than 20 mph, even the wind-protected building will sustain pressure effects.

The wind speed affecting the building generally correlates with the wind speed recorded at the local weather station. Wind speed has a profile from zero speed at the ground to a maximum value at a point above the terrain effects. Even the 10-m-high standard wind measurement sensor is placed in a changing wind speed regime within the boundary layer (Blomsterberg and Harrje 1979a, 1979b; ASHRAE 1985a). Wind effects are made complex by the nature of the terrain that surrounds the building and the shape of the building itself. Changes in the wind direction may establish entirely different wind paths, which may be further affected by trees or other buildings standing in the path of the wind (Buckley et al. 1978; Harrje, Mattingly, and Heisler 1979).

Because of openings in the building envelope and the profiles of pressure on the building surfaces, various levels of local pressurization or depressurization may take place at any opening. Thus, opening a window may allow air to enter or exit the building just as flow over the chimney may force the chimney to backflow or at the other extreme, may cause a higher exhaust flow. Zones of high and low pressure on the building surface vary in position with wind direction and speed and with stack effects. Similar pressure increases and decreases occur on the surrounding ground surface and can influence the flow of soil gases into the building (Harrje, Hubbard, and Sanchez 1987).

## EQUIPMENT AND APPLIANCES FOR VENTILATION

Although most prevalent in larger buildings, mechanical ventilation is becoming more common in the advanced design homes of the past few years such as the R–2000 homes in Canada. A heat recovery ventilator (HRV, air-to-air heat exchanger) is central to the ventilation design of these homes and provides controlled ventilation during all seasons (Riley 1985). By generating its own pressure and flow conditions, mechanical ventilation systems can overwhelm the pressures developed by stack and wind effects.

Many of the ventilation-related components in buildings use balanced flow operation: Supply air and return air are equal or have a known relationship to each other to maintain a desired pressure condition and flow distribution. Turning on an exhaust fan, however, produces local depressurization in a large office building or in a home kitchen or bathroom. The depressurization can draw air from other spaces in the building to the exhausted room or zone or suck air and soil gas in from the outside. The depressurization can also cause backdrafting of combustion exhaust systems (ASHRAE 1985a; Harrje, Hubbard, and Sanchez 1987, 1988).

Heating, ventilating, and air-conditioning (HVAC) equipment commonly leads to locally pressurized and depressurized zones, particularly if the system is not balanced. The system may be balanced initially, but changes over time and "adjustments" by operations personnel or occupants may greatly alter it. System designs that provide adequate air supplies but insufficient air returns may also produce localized inhomogeneity of pressure in all types of buildings (Harrje, Gadsby, and Comer 1986). The home with conditioned air supplies in every room but only one (or at the most two) return grills is a simple but common example. Each time the furnace, air conditioner, or heat pump operates, certain rooms are pressurized, causing higher than normal air exfiltration, while others are depressurized, increasing air infiltration locally. Thus, operation of the HVAC system increases air infiltration to sometimes more than double the rate observed with the system off or adequately balanced. In the basement, where the HVAC equipment is located, basement air is sucked into leaks in the return ducts and air handler fan housing because of inadequate returns. A depressurized basement can suck in soil gas (Harrje 1986; Harrje and Gadsby 1986; Harrje, Hubbard, and Sanchez 1987, 1988) and cause backdrafting from combustion devices into the home (Harrje, Hubbard, and Sanchez 1987, 1988).

Throughout the house, dryer vent fans, kitchen fans, bathroom fans, and even attic fans can cause negative pressures to exist for short or long periods of time and increase entry of unwanted soil gas or exhaust products into living areas.

## THE ROLE OF THE OCCUPANTS

Although the building characteristics, ventilation equipment, and meteorology all affect building dynamics, the most important factor influencing air movements is often the actions of the occupants themselves. The occupants may directly influence ventilation through use of doors, vents, and windows. This effect on ventilation may be manifest in energy use. For example, studies of energy use typically show a twofold variation in energy use for identical homes (Fracastoro and Lyberg 1983).

Although the importance of occupant behavior has been mostly studied in single-family housing, larger buildings may also be affected by it. Studies in multifamily homes have pointed to ten-fold variations in window ventilation levels for interior temperature control—residents open windows to lower temperatures in overheated rooms (Harrje and Kempton 1986; Bohac, Dutt, and Feuermann 1987).

## MODELING POLLUTANT FLOWS

Modeling of pollutant flows within buildings, taking into account pressure differences from exterior and interior sources, building geometry, and interior events, has been achieved with equations based on the work of Walton (ASHRAE 1985b; Walton 1985; Grot and Axley 1987). The building airflow patterns are described by the program AIRMOV, using PC-sized computers. The measurement techniques discussed previously in this chapter are useful in providing a data base for validating the computer program solutions.

Two classes of flow elements have been developed in models from the National Institute of Standards and Technology: flow-resistant elements and fan/pump elements. The flow resistant element may be used to model a large variety of flow paths, from ducting to envelope or interior surface openings. The fan/pump elements model the HVAC system where appropriate. Currently, detailed time histories of airborne contaminants are being modeled using these procedures (Grot and Axley 1987).

## SUMMARY

In all buildings, from the most sophisticated to the simple one-family home, understanding the dynamics of air entry into the building and air flow within the building is vitally important if acceptable air quality is to be maintained. To this end, the education of building occupants, builders, and maintenance staff is highly important. Monitoring, which is more than a research tool, plays a key role in maintaining indoor air quality and can allow near-optimum building function, with individual building dynamics and occupancy factors as part of the total equation.

## REFERENCES

American Society of Heating, Refrigerating, and Air-Conditioning Engineers. 1985a. Natural ventilation. In *ASHRAE Handbook of Fundamentals;* 22.1–51. Atlanta, Ga.: ASHRAE.

American Society of Heating, Refrigerating, and Air-Conditioning Engineers. 1985b. Duct design. In *ASHRAE Handbook of Fundamentals,* Atlanta, Ga.: ASHRAE.

American Society of Heating, Refrigerating, and Air-Conditioning Engineers. 1989. *ASHRAE Standard 62-1989. Ventilation for acceptable indoor air quality.* Atlanta, Ga.: ASHRAE.

ASTM. 1988a. *Standard E741-82.* Standard test method for determining air leakage rate by tracer dilution. *Annual Book of ASTM Standards,* 568–75. Philadelphia: ASTM.

ASTM. 1988b. *Standard E779-87.* Standard test method for determining air leakage rate by fan pressurization. *Annual Book of ASTM Standards,* 603–6. Philadelphia: ASTM.

ASTM. 1988c. *Standard E11-86.* Standard practice for air leakage site detection in building envelopes. *Annual Book of ASTM Standards,* 885–89. Philadelphia: ASTM.

Blomsterberg, A. K., and Harrje, D. T. 1979a. Approaches to evaluation of air infiltration energy losses in buildings. *ASHRAE Trans.* 85:797–815.

Blomsterberg, A. G., and Harrje, D. T. 1979b. Evaluating air infiltration energy losses. *ASHRAE J.* 21:25–32.

Bohac, D. L., and Harrje, D. T. 1987. The use of modified constant concentration techniques to measure infiltration and interzone air flow rates. *Proceedings of the eighth AIVC* conference: Ventilation technology, research and application, 129–52. Coventry, Great Britain: AIVC. Publication no. AIC-PROC-8-5-87.

Bohac, D. L.; Dutt, G. S.; and Feuermann, D. 1987. Approaches to estimating air flows in a large multifamily building. *ASHRAE Trans.* 93:1335–58.

Brunsell, J. T. 1987. The effect of vapor barrier thickness on air tightness. *Proceedings of the eighth AIVC conference: Ventilation technology, research and application,* 63–73. Coventry, Great Britain: AIVC. Publication no. AIC-PROC-8-5-87.

Buckley, C. E., et al. 1978. *The optimum use of coniferous trees in reducing home energy consumption.* Princeton, N.J.: Princeton University Center for Environmental Studies. Report no. 71.

Dietz, R. N., and Cote, E. A. 1982. Air infiltration measurements in a home using a convenient perfluorocarbon tracer technique? *Environ. Int.* 8:419–33.

Dietz, R. N.; D'Ottavio, T. W.; and Goodrich, R. W. 1985. Multizone infiltration measurements in homes and buildings using a passive perfluorocarbon tracer method. *ASHRAE Trans.* 91:1761–75.

Dietz, R. N., et al. 1986. Detailed description and performance of a passive perfluorocarbon tracer system for building ventilation and air exchange measurements. In *Measured air leakage of buildings.* Ed. H. R. Trechsel and P. L. Lagus, 203–64. Philadelphia: ASTM. Publication no. ASTM-STP/904.

Elmroth, A., and Levin, P., eds. 1983. *Air infiltration control in housing: A guide to international practice.* Stockholm, Sweden: Swedish Council for Building Research. Publication no. D2 1983.

Erickson, B. E. 1988. *Radon in housing.* Gavle, Sweden: Swedish National Institute for Building Research.

Fanger, P. O. 1987. A solution to the sick building mystery. In *Indoor air '87: Proceedings of the fourth international conference on indoor air quality and climate.* Ed. B. Seifert et al., Vol. 4, 49–55. Berlin: Institute for Water, Soil, and Air Hygiene.

Fanger, P. O., et al. 1988. Air pollution sources in offices and assembly halls quantified by the Olf unit. *Energy and buildings,* Vol. 12, 7–19. Lausanne, Switzerland: Elsevier Sequoia.

Fracastoro, G. V., and Lyberg, M. D., eds. 1983. *Guiding principles concerning design of experiments, instrumentation and measuring techniques.* Stockholm, Sweden: Swedish Council for Building Research. Publication no. D11.

Geiger, R. 1965. *The climate near the ground.* Cambridge, Mass.: Harvard University Press.

Grot, R. A., and Axley, R. 1987. The development of models for the prediction of indoor air quality in buildings. *Supplement to Proceedings of the eighth AIVC conference: Ventilation Technology and Application,* 171–97. Coventry, Great Britain: AIVC. Publication no. AIC-PROC-8-5-87.

Grot, R. A., and Clark, R. E. 1981. Air leakage characteristics and weatherization techniques for low-income housing. *Proceedings of the ASHRAE/DOE-ORNL conference: Thermal performance of the exterior envelopes of buildings,* 178–94. Atlanta, Ga.: ASHRAE.

Grot, R. A., and Persily, A. K. 1986. Measured air infiltration and ventilation rates in eight large office buildings. In *Measured air infiltration in buildings.* Ed. H. R. Trechsel and P. L. Lagus, 151–83. Philadelphia, Pa.: ASTM. Publication no. ASTM STP-904.

Harrje, D. T. 1985. Air exchange in buildings. *Proceedings of the indoor air quality seminar: Implications for electric utility conservation programs,* 3.1–10. Palo Alto,

Calif.: Electric Power Research Institute. Publication no. EPRI-EA/EM/3824.

Harrje, D. T. 1986. Clean and economical air in houses. *Architect. Technol.* July/August: 33–36.

Harrje, D. T., and Born, G. J. 1982. Cataloguing air leakage components in houses. *Proceedings of the ACEEE 1982 summer study: Existing residences.* Washington, D.C.: American Council for an Energy Efficient Economy.

Harrje, D. T., and Gadsby, K. J. 1986. Practical engineering solutions for optimizing energy conservation and indoor air quality in residential buildings. *Proceedings of the international conference on indoor air quality and climate,* IAQ 1986. Atlanta, Ga.: ASHRAE.

Harrje, D. T., and Kempton, W. M. 1986. Ventilation, air infiltration and building occupant behavior. *Proceedings of the seventh AIC conference: Occupant interaction with ventilation systems* 2.1–16. Coventry, Great Britain: AIVC. Publication no. AIC-PROC-7-86.

Harrje, D. T.; Bohac, D. L.; and Fortmann, R. C. 1987. Measurement of seasonal air flow rates in an unoccupied single-family house. *Proceedings of the eighth AIC Conference: Ventilation Technology, Research and Application,* 15.1–15. Coventry, Great Britain: AIVC. Publication no. AIC-PROC-8-87.

Harrje, D. T.; Bohac, D. L.; and Nagda, N. L. 1985. Air exchange rates based upon individual room and single cell measurements. *Proceedings of the sixth AIC conference: Ventilation strategies and measurement techniques,* 7.1–14. Coventry, Great Britain: AIVC. Publication no. AIC-PROC-6-85;

Harrje, D. T.; Dutt, G. S.; and Beyea, J. 1979. Locating and eliminating obscure but major energy losses in residential housing. *ASHRAE Trans.* 85:521–34.

Harrje, D. T.; Gadsby, K. J.; and Comer, C. J. 1986. Transients and physics of return air. In *Proceedings of the air movement and distribution conference.* Ed. C. G. Marsh and V. W. Goldschmidt, Vol. 2, 10–16. Lafayette, Ind.: Purdue University.

Harrje, D. T.; Gadsby, K. J.; and Linteris, G. T. 1982. Sampling for air exchange rates in a variety of buildings. *ASHRAE Trans.* 88:1373–84.

Harrje, D. T.; Grot, R. A.; and Grimsrud, D. T. 1981. Air infiltration—site measurement techniques. *Proceedings of the 2nd AIC conference: Building design for minimum air infiltration,* 113–33. Coventry, Great Britain: AIVC. Publication no. AIC-PROC-2-81.

Harrje, D. T.; Hubbard, L. M.; and Sanchez, D. C. 1987. *Proceedings of the radon diagnostics workshop.* Princeton, N.J.: Princeton University Center for Energy and Environmental Studies. Report no. 233.

Harrje, D. T.; Hubbard, L. M.; and Sanchez, D. C. 1988. Diagnostic approaches to better solutions of radon IAQ problems. *Proceedings of healthy buildings.* Stockholm, Sweden: Swedish Council of Building Research.

Harrje, D. T.; Mattingly, G.; and Heisler, G. 1979. The effectiveness of an evergreen windbreak for reducing residential energy consumption. *ASHRAE Trans.* 85:428–44.

Harrje, D. T., et al. 1985. Documenting air movements and air infiltration in multicell buildings using various tracer techniques. *ASHRAE Trans.* 91:2012–26.

Highland, J. H., et al. 1985. The impact of groundwater contaminants on indoor air quality. *Proceedings of the twelfth energy technology conference,* 728–40. Rockville, Md.: Government Institutes.

I'Anson, S. J.; Irwin, C.; and Howarth, A. T. 1982. Air flow measurement using three tracer gases. *Building Environ.* 17:245–52.

Jun, G., and Sheng, L. M. 1987. The effective and ineffective heat loss by infiltration: Field measurement in a dormitory. *Proceedings of the third international congress on building energy management, Vol. 3: Ventilation air movement and air quality,* 52–57. Lausanne, Switzerland: École Polytechnique Federale de Lausanne.

Kronvall, J. 1980. *Airtightness: Measurements and measurement methods.* Stockholm, Sweden: Swedish Council of Building Research. Report D8.

Liddament, M. W. 1986. A review of European research into airtightness and air infiltration measurement techniques. In *Measured air leakage of buildings.* Ed. H. R. Trechsel and P. L. Lagus, 407–15. Philadelphia: ASTM. Publication no. ASTM-STP/904.

Nazaroff, W. W., et al. 1985. Radon transport into a detached one-story house with a basement. *Atmos. Environ.* 19:31–46.

Persily, A. K. 1982. Understanding air infiltration in homes. Ph.D. diss., Princeton University Center for Energy and Environmental Studies, Princeton, N.J. Report 129.

Reinhold, C., and Sonderegger, R. 1983. Component leakage areas in residential buildings. *Proceedings of the fourth AIC conference: Air infiltration reduction in existing buildings,* 16.1–30. Bracknell, Berkshire, Great Britain: AIVC. Publication no. AIC-PROC-11-83.

Riley, M. 1985. Mechanical ventilation system requirements and measured results for homes constructed under the R-2000 Super Energy-Efficient Home Program. *Proceedings of the sixth AIC conference: Ventilation strategies and measurement techniques,* 16.1–21. Coventry, Great Britain: AIVC. Publication no. AIC-PROC-6-85.

Sinden, F. W. 1978. Multi-chamber theory of air infiltration. *Building Environ.* 13:21–28.

Walton, G. 1985. *Estimating interroom contaminant movements.* Washington, D.C.: U.S. Department of Commerce, National Bureau of Standards. Publication no. NBSIR 85-3229.

# 4

# ASSESSMENT OF
# INDOOR AIR QUALITY

John F. McCarthy, Sc.D., David W. Bearg, M.S.,
John D. Spengler, Ph.D., M.S.

Environmental monitoring is conducted for a variety of purposes, including determination of compliance and enforcement, detection and diagnosis of unusual conditions, and research. The particular purpose of the investigation determines the contaminants to be sampled, the sampling locations, the instrumentation used, the frequency of measurements, and the required sensitivity of detection. This chapter begins by providing a systematic approach to investigating buildings. It focuses primarily on buildings whose occupants have experienced complaints potentially related to conditions in the indoor environment. The chapter then discusses air sampling equipment for measuring concentrations of gases and of particulate matter. The review is not comprehensive but illustrates the current options for assessing indoor air quality. More detailed descriptions of sampling strategies, methods, and equipment are available in recent books (Lioy and Lioy 1983; Nagda, Rector, and Koontz 1987; Lodge 1989; American Conference of Governmental and Industrial Hygienists [ACGIH] 1989). Chapter 3 addresses the dynamics of air exchange in homes and buildings and describes the commonly used methods for measuring airflow within buildings and the air exchange rates with outside air.

The growing recognition of indoor air quality problems in both homes and buildings has prompted the development of strategies for investigating these problems and for measuring indoor air quality. Investigations of indoor air quality problems may include engineering tests, physical or chemical measurements, health and comfort surveys of the occupants, and medical evaluation tests of the occupants (Lioy and Lioy 1983; Thorsen and Molhave 1987; Woods, Morey, and Rask 1987; Quinlan et al. 1989; Wallingford and Carpenter 1986). Typically, investigations are initiated (a) to demonstrate compliance with federal or state regulations; (b) to respond to complaints of poor air quality by building occupants;

(c) to audit the space before occupancy, change of use of the space, or design modifications that may vary the physical layout; and (d) to evaluate the operating performance of systems. At present, complaints by occupants lead to the initiation of most investigations.

Occupants of buildings receive a large number of sensory stimuli that determine perceptions of the indoor environment (Baker 1989) (see Chapter 1). Each occupant integrates the many physical, chemical, and psychological inputs that together determine subjective judgment of the acceptability of the space. In achieving an acceptable indoor environment, those involved in the construction and subsequent operation of buildings must understand the complex nature not only of the structure and its operation but also of occupant responses. In addressing indoor air quality problems, investigators must also understand the complex interface between the occupants and the building environment.

Thus, many factors can cause complaints to be initiated by occupants, and a multidisciplinary approach, often involving building engineers, health professionals, and experts in indoor air quality assessment, is needed in investigating occupant complaints. A systematic approach should be taken to integrate the efforts of the team in order to resolve "problem buildings." Typically, a building survey includes four types of activity: communication, engineering analysis, instrumental surveys, and quality assurance. This chapter will discuss these aspects of building investigations and provide a condensed summary of some available instruments. Persons suspecting that their illness may be related to the building they occupy should be encouraged to undergo evaluation by appropriate medical personnel.

As environmental problems in buildings were initially recognized during the 1970s and early 1980s, traditional industrial hygiene measurement techniques were employed to evaluate indoor air quality. However, these methods generally do not have sufficient sensitivity to measure accurately the contaminant levels that are encountered indoors. To evaluate the indoor environment effectively requires a different perspective from that of traditional industrial hygiene. Regulatory compliance in the industrial environment is generally based upon meeting specific limits of individual exposures, that is, permissible exposure limits (PEL) (Occupational Safety and Health Administration [OSHA] 1989). Industrial hygiene surveys are directed at improved contaminant control or maintaining worker protection. Acceptable indoor air quality, on the other hand, is generally achieved through reliance on prescriptive criteria (e.g., outdoor air ventilation rates) to limit contaminant levels (American Society of Heating, Refrigerating, and Air-Conditioning Engineers [ASHRAE] 1989). These criteria, developed primarily for design purposes, recognize the numerous, nonspecific sources that may impact the indoor environment. New approaches designed for assessing the indoor environment are needed to investigate problem buildings, since the conventional industrial hygiene approach is not suitable (Woods, Morey, and Stolwijk 1988).

DESCRIBING THE PROBLEM: THE FIRST STAGE OF INVESTIGATION

The first step in conducting an investigation is to describe the scope of the problem; this first step often sets the tone for the entire assessment. An outside investigator may have difficulty in describing the full scope of the problem, however, because building occupants, management, owners, and facility operators often do not share a common level of concern. The responsibilities of these groups are different, and the actual or perceived consequences of the problem may vary among them. The threat of litigation may also impact decisions. However, the information gathered by the investigator at this time must be sufficient to describe the characteristics of the problem and to develop hypotheses concerning its source (National Institute for Occupational Safety and Health [NIOSH] 1987). This first stage might consist of a detailed walk-through survey of the building; a screening questionnaire for the occupants of the space; and interviews with management, employees, and other concerned parties such as involved medical and facilities personnel and industrial hygienists.

The health and comfort effects of concern should be described in this first stage. The populations at risk should be characterized by location, employment status, age, gender, or other potentially important attributes. Table 4.1 provides a brief guide for characterizing complaints; the description should cover the symptoms, the timing of occurrence in relation to entering and leaving the workplace, the severity, and the locations of affected persons. This information may provide links to changes in the operation of the heating, ventilating, and air-conditioning (HVAC) systems, to renovations, relocations, and equipment use, and to other factors.

Table 4.1   Initial Characterization
of Complaints

Nature of complaints/symptom
　　Site or organ system affected (e.g., respiratory)
　　Severity
　　Duration
　　Associations
　　Treatment/confirmations
Timing of complaints
　　Long-term (continuing, periodic, seasonal, week-
　　　ly, daily)
　　Short-term (isolated events)
Location of affected and not-affected groups
Numbers affected
Demographics of occupants with and without com-
　　plaints
　　Age
　　Gender
　　Employment status

Table 4.2    Survey of Facilities

Physical layout of building
    Work stations
    Location of air supplies and returns
    HVAC zones
HVAC inspection
    Coils
    Filters
    Fans
    Drip pans
    Condensers
    Air intakes
    Distribution ductwork
HVAC operation
    Load analysis
    Control analysis
    Assessment of modifications


Table 4.3    Potential Sources Impacting
Air Quality

Exterior sources impacting air intakes
    Loading docks
    Roadways
    Cooling towers
    Other external sources
    Locations of intake and exhaust vents
Interior sources
    Insulation (man-made fibers, asbestos)
    Equipment
    Cleaning compounds
    Office furnishings
    Areas damaged by floods, high humidity, or other
      agents

During this initial survey, potential sources of contaminants in the space should also be identified. This characterization should assess whether the contaminants are continuously or intermittently present; whether specific point sources or area releases contaminate individual spaces; and whether the sources originate indoors or outdoors.

Finally, a history of the building should be developed. The history of the building mechanical system and its functioning should be reviewed, as should records of construction/renovation and building occupation. Any modifications to the HVAC system or the physical plan should be noted. An initial evaluation of the system's performance relative to its design goals should also be made. Table 4.2 outlines the principal components of a building which should be surveyed both at the time of initial inspection and in subsequent detailed follow-up. Table 4.3 details potential sources, both inside and outside, that may affect indoor air quality in

Table 4.4   Indoor Environmental Climate
and Comfort Factors[a]

| Factor | Parameters |
|--------|------------|
| Thermal | Dry-bulb temperature |
| | Wet-bulb temperature |
| | Vertical temperature gradient |
| | Plane-radiation temperature |
| | Omnidirectional air velocity (drafts) |
| Acoustic | Full bank sound level |
| | Frequency, intensity, type |
| Vibration | Frequency and amplitude |
| Lighting | Full-spectrum analysis |
| | Quantity (intensity) |
| | Quality (flickering, color, glare, or |
| | other problems) |

[a]For further guidance, see ASHRAE (1985).

structures. Table 4.4 lists indoor environmental, climate, and comfort factors that can affect the occupants of a space.

After this first-stage assessment, an experienced investigator may detect the source of the problem. If remedial steps cannot be identified, then a more detailed investigation must be undertaken. However, at this point, the problem should have received sufficient description to permit development of a hypothesis and specification of the protocols necessary for further exploration.

SURVEY MONITORING: THE SECOND STAGE OF INVESTIGATION

The second stage of investigation often has three components: system evaluation, definition of microenvironments, and environmental screening. A system evaluation usually begins with a review of specifications, interviews with relevant personnel, and direct inspection of the premises. The evaluation also covers comfort controls in terms of sensor location, set points, and access. It is also important to establish the lines of responsibility for comfort conditions and the actions of facility operators in response to occupant requests. A more thorough system evaluation consists of analyzing (measuring) airflow through diffusers and other mechanical devices, both for supply and exhaust. Heating and cooling coils, drip pans, and filters should be inspected and maintenance schedules reviewed. The evaluation should also address the thermal loads of the building as originally designed and subsequent changes that could affect building load.

The concept of microenvironments is essential to building investigations (see Chapter 5). For the protocol circumstances of a building investigation, microenvironments may be defined as spaces sharing a common HVAC system, a ducted air supply, a zone, or a floor of a building. Microenvironments could also be defined as locations in which employees experiencing similar complaints are located. The concept of microenvironments should drive the sampling plan since each sampling location is generally assumed to be representative of a homogeneous environment. Therefore, variation of measurements within a microenvironment must be less than the variance between different microenvironments. The outdoors also represents one or more microenvironments and may be sampled to establish background levels. However, a close inspection, and possibly sampling, of external sources that may impact a building may be required. There may be substantial variation in the air of various external areas of the building, which should be accounted for in the sampling scheme.

Five types of areas should be considered in developing a sampling strategy: (a) areas with the most susceptible occupants; (b) areas with potential sources; (c) areas with the least effective ventilation; (d) control areas having the least problems; and (e) outdoor air.

Environmental screening describes potential contaminant levels or other physical conditions in the space. Data can be collected with real-time survey monitors, such as those for carbon monoxide, carbon dioxide, temperature, humidity, and light levels, or integrated measurements can be used for respirable particulate matter or volatile organic compounds. For some contaminants (e.g., asbestos or microorganisms), bulk samples or surface samples are the most cost-effective means of identifying potential sources. The equipment used for making measurements should be calibrated in the anticipated range of field measurements both before and after sampling. The calibration procedures should be traceable to primary standards. (See Tables 4.6 through 4.11 for selected instrumentation suitable for building surveys.)

Depending on the results of the initial screening survey, additional information may be required to characterize fully the problem building. Table 4.5 summarizes additional considerations in planning a more detailed environmental survey.

*Selection of Parameters to Be Measured*    Information gathered during the initial stages of investigation can define a set of contaminants and/or environmental conditions (i.e., temperature, relative humidity, drafts, air exchange rate, and other factors) which need to be monitored. These parameters can usually be obtained from a history of the building, an inventory of products used in the building, locations of potential sources, and a history of occupant complaints.

Table 4.5    Survey Design

Selection of physical/chemical contaminants to be
   measured
Time scale of measurements, duration, frequency
Establishment of required level of detection
Selection of instrumentation
Selection of sampling locations
Quality assurance program
Data analysis and presentation

*Time Scale of Measurements* The time scale of environmental measurements should be related to the potential health effects of interest. This can be refined further to reflect individual time and activity patterns that may have an important impact on overall exposures. Guidance in deciding on an appropriate sample duration to assess the impact of specific contaminants can come from relevant medical and toxicologic literature. For example, if there are short-term exposure limits for specific pollutants, the pollutants may have a significant short-term toxic effect and therefore should be evaluated with this concern in mind. Long-term integrated samplers can be used to characterize exposures to pollutants that cause toxic effects after chronic exposure.

Since integrated sampling methods average the concentrations of pollutants over the duration of the sample, they do not provide information on short-term excursions and peak concentrations which may be an important consideration in assessing individual exposures to pollutants. Furthermore, integrated samples generally do not capture information on cyclic exposures or variations that can occur throughout the sampling period. The critical concern in developing any sampling strategy is that samples are collected during the entire anticipated exposure period. The intermittent nature of many exposures requires that short-term sampling does not replace carefully formulated protocols for assessing individual exposures. Frequently the duration of sampling is limited by the collection media employed. For such methods it may be necessary to collect successive samples to ensure that any exposure events are effectively captured. For some pollutants, continuous sampling and analytical instruments with strip chart recorders or data loggers may be needed, as used for outdoor monitoring.

Time scales of interest can be seasonal, weekly, daily, or of shorter duration. The episodes of exposure may fall into a regular pattern, or they may be sporadic and unpredictable. External sources may impact pollutant levels, and meteorologic factors may have important influences on overall exposures. A historical review of complaints can help in determining the appropriate time scale for measurement.

The evaluation should consider that complaints by building residents or occupants may precede the monitoring and environmental assessment of the building by several weeks or more. The environmental conditions that produced the symptoms among occupants may have been transient or altered after complaints were made, and thus relating current measurements to past symptoms may be misleading.

The adverse effects experienced by occupants may be displaced from the relevant exposures or conditions in place and in time. For example, an individual may become sensitized to a contaminant over a period of time and then respond to much lower levels than had been encountered initially; cancer may follow the onset of an exposure by many years; asthmatics may experience bronchoconstriction hours after exposure to an agent rather than immediately; exposure that affects the fetus during the first trimester of pregnancy may be manifest only after birth. The investigator must understand the temporal relationship between exposures to various agents and the temporal evolution of injury, symptoms, and disease and the limitations of extrapolating measurements over time and place, particularly if changes of occupancy, function, material, ventilation, or external conditions have taken place.

*Required Level of Detection*  Ideally the level of detection for instrumentation and analytical methods should be determined by the level of a particular contaminant expected to impact health or well-being. However, for many indoor pollutants, the needed scientific evidence is unavailable, particularly across the entire spectrum of sensitivity. At times trade-offs must be made among availability of instrumentation, portability, degree of obtrusiveness, and cost of analysis. To conduct a valid sampling program, the lower limit of detection must be assessed before going into the field; ideally it should be 10 percent of the desired change, whether in relation to levels associated with a health response or to an environmental standard. As general guidance, setting a lower detection limit of 1 percent of the occupational threshold limit value (TLV) or permissible exposure limit should be encouraged.

*Selection of Instrumentation*  Tables 4.6 through 4.11 list selected methods and techniques for measuring air pollutants which are suitable for indoor air quality investigations. These can be divided into the categories of direct measurement techniques, passive sampling with active analysis procedures, and active sampling with active analysis procedures. Often the choice of instrumentation depends upon the required level of detection and the time scales of interest.

*Selection of Sampling Locations*  Indoor monitoring always occurs in a dynamic environment, and the design of measurement surveys and the interpretation of results should appropriately consider the complex and changing nature of the monitored environment. Building occupants are not typically confined to a single location, and fixed location monitoring might not adequately represent personal exposures. For example, exposure to asbestos may be very low for most occupants in a building that has asbestos-containing materials, but maintenance and services employees, while running computer and telephone cables above the acoustical ceiling tile, could experience substantially higher fiber exposure as the material is disrupted. Similarly, higher radon levels are often found in basements, whereas in upstairs living areas the concentration can often be one-half to one-quarter of the basement concentration. Observation of occupant activity patterns, understanding of the ventilation system and air movement, and knowing the location of potential pollutant sources should guide investigators in selecting the sampling locations. It may be necessary to monitor in "control" areas or in other buildings for comparison. Depending upon the contaminants and conditions being examined, outdoor (upwind and downwind) monitoring might be required.

*Quality Assurance and Control*  Adequate quality assurance and quality control procedures should be employed to ensure the accuracy of the data collected (Corn

1985; NIOSH 1984). The foremost consideration must be whether or not an adequate number of samples has been collected. Sampling statistics can be used for this purpose, and a pilot study may be needed. An evaluation of the variation among results is an important consideration in assessing how many additional samples must be collected to characterize the environment fully. Consideration should be given to the possible variation of contaminant concentrations over both time and space.

The quality assurance and control program should include field blanks, replicates, split samples, and spiked samples as appropriate. A certain number of replicate samples should be collected to assess the precision of sampling and analysis methods. Furthermore, an appropriate number of field blanks should be collected, generally two for each of ten actual samples. The field blanks should be retained independently of media blanks, which can be used by the laboratory to assess extraction efficiency or media contamination. Samples sent to a laboratory should be randomly numbered and presented in a blind manner to avoid potential conflicts and to ensure against bias by the analysts. It may be advisable to "split" samples and send them to the same and another independent laboratory for analysis; this approach uncovers systematic bias in the results of a particular laboratory. Any laboratory used for an investigation should have an internal, documented quality assurance and control program. For some types of samples, such as organic vapors collected on adsorbents or metals collected on filters, the recovery efficiencies of the analyses should be reported. If there is potential litigation, the laboratories should maintain records of instrumentation and calibration and of raw output for each analysis.

HEALTH AND COMFORT ASSESSMENT: THE THIRD STAGE OF INVESTIGATION

Environmental monitoring may fail to provide clear evidence of an agent or condition that can be causally associated with the reported symptoms or complaints. Measurements are performed after complaints have been made, and the originally inciting conditions may have been changed in response to concerns about particular pollutants. The monitoring methods may not have been sufficiently sensitive at the levels actually associated with the reported problem or may have failed to detect an unusual temporal pattern.

Therefore, it might be necessary to formulate a third, more comprehensive, stage of investigation, which includes a more thorough inquiry on symptoms and complaints. To correlate the subjective responses of building occupants with the objective measurements obtained during the investigation, a detailed occupant evaluation should be conducted. The evaluation might include collection of medical and symptom information related to the workplace and to all other environments. Various clinical diagnostic tests may be indicated, such as serum precipitins against antigens associated with hypersensitivity pneumonitis, or spirometry, a test of pulmonary function.

In some cases, the investigation may require documentation of symptom rates and thus, addition of an epidemiologist to the investigating team. Self-administered questionnaires have been used in many building investigations. The technique can be useful for identifying clustering of symptoms by location or in groups of employees categorized by time of occurrence and other factors. Although the approach of administering questionnaires to measure symptom occurrence appears straightforward, the responses are prone to bias and cannot be validated readily. Data collection from nonexposed control subjects may facilitate interpretation of the response by exposed persons.

Evaluations are usually conducted among occupants who are aware of potential health and comfort concerns. Job action and/or litigation may be pending. In such emotionally charged situations, there is a strong potential for reporting bias. Even without such obviously stressful conditions, reporting bias may occur. For example, women may have higher complaint rates than men, and complaint rates from public sector employees may tend to be higher than from private sector employees (Finnegan and Pickering 1987). Work status, dissatisfaction with the work station, and work pressures may be reflected in complaints obtained with self-completed questionnaires. Consultation with a psychologist may be warranted.

Investigations are often begun well after the onset of complaints. Environmental monitoring and/or contemporary comfort conditions can suggest a situation quite different from that initiating the original occupant complaints. However, retrospective reconstruction of exposures and symptoms by questionnaire is difficult, and therefore failure to find clear associations among symptoms, contaminant levels, and environmental conditions is not unexpected. Facility managers may have already adjusted HVAC systems or made other modifications in response to occupant complaints. In new or modified buildings, high emission rates of contaminants from building materials or furnishings may have led to the onset of complaints whereas months later, measurements may fail to detect high concentrations as emission rates drop.

Buildings are complex and often house multiple functions. A school building, for example, may have laboratories, classrooms, offices, and vocational education shops. Investigators should not search for a single causative condition but should consider causative agents in each type of environment. For example, some occupants might work in an area in which water damage has caused mold to grow; others may sense the uncomfortable vibrations caused by heavy equipment; and others may have inadequate ventilation. Nonspecificity of symptoms may make identification and resolution of all independent problems an impossible task.

Even in light of these limitations, further environmental monitoring in the occupied space is warranted at this phase of the investigation. However, measurements made to characterize conditions in the space in earlier phases of an investigation should now be performed in conjunction with a dynamic HVAC system evaluation in order to assess the occupied space as changes are made in the operating parameters of the building. In addition to monitoring potential contaminants in the space, objective measurements of other environmental parameters such as thermal, acoustic, vibration, and lighting conditions may also be indicated (Table 4.4).

This portion of the study requires a detailed understanding of the measurement systems available, the use of surrogate measurements such as tracer gases when appropriate, and the relationship of measurements to overall building operations and occupant activities. The conditions present during a building investigation may not be the same as those during the periods of maximum complaints. From the data gathered in earlier phases of the study, an understanding of how the system operates will have been obtained. Using this information, the investigator may artificially manipulate the HVAC system controls to create a "worst case" situation while correlating real-time measurements with system operations. This same approach can be used in a proactive approach to optimize system performance.

## MEASUREMENT OF INDOOR AIR POLLUTION

The remaining sections of this chapter provide a guide to the tables (Tables 4.6 to 4.11) summarizing indoor air monitoring equipment. Although the tables are not comprehensive, they do contain brief descriptions of examples of the more common types of equipment currently used for building investigations and indoor air quality research (Lioy and Lioy 1983; ACGIH 1989). Earlier in this chapter, the factors to be considered in the selection of instruments and/or analytical methods were reviewed. Equally important choices must be made on the required frequency of sampling, location, sample duration, level of detection, ancillary measurements such as ventilation rates, and quality assurance protocols.

Often, a choice must be made between continuous measurements from direct reading instruments and integrated measurements. Both types have advantages and disadvantages, and the selection should reflect the purpose of the investigation. Some human responses are likely to be associated with short-term excursions, even as short as seconds or minutes. For example, odor, taste, and allergic responses can follow a single breath containing some contaminants. Obviously, direct reading or very short-term integration would be more appropriate for characterizing pollutants that so quickly produce responses. On the other hand, for contaminants that are associated with chronic effects on health, the long-term integration of measurements is more relevant. For contaminants such as chlorinated volatile organic compounds and radon, it is more appropriate to measure over weeks to months to smooth out the short-term fluctuations and to provide a more biologically appropriate measure of exposure. Nevertheless, even short-term continuous measurements of radon and pesticides can be very helpful in studying sources and factors influencing concentration such as subslab and/or basement depressurization.

### DIRECT MEASUREMENT TECHNIQUES

These instruments can provide continuous or short-term integrated (over minutes) on-site measurements. They are direct reading and do not require that samples be taken to a laboratory. The pollutants for which direct measurement techniques are available include respirable suspended particulate matter (RSP), fibers, carbon monoxide, carbon dioxide, nitrogen dioxide, volatile organic compounds, $SO_2$, and radon.

*Respirable Suspended Particulate Matter*    A variety of devices are currently available for the direct measurement of particulate matter in the respirable size range (Table 4.6). Many of the devices collect particles on filters and typically provide results as milligrams or micrograms per cubic meter of air sampled. Other equipment uses optical techniques to assess the number of particles. The optical approaches for the direct measurement of RSP in air are often based on the near-forward light-scattering properties of fine particulate matter.

The mass of RSP can be measured directly with several innovative techniques. In the early 1970s, the bureau of mines directed the development of direct reading gravimetric dust monitors, which are no longer made. These devices measure the reduction in β-rays (high-energy electrons) from a safe radioactive source; the β-energy detected is reduced by the mass of dust deposited on a filter or impactor plate separating the source from the detector. Because the dust mass must build up to a measurable level, these devices measure a time-averaged value, but the measurement times can be as short as several minutes in very dusty areas or longer in less dusty areas. Since β-absorption by matter is relatively independent of the elemental nature of the dust for light elements, the measurement provides a good representation of total levels of dust mass.

Other techniques for RSP measurement involve the combination of impaction or electrostatic precipitation and piezoelectric resonance. An airstream first passes through an impactor or cyclone to remove the nonrespirable particles. The respirable particles are deposited by an electrostatic precipitator onto the quartz crystal sensor. The difference in oscillating frequency between the sensing and reference crystals is monitored and displayed during the measurement. At the end of the measurement period the actual concentration in $mg/m^3$ is displayed. Impactors with cutoff diameters are available for these devices in the range of $0.5-10.0 \mu m$. In evaluating results obtained by this device it should be noted that semivolatile compounds that have been adsorbed onto the surface of the collected particulate material will be included in the total measured mass. This approach contrasts with the filter sampling technique in which continued sampling may drive off these semivolatile compounds from particle surfaces.

An additional technology currently available for the real-time direct measurement of RSP mass incorporates a tapered tubular element that is set into oscillation by a feedback amplifier. A vacuum pump attached to the tube's base draws the gas through a filter mounted on top of the tube. Particles become trapped in the filter. A microcomputer calculates the mass of the particles based on the change in frequency of vibration. This device can provide continuous mass measurement at flow rates ranging from 1 to 5 liters/min and can compute total mass, mass rate, or mass concentrations.

| Sampler | Source | Comments |
|---|---|---|
| Integrated gravimetric collection on filters | Several manufacturers, cyclones, preseparators, filters, and pumps | Detection limit depends on flow rates, duration, balance and preconditioning of filters before weighing[b] |
| Impactors and filters | Personal exposure monitor MSP Corporation 7949 Country Road 11 Maple Plains, MN  55359 | 4 liters/min flow rates. Cut size variable but available at 2.5 and 10 μm |
| Integrated gravimetric; particles <10-μm or <2.5-μm diameter | MS & T Impactor Air Diagnostics Inc. RR 1, Box 445 Naple, ME  04055 (207)583–4834 | 4 and 10 liters/m; mass flow controller for 14-day timer, double impactor for sharp cut; fixed location |
| Instantaneous (2/10 s); TSP or RSP; 0.1-10-μm forward light scattering | Miniram (personal aerosol monitor) Ram-1 larger device MIE, Inc. 213 Burlington Road Bedford, MA  01730 (617)275–5444 | Miniram, range 0.01–10 mg/m$^3$ or 0.1–100 mg/m$^3$. Averaging times, 10 s to 8 h TWA[c], Ram-1 range, 0.001–200 mg/m$^3$ calibrated with Freon-12 or by reference to gravimetric method |
| Semi-instantaneous; RSP fraction using piezoelectric balance | Piezobalance (model 3500) TSI, Inc. P.O. Box 64394 St. Paul, MN  55164 (612)483–0900 | Less reliable for concentration <10 μg/m$^3$ at 2-min averaging. Averaging time is variable. Difficult to calibrate (needs chamber tests or comparison to other methods) |
| Continuous; RSP sub-micron light-scattering multisensor monitor | Handheld aerosol monitor (HAM) PPM, Inc. 11428 Kingston Pike Knoxville, TN  37922 (615)966–8796 HUND 401 Broadway New York, NY  10013 (212)219–2468 | Lower detection limit about 10 μg/m$^3$. Can set zero and check span point in field but is calibrated by comparison with other methods |
| Light scattering for fiber detection | Fibrous aerosol monitor (FAM-1) MIE, Inc. 213 Burlington Road Bedford, MA  01730 (617)275–5444 | Counts all fiber types per cm$^3$ by detecting scattered light from fibers rotating in oscillating electric field. Detection, 0.1 f/cm$^3$ for 1 min, 0.001 f/cm$^3$ for 100 min, 0.0001 f/cm$^3$ for 1,000 min |

[a]Particles can be measured using a variety of techniques. Using cyclone or impactor separators, smaller size fractions can be collected on filters. Mass can also be measured using the optical properties of particles. For the most part, measuring particles requires equipment costing several hundred to a few thousand dollars. Equipment using filters require that they be preweighted and postweighted in a temperature- and humidity-controlled room. Particle sizes are commonly referred to as TSP (total suspended particulate matter), RSP (respirable suspended particulate matter), PM$_{10}$ (particles <10-μm aerodynamic diameter), submicron sizes (<1 μm aerodynamic diameter). RSP size refers to a specific ACGIH cut curve where 90 percent of >10-μm, 50 percent of 3.5-μm, and 10 percent of 2-μm size particles are excluded.
[b]Filters can be Teflon, Nuclearpore, glass-fiber, or quartz, among other types. They can be analyzed for mass, particulate phase organics, pH, nitrates, sulfates, fibers, metals, and other contaminants with proper attention to handling.
[c]Time-weighted average.

*Fibers* Real-time monitoring of airborne fibers, including asbestos, can be achieved by a technique similar to that used for optically measuring respirable particulates (Table 4.6). A two-step sensing procedure is used to count fibers independent of the presence of nonfibrous particles; the fibers are induced to rotate rapidly by the application of a rotating electric field, and the resulting light-scattering signature from the oscillation of the fibers is detected during illumination by a helium-neon laser-generated light beam.

*Carbon Monoxide* Carbon monoxide (CO), a fairly nonreactive chemical, oxidizes to form the more stable carbon dioxide. Several detectors make measurements using the principle of electrochemical oxidation (Table 4.7). Although other air pollutants can interfere with the detection of CO by this approach, these pollutants can be removed by an inlet scrubber such as a Purafil filter. Ambient air is actively drawn past a catalytically active electrode or, in other devices, is allowed to diffuse passively across an electrochemical cell that oxidizes CO and produces a signal proportional to the CO concentration in the sample airstream.

*Carbon Dioxide* The measurement of carbon dioxide ($CO_2$) concentration is based upon this compound's characteristic absorptive band in the infrared range (at a wavelength of 4.25 $\mu$m) (Table 4.7). Monitors used for $CO_2$ can be either dedicated units set up specifically and only for $CO_2$ or other general purpose instruments that can be adjusted for $CO_2$ but are also used for other chemicals such as CO, formaldehyde, or total hydrocarbons. The amount of infrared energy absorbed is proportional to the concentration of the compound being analyzed.

*Nitrogen Dioxide* The instrumentation available for the real-time measurement of nitrogen dioxide ($NO_2$) is similar in principle of operation to that for measuring CO (Table 4.7). Filters are required, however, to provide specificity and to remove interference from other oxidizable chemicals such as methane and CO. Gas scrubbers are needed to remove potential interference from such agents as chlorine, ethyl mercaptans, methyl mercaptans, sulfur dioxide, ozone, and hydrogen sulfide when these chemicals are at concentrations equivalent to the $NO_2$.

*Volatile Organic Compounds* This topic is covered in more detail in Chapter 11. The measurement of many volatile organic compounds can be achieved by the same infrared absorbance technique described for $CO_2$ (Table 4.8). Infrared analyzers detect individual compounds by varying the analytical wavelength and path length of the device.

Other devices are less specific (Table 4.8). Many organic chemicals have ionization potentials of less than 10.6 electron volts (eV) whereas the normal air gases such as nitrogen and oxygen have ionization potentials of 12 eV or greater. *Ionization* refers to the formation of ions due to the absorbance of energy. In one device employing ionization, a miniature lamp emits very short wavelength ultraviolet (UV) radiation that has sufficient energy to cause "photoionization" when it strikes

Table 4.7   Selected Examples of Sampling Equipment for Indoor CO,
$CO_2$, and $NO_2$ Pollutants

| Sampler | Source | Comments |
|---|---|---|
| CO: continuous electrochemical | ECOlyzer 2000, 6000 Energetic Sciences, Inc. Division of Becton Dickinson and Co. 6 Skyline Drive Hawthorne, NY   10532 (914)592-3010 | Various ranges 0–50 ppm, 0–100 ppm, etc.; portable and personal versions available; alarm option, cells expendable, LOD[a] ~2 ppm |
| CO: continuous electrochemical | Interscan Corporation P.O. Box 2496 21700 Nordhoff Street Chatsworth, CA   91311 (213)882-2331 | Various ranges; cells expendable, LOD[a] ~1 ppm |
| CO: passive diffusion | Lab Safety Supply Co. P.O. Box 1368 Janesville, WI   53547 (608)754-2345 | LOD[a] 50 ppm for 8 h; will produce color change |
| CO: passive diffusion detector | Quantum Eye Quantum Group, Inc. 11211 Sorrento Valley Road Suite D San Diego, CA   92121 (619)457-3048 | Simple color change detector, not for permanent use, not quantitative |
| CO: detector tube, grab sample | National Draeger, Inc. P.O. Box 120 Pittsburgh, PA   15230 (412)787-8383 | Range 5–700 ppm by color change; semiquantitative |
| CO: detector tube, grab sample | Toxic gas detector system Matheson-Kitagawa P.O. Box 85 932 Paterson Plank Road East Rutherford, NJ   07073 (201)933-2400 | Range 5–50 ppm by color change on stain tube; semiquantitative |
| $CO_2$: continuous infrared | Portable infrared $CO_2$ monitor 4776 GasTech, Inc. 8445 Central Avenue Newark, CA   94560 (415)794-6200 | Range 300 to >5000 ppm; ambient levels typically 350–450 ppm |
| $NO_2$: continuous electrochemical | Interscan Corporation P.O. Box 2496 21700 Nordhoff Street Chatsworth, CA   91311 (213)882-2331 | Various ranges; cells expendable; >20 ppm |
| $NO_2$: continuous electrochemical | Transducer Research, Inc. 1228 Olympus Drive Naperville, IL   60540 (708)369-1336 | Introduced 1989; >2 ppb, built-in data logger, zero |
| $NO_2$: personal and alarm | MDA Scientific 405 Barclay Boulevard Lincolnshire, IL   60069 (800)323-2000 | 2–3 ppm; 1/3 TLV electrochemical cell based 15 min to 8 h; TWA |

(*continued*)

Table 4.7  (*Continued*)

| Sampler | Source | Comments |
|---|---|---|
| NO$_2$: passive diffusion tubes | Environmental Sciences and Physiology Harvard School of Public Health 665 Huntington Avenue Boston, MA   02115 (617)432-1165 | LOD$^a$ 500 ppb for a 1-h exposure (5 ppb for 100 h) |
| NO$_2$: passive tubes and badges | Micro Filtration Systems 6800 Sierra Court Dublin, CA   94568 (415)828-6010 | Contact manufacturer |
| NO$_2$: diffusion badge | Environmental Sciences and Physiology Harvard School of Public Health 665 Huntington Avenue Boston, MA   02115 (617)432-1165 | LOD 50 ppb for a 1-h exposure (5 ppb for 10 h) |

$^a$Limit of detection.

the molecules of certain chemicals. The instrument continuously draws air into a tiny ionization chamber that is flooded with UV light. As ions are formed, they migrate to the electrodes and cause a measurable change in the electric current, which is indicated in the LCD display. These devices cannot distinguish between different pollutants; the signal produced represents a composite of all different ionizable pollutants. However, the instrument response may be calibrated for a particular compound.

*Radon*   The direct measurement of radon relies on the interaction of emitted α-particles with a coating of ZnS(Ag) on a glass tube, which causes a flash of light (scintillation) detectable by a photomultiplier tube (Table 4.9). The response of this tube to the light is an electrical signal. This type of device, called a *continuous radon monitor,* samples the ambient air by pumping air into a scintillation cell after passing it through a particulate filter that removes dust and radon decay products. As the radon in the air decays, the ionized radon decay products plate out on the interior surface of the scintillation cell. The continuous radon monitor may have continuous flow through the cell or fill it periodically. In either case, the instrument must be calibrated at known radon concentrations to obtain the conversion factor used electronically to convert count rate to radon concentration.

INTEGRATING DEVICES: PASSIVE SAMPLING

The pollutants for which passive sampling techniques are available include NO$_2$, formaldehyde, and radon. Exposure must be determined by an estimate of concentration and duration with respect to the detection limit for each device.

Table 4.8 Selected Examples of Available Equipment
for Indoor Organic Air Pollutants

| Sampler | Source | Comments |
|---|---|---|
| Organic vapors | Industrial Scientific Corporation<br>355 Steubenville Pike<br>Oakdale, PA 15071<br>(412)758–4353 | |
| Organic vapors | OVM Logger (model 580A)<br>Thermo Environmental Instruments, Inc.<br>8 West Forge Parkway<br>Franklin, MA 02038<br>(508)520–0430 | General organic vapor monitor detects by photoionization. Detects down to 0.1 ppm benzene in air |
| Organic vapors | Portable gas chromatographs<br>Thermo Environmental Instruments, Inc.<br>8 West Forge Parkway<br>Franklin, MA 02038<br>(508)520–0430 | Four detectors possible:<br>electron capture<br>flame ionization<br>thermal conductivity<br>photoionization |
| Organic vapors: portable gas chromatograph | Century OVA (portable organic vapor analyzer)<br>Foxboro Company<br>Foxboro, MA 02035<br>(203)853–1616 | Total organic vapor detector ($\sim$0.2 ppm); selected organic vapor detector |
| Organic vapors: portable gas chromatograph | Photovac IOS (portable air analyzer)<br>Photovac International, Inc.<br>741 Park Avenue<br>Huntington, NY 11743<br>(516)351–5809 | Total organic vapor detector; selected organic vapor detector including benzene, C4-C8 hydrocarbons, mercaptans, halocarbons |
| Organic vapors: hydrocarbon chemical reaction tubes | National Draeger, Inc.<br>P.O. Box 120<br>Pittsburgh, PA 15230<br>(412)787–8383 | Stain-tube detectors; semiquantitative |
| Organic vapors: charcoal badges | 3M Corporation<br>Technical Service Department<br>3M Center<br>St. Paul, MN 55144<br>(612)733–1110 | Depends on vapors and sampling times; minimum level, 10/mg, requires lab analysis |
| Organic vapors: thermal ionization | TIP Air Analyzers<br>Photovac International, Inc.<br>741 Park Avenue<br>Huntington, NY 11743<br>(800)387–5700 | Semiquantitative response to several compounds. Can be calibrated to respond relative to that compound |
| Organic vapors and other gases: infrared detector | MIRAN portable air analyzers<br>Foxboro Company<br>South Norwalk, CT 06856<br>(203)853–1616 | Tunable infrared wavelength, needs separate calibration for each gas |
| Formaldehyde: passive samplers | GMD Systems, Inc.<br>Old Route 519<br>Hendersonville, PA 15339<br>(412)746–1359 | LOD[a] 0.2 ppm for 15 min; 0.005 ppm for 8 h |

*(continued)*

Table 4.8  (*continued*)

| Sampler | Source | Comments |
|---|---|---|
| Formaldehyde: diffusion tube | Air Quality Research, Inc.<br>901 Grayson Street<br>Berkeley, CA   94710<br>(415)644–2097 | LOD[a] 0.01 ppm for 7-day exposure; 1.68 ppm for 1 h |
| Formaldehyde: Pro-tek adsorption badge | E.I. Dupont Company<br>Applied Technical Division<br>North Walnut Road<br>P.O. Box 110<br>Kennett Square, PA   19348<br>(800)344–4900 | 1.6 to 54 ppm/h up to 7 days or 0.2 to 6.75 ppm for 8-h exposure |
| Formaldehyde: diffusion monitor | 3M Corporation<br>Technical Service Department<br>Building 260-3-2<br>3M Center<br>St. Paul, MN   55144<br>(612)733–1110 | LOD[a] low as 0.8 ppm for 1 h, equal to 0.1 ppm for 8 h, and 0.005 ppm for 1 week |
| Formaldehyde: automated wet chemistry/colorimetry | CEA TGM 555<br>CEA Instruments, Inc.<br>16 Chestnut Street<br>P.O. Box 303<br>Emerson, NJ   07630<br>(201)967–5660 | Wet chemistry colorimetric sampler. Detection limit 0.002 up to 5 or 10 ppm, depending on range setting |

[a]Limit of detection.

*Nitrogen Dioxide*   Several passive monitoring devices for the measurement of oxides of nitrogen have been developed (Palmes 1981; Woebkenberg 1981) (Table 4.7). The Palmes tube, which consists of an acrylic tube with one fixed cap and one removable cap, contains stainless steel screens impregnated with triethanolamine that absorbs $NO_2$. Spectrophotometric analysis is carried out in the laboratory to determine the concentration of $NO_2$. These tubes have a detection limit of about 500 ppb-h. A one-week exposure should detect levels less than 5 ppb. An $NO_2$ filter badge, which uses the same absorbing material but with a larger surface area, has a detection limit of about 50 ppb-h.

*Formaldehyde*   Passive diffusion monitors for the measurement of formaldehyde (HCHO) work on a principle similar to that for $NO_2$. For this air contaminant, however, a glass-fiber filter treated with sodium bisulfite at the fixed end of the tube reacts with and removes the HCHO. Collected HCHO is quantified in the laboratory using the chromotropic acid procedure.

*Radon*   Three passive sampling techniques are available for the measurement of radon (Table 4.9). Charcoal canisters can be used for short-term average measurements (two to five days), and $\alpha$-track detectors (ATD) can be used for longer term measurements of up to weeks or months. A third type of passive radon detector is the Electret Passive Environmental Radon Monitor "E-PERM," available from Rad-Elec, Inc.

Table 4.9  Radon Gas $^{222}$Rn Detectors

| Device | Description | Manufacturer | Manufacturer Specifications Sensitivity | Manufacturer Specifications Averaging Time | Sampling Features Passive (P) or Active (A) | Sampling Features Integrating (I) or Continuous (C) |
|---|---|---|---|---|---|---|
| Charcoal canister detector | Radon adsorption/γ-scintillation (NaI crystal) | F & J Specialty Products Inc.[a] P.O. Box 660065 Miami Springs, FL  33266 (305)888–0383 (charcoal canister maker) | 0.2 pCi/liter[b] | 2–7 days | P | I |
| Charcoal vial detector | Radon adsorption/α-scintillation (liquid) | Niton Corporation 74 Loomis Street Bedford, MA 01730 (617)275–9275 | 0.1 pCi/liter[b] | 2–7 days | P | I |
| ATE (e.g., Track Etch® Radtrak®) | CR-39/plastic/microscopy | TERRADEX Corporation[a] (a Tech/OPS Company) 3 Science Road Glenwood, IL  60425 (800)528–8327 | 0.4 pCi/liter | ≥3 months to 1 year | P | I |
| E-PERM® | Electret ion detector | Rad Elec, Inc. 5330J Spectrum Drive Frederick, MD  21701 (301)694–0011 | 1 pCi/liter | 2–7 days; 2–52 weeks | P | I |
| AT EASE® detector | Solid-state detector | Sun Nuclear Corporation 415-C Pineda Court Melbourne, FL  32940 (305)259–6862 | $60 \dfrac{\text{cpm}}{\text{pCi/liter}}$ | 4, 8, 12, or 24 h | P | C |
| Survivor 2® | Ion chamber | Threshold Technical Products, Inc. 11325 Reed Hartman Highway Cincinnati, OH  45241 (800)458–4931 | 0.1 pCi/liter (minimum reading) | 12 h | P | C |

| Device | Detection method | Manufacturer | Sensitivity | Count time | | |
|---|---|---|---|---|---|---|
| femto-TECH® radon monitor (model R210F) | Pulsed ion chamber | femto-TECH, Inc. P.O. Box 8257 1325 Industry Drive Carlisle, OH 45005 (513)746–4427 | $0.3\ \frac{\text{cpm}}{\text{pCi/liter}}$ | ~3 min | P | C |
| Radon Tracker® (model RGM-2) | | | N/A | N/A | A | C |
| Eberline® radon gas monitor (model RGM-2) | α-Scintillation | Eberline Instrument Corp. P.O. Box 2108 Santa Fe, NM 87504 (505)471–3232 | $4\ \frac{\text{cpm}}{\text{pCi/liter}}$ | 1 h | A | C |
| EDA® PERM (model RDT-310) | Thermoluminescent detector (TLD) | EDA Instruments, Inc. 4 Thorncliffe Park Drive Toronto, Ontario M4H 1H1 Canada (416)425–7800 | N/A | N/A | P | I |
| PYLON® portable radiation monitor (model AB-5) and either | | Pylon Electric Development Company, Ltd. 147 Colonnade Road Ottawa, Ontario K2E 7L9 Canada (613)226–7920 | | | | |
| PYLON® Lucas cell (models 300 and LCA-2) | α-Scintillation | | 0.3 pCi/liter | 1–99 s, min, or h | A | C |
| or | | | | | | |
| PYLON® passive gas monitor (model PRD-1) | α-Scintillation | | $1.1\ \frac{\text{cpm}}{\text{pCi/liter}}$ | 1–99 s, min, or h | P | C |

Source: "Radon/Radon Progeny Measurement Proficiency Program Cumulative Report" (updated periodically), Office of Radiation Programs, U.S. EPA, Washington, D.C., 1988. Lists laboratories that are certified to do these tests.

[a]Many companies provide measurement service; see source footnote.
[b]Estimated.

Charcoal canisters are passive integrating detectors that can be used to determine the average radon concentration over a short sampling interval. At the laboratory, the canisters are analyzed for radon decay products by placing the canister directly on a $\gamma$-detector to count $\gamma$-rays of energies between 0.25 and 0.61 MeV. The charcoal canister system can be calibrated by analyzing canisters exposed to known concentrations of radon in a calibration facility.

An ATD consists of a small piece of plastic enclosed in a container with a filter-covered opening. $\alpha$-Particles emitted by the radon decay products in air strike the plastic and produce submicroscopic damage tracks. At the end of the measurement period, the detectors are returned to a laboratory, and the plastic is placed in a caustic solution that accentuates the damage tracks, which are then counted using a microscope or an automated counting system. The number of tracks per unit area estimates the radon concentration in the air; a conversion factor derived from data generated at a calibration facility is used for the calculation.

In the E-PERM detector, an electret (a material with a permanently embedded electric field) is placed in an air chamber. A filter on the chamber allows air and radon to enter but blocks already existing ions. When the chamber is opened, radon enters and creates ions (charged particles) during decay. When the ions strike the electret, its charge is reduced, and the charge on the electret is subsequently analyzed to calculate the radon level.

Tables 4.9 and 4.10 list the many radon and radon progeny detectors that are currently available. The Environmental Protection Agency (EPA) has tested several devices in its radon measurement proficiency program. Information on commercial radon testing can be obtained from EPA Office of Radiation Programs in Washington, D.C., or from regional EPA or state offices.

INTEGRATING DEVICES: ACTIVE SAMPLING

The pollutants for which active sampling techniques are available include RSP, asbestos, formaldehyde, volatile organic compounds, and microbiologicals. Active sampling involves the use of a sampling train with a collection medium (solution, filter, or other absorbing bed) and a pump. The pump draws the air sample into the detector.

*Respirable Suspended Particulate Matter*   RSP can be measured in air by filtration to collect the sample with subsequent analysis for mass or composition (Table 4.6). Particles can be size fractionated by utilizing specially designed inlets. The filters used to collect the RSP must be preweighed and then reconditioned and reweighed in a controlled humidity environment to control for the uptake of water vapor during sampling. Sampling must be performed at a calibrated volumetric rate in order for the results to be presented in terms of mass per unit volume of air sampled.

*Asbestos*   The Asbestos Hazard Emergency Response Act (AHERA) of 1986 (U.S. EPA 1987) provides for the establishment of federal regulations for the inspection, sampling, and assessment of asbestos-containing materials. In monitoring for asbestos hazards, four types of microscopic analysis techniques are commonly used. Various state and federal accreditation programs have been established to ensure competence. Polarized light microscopy allows identification of asbestos by viewing the morphology of fibers directly, using stereoscopic polarized light examination. Phase-contrast microscopy is widely used for assessing worker exposure to airborne fibers, using the NIOSH 7400 method and the OSHA reference method. Transmission electron microscopy (TEM) embodies state-of-the-art technology for analyzing airborne concentrations of asbestos fibers. Fibers as small as 0.1 $\mu$m in length are discernible. Asbestos fiber types can also be identified positively through the use of TEM or scanning electron microscopy (SEM) analysis.

The traditional technique for the assessment of asbestos in the workplace has been optical microscopy. This approach typically uses a microscope setup to utilize phase contrast and requires a trained operator. Analysis can be performed on suspect materials, wipe samples, or air samples collected on an appropriate filter substrate.

*Formaldehyde*  The measurement of formaldehyde in air can be achieved by using impingers for collection in an absorbing reagent followed by spectrophotometric analysis in a laboratory. Absorbing reagents are either deionized distilled water that is kept chilled during sampling or a 1 percent solution of sodium bisulfite. Analysis can be performed by the chromotropic acid method or the pararosaniline method.

*Volatile Organic Compounds*  The diverse properties of organic compounds, including less volatile insecticides and pesticides, pose a difficult challenge for making measurements (see also Chapter 11). A suitable collection medium, such as Tenax, Sphericarb, and activated carbon, traps or adsorbs these molecules without permitting reactions, backdiffusion, or breaking through (Table 9.8). Whole air samples can be collected in evacuated stainless steel cylinders or in nonreactive bags. Organic compounds are recovered from these collection devices and analyzed usually by gas chromatography and mass spectrometry or gas chromatography with other types of detectors.

*Microbiologicals*  The measurement of microbiologically active organisms in the air can be achieved by using impinger samplers that draw known volumes of air past plates of growth media (Table 4.11). The plates can then be incubated at appropriate temperatures to foster the growth of the specific organisms of interest, whether bacteria or fungi. Counting the number of colonies formed yields results in terms of colony-forming units per volume of air sampled. The sample can be cultured to determine the particular organisms present.

Table 4.10  Radon Progeny Detector

| Device | Description | Manufacturer | Manufacturer Specifications | | Sampling Features | |
|---|---|---|---|---|---|---|
| | | | Sensitivity | Averaging Time | Passive (P) or Active (A) | Integrating (I) or Continuous (C) |
| RAD® radon/thoron daughter monitor (model M-1) | Filter and CR-39 plastic (RPISU[a])/ microscopy | R.A.D. Service & Instruments, Ltd. 50 Silver Star Boulevard Scarborough, Ontario M1V 3L3 Canada (416)298–9200 | 0.1 mWL[b] | 3 days to 2 weeks | A | I |
| "Radon Sniffer" working level meter | Filter/solid-state detector | Thomson & Nielsen Electronics, Ltd. 4019 Carling Avenue Kanata, Ontario K2K 2A3 Canada (613)592–3019 | 1 mWL[b] (minimum reading) | | A | C |
| EBERLINE® radon working level systems (models | Filter/solid-state detector | Eberline Instrument Corporation P.O. Box 2108 | 0.02 mWL[b] is lowest detectable | 1 h | A | C |

| | | | | | | |
|---|---|---|---|---|---|---|
| WLM-1 and WLR-1 | | Santa Fe, NM 87504 (505)471–3232 | level | | | C |
| EDA® working level monitor (model WLM-30) | Filter/solid-state detector | EDA Instruments, Inc. 4 Thorncliffe Park Drive Toronto, Ontario M4H 1H1 Canada (416)425–7800 | 1 mWL[b] | Programmable | A | C |
| EDA® RPISU[a] (model 225) | Filter/TLD | | N/A | ≥3 days[c] | A | I |
| alphaNUCLEAR® alphaSMART® (model 760) | Filter/solid-state detector | alphaNUCLEAR company 1125 Derry Road East Mississauga, Ontario L5T 1P3 Canada (416)676–1364 | 0.05 mWL[b] | Programmable | A | C |
| PYLON® portable radiation monitor (model AB-5) plus α-Detection assembly (model AEP) | Filter/α-scintillation | PYLON Electronic Development Company, Ltd. 147 Colonnade Road Ottawa, Ontario K2E 7L9 Canada (613)226–7920 | 0.2 mWL[b] | 1,699 s, min, or h | A | C |

[a]Radon Progeny Integrating Sampling Unit.
[b]Milli working level.
[c]Rough estimate.

Table 4.11   Selected Examples of Sampling Equipment
for Indoor Microbiologic Pollutants

| Sampler | Source | Comments |
|---|---|---|
| Slit impactor rotating agar | Casella Bacteria Sampler Casella London, Ltd. Regent House Britannia Walk London N1 7ND England | Rotating disc containing agar; heated 37°C for 24 h; different agar for different organisms; need laboratory for culturing and identification |
| Impaction into agar dish | Andersen 1-cubic ft/min viable (microbial) sampler Andersen Samplers, Inc. 4215-C Wendell Drive Atlanta, GA   30336 | Typically operating with last stage only of a multiple-stage impactor; air accelerated through jets to impact on agar (nutrient) dish; organisms must grow into colonies for identification. Note: adjustment of colony-forming units/m$^3$ required |
| Slit impactor on rotating drum | 7-day volumetric spore trap Burkard Manufacturing Company Woodcock Hill Industrial Estates Rockmansworth Hertfordshire WDS 1PL England | Samples for fungus spores and pollens by impaction onto adhesive-coated strip; rotating drum provides 24-h to 7-day sampling; viable and nonviable organisms must be microscopically identified. |

## SUMMARY

Problem buildings generally require rapid investigation to uncover the causes of the problems and effectively remedy them. Any obvious defects of the building or mechanical system should be identified in the first phase of the investigation. Measurements made during the subsequent stage of investigation should indicate whether an eminent hazard exists in the building. Underlying problems may often be identified and resolved at this point in the investigation. However, because a building is complex and several factors may simultaneously impact a space, an investigation must often enter into a more extensive phase. Through the manipulation of many parameters controlling building systems, review of the building's history regarding occupant activities, furnishings and other aspects of use, and correlation of this information with the complaint history of the occupants, the investigator should gain an understanding of the building, its actual and expected performance, and its potential impacts on the occupants. At this point the effective resolution of the problem should be possible.

As a component of all building investigations, the investigators must communicate their findings to both building management and the occupants. A report should be sufficiently detailed to include design, methods, results, and limitations of interpretation. Definitive causal associations are often impossible to make in building investigations; however, remedial steps can many times be inferred. The recommendations should include corrective and preventive measures.

## REFERENCES

American Conference of Governmental and Industrial Hygienists. 1989. *Air sampling manual.* 7th ed. Ed. S. W. Hering. Cincinnati, Ohio: ACGIH.

American Society of Heating, Refrigerating, and Air-Conditioning Engineers. *ASHRAE Standard 55-1981. Thermal environmental conditions for human occupancy.* Atlanta, Ga.: ASHRAE.

American Society of Heating, Refrigerating, and Air-Conditioning Engineers. 1989. *ASHRAE Standard 62-1989. Ventilation for acceptable indoor air quality.* Atlanta, Ga.: ASHRAE.

Baker, D. B. 1989. Social and organizational factors in office building-associated illness. In *Occupational medicine: State-of-the-art reviews.* Ed. J. E. Cone and M. J. Hodgson, Vol. 4, 607–24. Philadelphia: Hanley & Belfus.

Corn, M. 1985. Strategies of air sampling. *Scand. J. Work Environ. Health* 11:173–80.

Finnegan, M. J., and Pickering, A. C. 1987. Prevalence of symptoms of the sick building syndrome in buildings without expressed dissatisfaction. *Proceedings of the fourth international conference on indoor air quality and climate: Vol. 2,* 17–21 August, Berlin.

Lioy, P. J., and Lioy, M. J. Y. 1983. *Air sampling instruments for evaluation of atmospheric contaminants.* 6th ed. Cincinnati, Ohio: ACGIH.

Lodge, J. P., Jr. 1989. *Methods of air sampling and analysis.* 3d ed. Chelsea, Mich.: Lewis Publishing.

Nagda, N. L.; Rector, H. E.; and Koontz, M. D. 1987. *Guidelines for monitoring indoor air quality.* New York: Hemisphere Publishing Corporation.

National Institute for Occupational Safety and Health. 1984. *Manual of analytical methods.* 3d ed., Vol. 1, 15–28. Cincinnati, Ohio: U.S. Government Printing Office. NIOSH Publication no. 84-100.

National Institute for Occupational Safety and Health. 1987. *Guidance for indoor air quality investigations, hazard evaluations and technical assistance, branch division of surveillance, hazard evaluations and field studies.* Cincinnati, Ohio: U.S. Government Printing Office.

Occupational Safety and Health Administration. 1989. *Air contaminants: Permissible exposure limits.* Title 29, Code of Federal Regulations, Part 1910.1000. Washington, D.C.: U.S. Government Printing Office. USDL Publication no. (OSHA) 3112.

Palmes, E. D. 1981. $NO_2$ and $NO_x$ diffusion techniques. *Ann. Am. Conf. Ind. Hyg.* 1:263–66.

Quinlan, P., et al. 1989. Protocol for comprehensive evaluation of building-associated illness. In *Occupational Medicine: State-of-the-art reviews.* Ed. J. E. Cone and M. J. Hodgson, Vol. 4, 771–98. Philadelphia: Hanley & Belfus.

Thorsen, M. A., and Molhave, L. 1987. Elements of standard protocol for measurements in the indoor atmospheric environment. *Atmos. Environ.* 21:1411–16.

U.S. Environmental Protection Agency. 1987. Asbestos-containing materials in school: Final rule and notice. *Fed. Reg.* 52:41826–900.

Wallingford, K. M., and Carpenter, J. 1986. Field experience overview: Investigating sources of indoor air quality problems in office buildings. In *Proceedings, IAQ '86:*

*Managing indoor air for health and energy conservation.* Atlanta, Ga.: American Society of Heating, Refrigerating, and Air-Conditioning Engineers.

Woebkenberg, M. L. 1981. Personal passive monitors for chemical agents. *Ann. Am. Conf. Ind. Hyg.* 1:107–15.

Woods, J. E.; Morey, P. R.; and Rask, D. R. 1987. Indoor air quality diagnostics: Qualitative and quantitative procedures to improve environmental conditions. Presented at symposium on design and protocol for monitoring indoor air quality, sponsored by ASTM, 26–29 April, Cincinnati, Ohio.

Woods, J. E.; Morey, P. R.; and Stolwijk, J. A. J. 1988. Indoor air quality and the sick building syndrome: A view from the United States. Presented at the Chartered Institute of Building Services Engineers advances in air conditioning conference, 7 October, London.

# 5

# PERSONAL EXPOSURE TO INDOOR AIR POLLUTION

P. Barry Ryan, B.S., M.D., Ph.D.
William E. Lambert, Ph.D.

## INTRODUCTION

The term *personal exposure* refers to pollutant contact with an individual as he or she moves through various environmental settings, and is represented by the concentration at the boundary prior to ingestion, dermal uptake, and/or inhalation of that contaminant by the individual.

Accurate characterization of personal exposure is needed for valid assessment of health effects and the design of more effective intervention strategies. Misclassified exposures reduce the sensitivity of epidemiologic studies to detect the effects of pollutants or lead to spurious associations. For example, use of ambient air pollution levels to characterize exposures for residents of a community will not classify personal exposures accurately if there are indoor sources of the same pollutant and/or a large proportion of time is spent indoors. Further, exposure to pollutants of outdoor origin will be modified by infiltration and reaction indoors. In the context of an epidemiologic study, if these factors are randomly distributed across communities (i.e., exposure groups), then the estimate of the magnitude of the health effect might be underestimated (Shy, Kleinbaum, and Morgenstern 1978; Ozkaynak et al. 1986). However, if there are systematic differences in the distribution of indoor sources, or mitigating factors, then it is possible that positive or negative associations might be incorrectly attributed to the "assumed" exposure variable.

Personal exposure data might improve the cost effectiveness of control and mitigation strategies. If a personal exposure study indicates that the major portion of the total exposure is attributable to automobiles, one control strategy would be to restrict motor vehicle emissions, reducing exposures to those people in transit or pursuing activities near traffic. Restrictions on stack emissions from a local power plant, although effective in reducing the total ambient pollutant burden of the community, might have little impact on total exposure to respirable particles inside residences. Investigations of personal exposures may also identify subgroups of the population whose particular behaviors would place them at risk for elevated exposures. Evaluation of activity patterns and exposures to specific sources may facilitate understanding of the determinants of the exposures and serve as a basis for intervention.

Several factors have contributed to the growing awareness of the importance of adequate estimation of personal exposure. The first is the development of new personal monitoring instrumentation, which is small and unobtrusive (Wallace and Ott 1982). The measurements using personal monitors have demonstrated clearly the inadequacies of assuming personal air pollution predicted by measurements made at outdoor sites, the usual approach for many community air pollutants. The error is particularly large for pollutants such as carbon monoxide (CO) and nitrogen dioxide ($NO_2$), which are emitted from localized sources such as automobiles, kerosene space heaters, and gas cooking ranges (Akland et al. 1985; Quackenboss et al. 1986), but also has been demonstrated for more uniformly distributed regional pollutants such as ozone ($O_3$) and fine particulate matter, whose concentrations in indoor settings are mediated by building structures and surfaces (Spengler and Soczek 1984; Spengler et al. 1985; Contant et al. 1987). Second, the complexities of human behavior and movement may play a major role in determining personal exposure. Yet it has proven difficult to develop mathematical models for estimating individual exposure based on outdoor fixed-site or area measurements. Further, even for modeling population exposures, there is a lack of population-based data on activity patterns suitable for exposure risk analysis (World Health Organization 1982; Ott 1985; Sexton and Ryan 1988). This chapter develops a conceptual framework for exposure assessment in the indoor setting. The current monitoring methods are reviewed as they relate to strategies for personal exposure assessment, and exemplary applications are described. A more detailed treatment of air pollution measurement is provided in Chapter 4.

## CONCEPTS AND DEFINITIONS

Figure 5.1 presents a conceptual framework for understanding personal exposure within the sequence of events between the emission of a pollutant from its source and the health effect experienced by a person who comes into contact with that pollutant. After release of a pollutant at a source, the pollutant moves through an environment in which it may be diluted and transformed by physical and chemical processes. As illustrated in the third component of the sequence, some of the pollutant (or the product of a transformation) eventually comes into contact with people, resulting in an "exposure." The link between the presence of a chemical contaminant in the environment and its contact with people is complex and in part determined by patterns of human behavior. The portion of exposure which is adsorbed, ingested, or inhaled into the body is termed the *dose*. It is this final

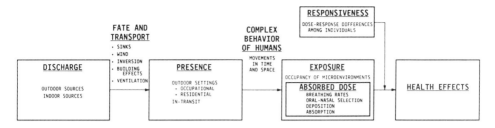

Figure 5.1. The biologic impact pathway.

amount of the chemical contaminant which produces the health effect. In the following sections, the terms *concentration, exposure,* and *dose* are more fully defined.

CONCENTRATION

The amount of a chemical contaminant at a particular location in a particular medium is termed the *concentration*. The concentration of an air pollutant is the amount of the material contained in a specified volume of air. Most air pollutant concentrations are expressed in mass per volume units (e.g., $\mu g/m^3$); however, gaseous pollutants may also be presented in units of a mixing ratio with air, typically in parts per million by volume (i.e., $ppm_v$). For certain particulate contaminants such as asbestos, the actual number of particles per unit volume is used (i.e., number count/$m^3$).

EXPOSURE

*Exposure* is defined as the contact of pollutant with a susceptible surface of the human body (Duan 1982; Ott 1985). For most air pollutants, this is the contact of pollutant with the skin, eyes, tissue in the nose, mouth, or throat, or the epithelium of the respiratory tract, the lining of the airways and alveoli. Thus, exposure can be simply defined as the simultaneous presence of a person and a pollutant in his or her immediate environment.

Exposure normally is considered to include within its definition an element of time. For example, exposures are typically given units of concentration multiplied by time (e.g., $\mu g/m^3$-h), connoting an equivalent exposure experienced by an individual subject to a fixed concentration for a period of time. This allows exposures to be placed on a scale and quantified. One may see from this that a complete description of exposure requires knowledge of three components: magnitude of pollutant concentration in the exposure environment; duration of the exposure; and the time pattern of the exposure. The first two components require little further explanation. The pattern of exposure is of importance because of possible differences in the effects of varying concentrations relative to fixed values. Further discussion can be found below.

Several commonly used means of characterizing exposure are presented in

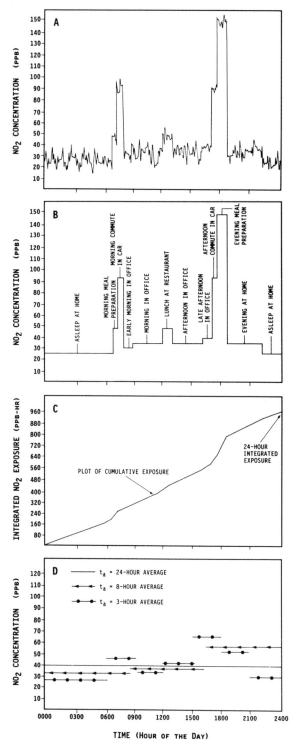

Figure 5.2. Examples of different ways to characterize an individual's personal NO$_2$ exposure profile. *Source:* Adapted from Sexton and Ryan (1988), with permission.

Figure 5.2. Graph A depicts the five-minute mean $NO_2$ concentrations (parts per billion or ppb) measured by a continuous monitor worn by an individual over a twenty-four-hour period. Some periods of the exposure profile are characterized by highly variable exposures to peak levels as high as 200 ppb, whereas other periods are characterized by fairly constant low levels of exposure. These exposures may be compartmentalized by averaging the concentrations within the time period of a specific activity. As graph B illustrates, an individual moves through several diverse exposure settings in the course of a day. Graph C shows the cumulative integrated exposure as the individual moves during the day. The rate of increase in integrated exposure is greater for certain exposure settings, such as cooking meals on a gas range. Note that the twenty-four-hour integrated exposure for this individual is 960 ppb-h. Graph D presents average exposure measurements for various lengths of averaging times. The longer averaging times effectively dampen the variation in personal exposure. Although the twenty-four-hour mean exposure was 40 ppb, mean exposure during the six-hour interval comprised of night sleep was 25 ppb, and the three-hour interval comprising the evening commute and meal preparation was 65 ppb. In this particular example of the different ways of averaging personal exposure, the biologically relevant measure of exposure is not known. Transient exposures to peak levels of $NO_2$ and/or long-term chronic exposures may be associated with oxidant damage and increased susceptibility to respiratory infection.

## DOSE

*Dose* refers to that amount of chemical contaminant which crosses a boundary of the body and reaches the site of toxic action. Time is implied in the concept because dose is typically expressed as mass or number of molecules. Dose, therefore, varies not only with the exposure profile (i.e., concentration and time course) but also with the physiologic state of the individual. For example, consider two individuals who are indoors at home. One sits in a chair and watches television, and the other rides an exercycle for one-half hour while also watching television. Although both individuals are equally exposed to radon present in the room air, the physically active person who is breathing faster, more deeply, and through the mouth receives a greater pulmonary dose relative to the person at rest.

If the site of toxic action is the lung epithelium, as for ozone, the amount of pollutant deposited on the lung epithelium is equivalent to the dose. If the pollutant is absorbed across the lung epithelium (see Chapter 8 on CO) into the blood, where it is transported to the target organ, the amount absorbed is the dose to the body, while the pollutant reaching the site of action is considered to be the biologically effective dose.

For particulate matter and water soluble gases, the route of breathing will affect the amount of chemical contaminant that reaches the lung. During nasal breathing, particles with an aerodynamic diameter of 2–5 μm are more likely to be filtered out in the nasal turbinates by impaction and adsorption onto mucus whereas particles of a smaller diameter pass through the nasal passageways of the head and on to the lower airways and alveoli where they may be deposited (Schlesinger 1988). Removal in the nasal passages is bypassed during mouth breathing. For nonreactive gases such as CO, the route of breathing does not affect the delivery of nonreactive gases to the deep lung. Therefore, for certain pollutants, estimates of pulmonary dose should consider ventilation and the route of inhalation along with the physical and chemical characteristics of the contaminant. Direct monitoring of breathing rates or level of physical exertion may be used to make a crude correction for oral breathing.

The definition of *biologically effective dose* can be refined further. Some inhaled contaminants undergo chemical transformation, and it is the metabolic products that are actually responsible for the toxic effect. Different metabolites may be formed depending upon the received dose, the rate of dosing, and the physiologic conditions. Hence, the effective biologic dose may be a fraction of the pollutant initially inhaled.

TIME-ACTIVITY PATTERNS

People encounter different concentrations in different settings, and depending upon source use and ventilation, among other factors, the concentrations in these settings will change over time. It may be important, therefore, to understand the patterns of human behavior relevant to exposures. Thus, an understanding of the settings and activities in which people spend their time could identify populations and/or behaviors at risk of high exposure. Such studies may reveal effective exposure mitigation opportunities, while providing the basis for modeling exposures which incorporate data from fixed location microenvironmental monitoring. For example, human behavior related to source use, such as the use of an exhaust fan while cooking, the use of a gas range for space heating, the substitution of microwave ovens for gas ranges will result in differential exposures for subgroups.

## MODELING PERSONAL EXPOSURE

Personal exposure may be modeled by considering a series of locations with air pollutant concentrations present. A person moves through these locations over time. A given location could be subdivided if activities, ventilation, or mixing cause changes in source use, strength, or dilution. In the generalized model (Ott 1985; Duan 1982; Fugas 1986), the mean concentrations experienced in successive settings, or *microenvironments*, are time weighted and summed to generate a total integrated exposure for some specified time interval, usually a twenty-four-hour period:

$$E = \Sigma \, f_i \, C_i$$

Where,

$\Sigma$ = Sum over all times and concentrations

$$E = \text{Total exposure}$$
$$C_i = \text{Concentration of pollutant in microenvironment } i$$
$$f_i = \text{Fractional time spent in microenvironment } i$$

When this model is applied to an individual's daily exposure profile, the total exposure is identical to the twenty-four-hour integrated exposure, or the cumulative exposure described in Figure 5.2, graph C. *Microenvironments* are specific situations of exposure, and as defined by Duan (1982), they are locations in space and time over which pollutant concentrations are assumed uniform and constant. Therefore, a kitchen location with cooking activity on a gas range is a microenvironment that is different and distinct from the same location before cooking began. Levels of pollutant concentration at certain locations (e.g., kitchen, garage, or traveling inside a car) may display high temporal variability, and therefore the choice of classification of the microenvironment, and hence averaging time, will influence the variability of the exposure measure. Quackenboss et al. (1986) suggested that although some variability in exposures may be lost by combining microenvironments into broad classes, the differences in variability within a class are likely to be smaller than those between microenvironmental classes (e.g., between indoor and outdoor locations or between residences and workplace). For certain pollutants, such as CO, continuous monitoring or a high resolution microenvironmental classification may be needed to characterize exposure adequately for accurate estimates of uptake by the body due to the time-exposure relationship for carboxyhemoglobin (COHb). In comparison, longer averaging times and more coarse characterization of microenvironments may be appropriate for pollutants such as lead, where body burden is the measure of interest.

The generalized model of total personal exposure may be applied to a specific group of people, or a *community*. The distribution of individual personal exposures made on a sample is combined with time-activity data on the population to estimate the distribution of total exposures for the population. The upper tail of the distribution for some pollutant exposures may identify a subgroup of the population with higher-than-average risk. This is of particular interest to decisionmakers concerned with public health. It should be recognized that this area of the distribution is somewhat more difficult to characterize than is the mean (Sexton and Ryan 1988), and many personal exposure measurements must be obtained to estimate accurately the frequency, magnitude, and duration of high-exposure events, which may be relatively rare. Examples of relatively lower frequency situations include faulty auto exhaust systems that result in high in-vehicle CO concentrations and the improper venting of furnaces that then leak emissions into residences.

### ASSESSMENT OF PERSONAL EXPOSURE

Techniques for the assessment of personal exposure to air pollution can be divided into two major classes. The first approach measures the concentrations of the pollutant using monitors worn on the person or located in specific settings frequented by the person (i.e., home, workplace, or car), and the second estimates exposures from measurements of biologic markers such as the pollutant concentrations in blood and breath samples (Sexton and Ryan 1988).

AIR POLLUTANT MONITORING

In his review of total exposure assessment, Ott (1985) separated exposure measurement into two general methodologies, direct and indirect.

*Direct Method*  In this approach, individuals wear personal monitors that measure the concentrations of pollutants in their breathing zone. While wearing the monitor, the subject maintains a diary record of locations visited and activities pursued. A variety of passive sampling devices that can provide integrated measurements of personal exposure is available, and continuous monitoring instrumentation with data-logging capacity continues to evolve (Wallace and Ott 1982; see Chapter 4 on environmental monitoring). However, implementing the direct method is labor intensive and time consuming, which may preclude its application to large samples, and personal monitors are not presently available for all pollutants of concern.

The direct method of personal exposure assessment has been applied in several surveys. The Environmental Protection Agency (EPA) obtained personal CO measurements on large probability samples of the residents of metropolitan Denver and Washington, D.C. (Akland et al. 1985; Wallace et al. 1988), which allowed the evaluation of the efficacy of outdoor monitoring networks to estimate actual population exposures. Personal exposures to CO have also been measured in a subgroup of Los Angeles men who have ischemic heart disease (Lambert 1990). The exposure patterns of these susceptible individuals were comparable to those measured in the general population at Denver and Washington, D.C. Nitrogen dioxide exposure has been characterized by direct monitoring carried out in conjunction with the Harvard six cities study (Quackenboss et al. 1986) and in probability samples of residents in Boston and Los Angeles (Ryan et al. 1989; Spengler et al. forthcoming). In the Total Exposure Assessment Methodology (TEAM) studies, the EPA surveyed personal exposure to various species including CO, volatile organic compounds (VOCs), pesticides, and particulate matter in several U.S. metropolitan areas (Wallace 1987; see also Chapter 11). The methodology of the EPA's carbon monoxide and VOC studies will be presented in detail in a later section of this chapter.

*Indirect Method*  This method avoids the practical and logistic constraints of direct monitoring. The indirect approach uses area or microenvironment monitors and time-activity data to estimate personal exposures. Ideally, a mathematical model relating personal exposure to area measurements and behavioral parameters should be developed and validated prior to the implementation of a large-scale monitoring program.

The indirect method has been applied to estimate the ozone exposure of asthmatics residing in Houston (Contant et al. 1987). This study will be discussed later under "Applications of Personal Exposure Monitoring Techniques." A simplified application of this method has also been used to study the exposures of infants to $NO_2$ in residences in Albuquerque, New Mexico (Harlos et al. 1987). Mothers reported the time-activity patterns of their children inside the residence, and total personal exposure to $NO_2$ was weighed according to the time that the child spent in the particular rooms in which the samplers were located (Table 5.1). The time-weighted estimate of personal exposure agreed closely ($R = .81$) with measurements made by a sampler worn on the child. This result supported the choice of area monitors for a larger scale study that will longitudinally measure the child's exposure from birth to age 18 months.

BIOLOGIC MONITORING

In performing a biologic assessment of exposure, samples of sputum, urine, blood, or expired breath are obtained and analyzed for the presence of the pollutant or its metabolite. Biologic monitoring is particularly useful if highly sensitive and specific markers of exposure are available, and it may be considered an indirect method of exposure assessment. Good markers of exposure are available for CO (Coburn, Forster, and Kane 1965; Joumard et al. 1981; Lambert, Colome, and Wojciechowski 1988), lead (Annest 1983; Billick 1983), and the nicotine component of environmental tobacco smoke (U.S. Department of Health and Human Services 1986). Biologic monitoring may be a more relevant measure than ambient concentrations for defining populations at risk or for conducting health effects research. However, although providing a surrogate measure of dose and an integrated measure of exposure, relating the biologic marker's level to personal exposure is often problematic for some contaminants due to the complex metabolic pathways involved and the variability in physiologic parameters affecting uptake

Table 5.1   Time-Weighted Contribution of Exposures to $NO_2$ in Several Residential Locations to Total (Twenty-Four-Hour) Exposures

| Location | Time[a] | | Mean $NO_2$[b] | | Exposure Contribution | |
|---|---|---|---|---|---|---|
| | Hours | S.D. | ppb | S.D. | ppb-hour | Percent Total |
| Bedroom | 14.1 | 6.2 | 42.9 | 15.3 | 604.9 | 61.4 |
| Living room | 6.3 | 4.5 | 50.2 | 22.4 | 316.3 | 32.1 |
| Kitchen | 0.78 | 0.73 | 65.5 | 31.5 | 51.1 | 5.2 |
| Outdoor[c] | 0.22 | 0.32 | 12.2 | 8.6 | 2.7 | 0.3 |
| Travel[c] | 0.80 | 0.98 | 12.2 | 8.6 | 9.8 | 1.3 |
| Total | 24.0 | | | | 948.8 | |

Estimated average infant exposure = 41 ppb

*Source*: Harlos et al. (1987), reprinted with permission.
[a]Time-location for all forty-six infants.
[b]$NO_2$ levels for twenty homes with complete data.
[c]Outdoor and travel levels are the seven-day average outdoor $NO_2$ values for the twenty homes.

and elimination (Wallace et al. 1988). Nevertheless, it must be recognized that environmental controls and mitigation strategies will be predicated upon reducing concentrations, and perhaps exposures. It is these more conventional measurements that lend themselves to the precise definitions necessary for enforcement. On the other hand, reduction of a biological marker like blood lead or COHb provides useful trends data and displays the effectiveness of source reduction.

TIME-ACTIVITY MONITORING

Human beings are not stationary, and the environments people inhabit may support several kinds of activities. Therefore, accurate estimates of exposure require assessments of the movements of people and the activities undertaken at various locations. Sociologists and geographers have collected information on activities and movement using self-administered diaries and recall interviews (Robinson 1988). With the diary method, subjects record activities and locations as they engage in activities through the day (Figure 5.3). If faithfully performed, this method can provide information with fine time resolution and good reliability (Michelson 1985). An alternative approach is the twenty-four-hour recall interview in which the respondent recalls the activities and locations of the preceding day within a structured line of questioning by an interviewer. Although providing a record of activities at a more coarse level of time than the diary approach, the interviewing process is generally regarded to produce a more complete and logical

| RID _ _ _ _ _    DATE _ _/_ _/_ _ | | | Nothing  Light      Heavy          Maximal<br>0   0.5   1   2   3   4   5   6   7   8   9   10 | |
|---|---|---|---|---|
| TIME<br>BEGAN | WHAT WERE YOU DOING?<br>(ANYTHING ELSE AT THE<br>SAME TIME?) | WHERE WERE YOU?<br>(ROOM IN HOUSE, OR<br>NEAREST INTERSECTION.) | WERE YOU NEAR ANY OF<br>THESE ACTIVITIES?<br>CHECK ($\checkmark$). | LEVEL OF<br>EXERTION |
| | | | (  )   Running autos<br>(  )   Gas stove/oven<br>(  )   Tobacco smoking<br>(  )   Woodburning<br>(  )   Running engines | |
| | | | (  )   Running autos<br>(  )   Gas stove/oven<br>(  )   Tobacco smoking<br>(  )   Woodburning<br>(  )   Running engines | |
| | | | (  )   Running autos<br>(  )   Gas stove/oven<br>(  )   Tobacco smoking<br>(  )   Woodburning<br>(  )   Running engine | |

Figure 5.3. Example of a page from a time-activity diary to monitor personal activity while wearing an air pollution monitor.

sequence of information (Michelson 1985). Standard formats for diaries and interviews have been described (Michelson 1985; Robinson 1988).

## APPLICATIONS OF PERSONAL EXPOSURE MONITORING TECHNIQUES

In this section, several study designs are presented to illustrate some specific methodologic aspects of the measurement of personal exposure. The first study is the Denver–Washington, D.C., CO study conducted by the EPA. This study represents the first large-scale application of the direct and indirect methods of population exposure assessment and creatively uses direct exposure measurement and biologic markers to characterize exposure. The second study presented uses the indirect method to estimate personal exposure to ozone for asthmatics living in Houston. The third study considers the measurement and modeling of personal exposure to nitrogen dioxide in Boston and Los Angeles. The fourth study is also one of the TEAM studies, conducted by the EPA to characterize population exposures. This chapter briefly focuses on the TEAM study of exposures to VOCs, although the EPA has conducted other exposure studies on pesticides and particulates that utilize the TEAM concepts.

### CARBON MONOXIDE

During the winters of 1982 and 1983, the EPA measured personal exposures to CO in statistically representative samples of the Denver and Washington, D.C., metropolitan areas (Akland et al. 1985). The goal of the research program was to generalize the direct measurement of personal exposures to the entire adult nonsmoking population residing in these areas. The sampling scheme was stratified and included disproportionately large numbers of individuals who commuted and who lived in residences with gas-fueled appliances or an attached garage. In each urban area, five hundred individuals were monitored; subjects wore a portable, continuously recording instrument and maintained a time-activity diary for one day in Washington, D.C., and two days in Denver. End-expired breath samples were collected from subjects at the end of each twenty-four-hour monitoring period to estimate blood COHb levels. The population estimates of personal exposure were derived from adjusted sampling weights. The results indicated that more than 10 percent of the personal exposures of residents of Denver, and 4 percent of the Washington, D.C., residents exceeded the eight-hour 9-ppm federal standard. Ambient fixed site monitoring data underestimated the distribution of these personal exposures (Figure 5.4). The exposures experienced in transit and outdoors near active roadways were identified as important contributors to total CO exposure. The observation that people spent more than one hour per day in transit and more than twenty-two hours per day indoors is important. The mean levels of CO measured in specific indoor microenvironments are presented in Chapter 9.

The breath samples were used to provide an additional measure of exposure for the Washington, D.C., sample (Wallace et al. 1988). Carbon monoxide levels in end-expired breath were used to estimate blood COHb concentration, a measure of

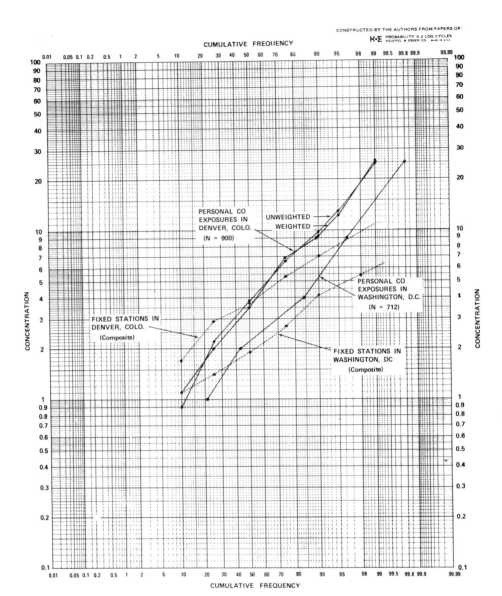

Figure 5.4. Frequency distribution of maximum eight-hour CO personal exposures and ambient concentrations for population samples in Denver, Colorado, and Washington, D.C., during the winters of 1982 and 1983. *Source:* Reprinted with permission from Akland G.G., et al. Measuring human exposure to carbon monoxide in Washington, D.C., and Denver, Colorado, during winter 1982–1983. *Environ Sci Technology* 19:911–18. Copyright 1985 American Chemical Society.

the cumulative exposure to CO. Exposure measurements from the continuous monitors were input into the pharmacokinetic model to calculate COHb levels at the end of the twenty-four-hour monitoring period (Coburn, Forster, and Kane 1965). The modeled COHb levels were 40–50 percent lower than those estimated from samples of end-expired breath. The availability of this alternative measure of exposure prompted the investigators to reevaluate the accuracy of the electronic monitors. Differences in the sensitivity of monitoring instrumentation, declining sensitivity with battery discharge, and improper calibration methods may have biased the measurements low in some monitors. Therefore, the investigators used the breath measurements to calculate individual correction factors to revise upwardly the distribution of personal exposures. Without the biologic marker data, the monitoring instrumentation would have underestimated the sample's exposures.

The efficacy of outdoor monitoring networks to estimate personal exposure was tested using the data derived from the Denver field survey. The exposure profiles were used to validate a population exposure model, the simulation of human activity and air pollution exposure (SHAPE) model (Ott 1988). Two days of personal monitoring data were available for each of 336 individuals living in Denver. The distributions of microenvironmental exposures and the ambient monitoring network data from the first day of monitoring of each individual were used to predict the personal exposures on the second day. The distribution of microenvironmental concentrations on the second day were calculated by adding microenvironmental source inputs onto the ambient background concentration measured on the second day. Using the actual time-activity data from the second day of monitoring, exposures in microenvironments were assigned by Monte Carlo sampling from the microenvironmental CO distributions. SHAPE was successful at predicting the mean of the cumulative distribution, but it tended to underestimate exposures in the tails of the distribution (Figure 5.5). Of particular concern was the underestimation of high exposures.

OZONE

Ideally, exposure models are constructed and validated with actual personal exposure data. It is not always necessary to perform this validation on a sample the size of that used in the EPA CO studies. For example, the $O_3$ exposure model developed by the University of Texas School of Public Health was validated in a community sample of relatively small size (Stock et al. 1985; Contant et al. 1987). Data to construct the model were obtained from twelve homes of asthmatics by measuring indoor and outdoor residential levels of $O_3$ with a mobile monitoring van and by measuring personal exposure with portable instruments carried by a field technician who followed the research subject. Fixed-site monitoring data were regressed on the indoor and outdoor residential measurements to define the relationship between levels of $O_3$ from the ambient monitoring network and the concentrations occurring at the residential sites. Hourly averages of $O_3$ concentration at indoor and outdoor residential sites were computed. The exposures of each individual were weighted according to records of personal activity maintained by

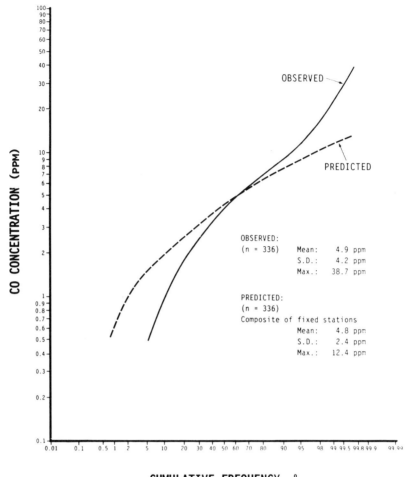

Figure 5.5. Logarithmic probability plot of cumulative frequency distributions of the maximum moving average eight-hour personal exposure to CO predicted by SHAPE using the ambient background concentration calculated from a composite measure from all fixed-site stations along with observed frequency distribution of the measured personal exposures for day 2 in Denver, Colorado. *Source:* Adapted from Ott et al. (1988), with permission.

the subjects. When compared with the actual hourly measurements of personal exposure, the model underestimated exposure by approximately 20 percent (Figure 5.6). However, use of the model to estimate personal exposure is considerably more accurate than using untransformed fixed-site measurements, for the indoor concentrations of $O_3$ were, on average, substantially less (<10%) than levels simultaneously measured at the nearest fixed site. Outdoor $O_3$ concentrations at homes were approximately 80 percent of those measured at fixed sites, but a

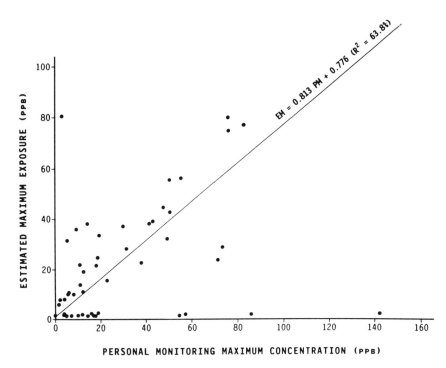

Figure 5.6. Scatter plot of $O_3$ exposure model estimate of maximum hourly average personal exposure versus maximum hourly average measurement of $O_3$ exposure by personal monitoring for forty-nine daytime monitoring periods between 7 A.M. and 7 P.M., with a mean duration of eight hours. *Source:* Adapted from Contant et al. (1987), with permission.

relatively small proportion of daily time is spent outdoors around the place of residence. This research demonstrated that large improvements in the accuracy of $O_3$ exposure assessments can be achieved by the simple weighting of personal activity patterns into indoor and outdoor classes.

NITROGEN DIOXIDE

Direct and indirect approaches to exposure assessment have been combined to strengthen the design of surveys to measure personal exposure to $NO_2$ in the community. The Harvard School of Public Health developed a model of personal exposure based on ambient monitoring information and coarse activity pattern information on time spent indoors at home, indoors at work, outdoors, and in transit (Ryan et al. 1988a, 1988b, 1989; Spengler et al. forthcoming). Comparison of the estimates of the initial model with actual personal monitoring data demonstrated the importance of refining the model to account explicitly for exposures in three other microenvironments with potentially elevated $NO_2$ concentrations: in-home cooking areas with unvented combustion appliances, travel on roadways during commuting hours, and certain occupational settings. Personal activity diaries were modified to collect information on the time spent in these special settings.

Personal exposure surveys on representative samples of urban residents were conducted to determine the population distributions of $NO_2$ exposures. Utilizing an integrating diffusion badge, personal exposures were quantified for approximately three hundred individuals in Boston and seven hundred residents in Los Angeles. Subjects wore one badge while indoors and a different badge when outdoors. Outdoor measurements were also made at each subject's residence. Ambient levels of $NO_2$ were higher in Los Angeles (30–70 ppb) than they were in Boston (20–30 ppb). Unlike Boston, in Los Angeles approximately 40 percent of the variance in personal exposures and 60 percent in indoor residential concentration was explained by ambient measurements made outside the residence. These results suggest that in areas of higher ambient pollution with substantial spatial variation, outdoor concentrations can influence exposure. This occurs through the contribution of outdoor concentrations to indoor concentrations because the modeled prediction does not improve when the fractional times spent outdoors are included as an independent variable.

VOLATILE ORGANIC COMPOUNDS

Wallace and co-workers at the EPA have measured personal exposures to VOCs in several metropolitan areas across the United States in a group of interrelated studies called the TEAM studies. In each metropolitan location, random stratified samples were selected on the basis of proximity to point sources and socioeconomic class, geographic area, and demographic characteristics including age, marital status, tobacco smoking status, and occupational class. Personal exposure to VOCs was measured with personal samplers; end-exposed breath samples were obtained at the end of each twenty-four-hour period; water samples from the homes were taken for VOC analysis; and outdoor sites were monitored (see Chapter 11 for further details). Sources of exposure were inferred by questionnaire data on personal activities and proximity to potential sources.

Table 5.2 presents a summary of the results of the TEAM survey in one urban location, the Bayonne and Elizabeth, New Jersey, survey. The exposures experienced outdoors and indoors were highly variable, both from compound to compound and within a compound. However, indoor concentrations were consistently higher than outdoor concentrations. The higher concentrations observed indoors were unexpected because this study site has many industrial sources of VOCs.

Breath measurements did not correlate well with ambient concentration measurements, further indicating that ambient data do not represent population exposures accurately. However, for some specific VOCs, elevated personal exposures as measured by breath samples were associated with certain types of activities. For example, personal exposure to benzene was correlated with visits to service stations, and tetrachloroethylene was correlated with visits to dry cleaning businesses.

The TEAM VOC studies have had a major impact on the way in which the research community views environmental exposures to VOCs. In a review of the

Table 5.2  Summary of Median and Maximum Concentrations
($\mu$g/m$^3$) for Elizabeth-Bayonne, New Jersey, *TEAM* Study
of Volatile Organic Compounds

| Compound | Outdoor[a] | Indoor[b] | Ratio[c] |
|---|---|---|---|
| Chloroform | 0.74[d] (21.5) | 2.94 (215) | 3.97 (10.0) |
| 1,1,1-Trichloroethane | 4.20 (40.0) | 15.60 (880) | 3.71 (22.0) |
| Benzene | 7.00 (91.0) | 13.00 (120) | 1.86 (1.32) |
| Carbon tetrachloride | 0.81 (14.0) | 1.38 (14.0) | 1.70 (1.00) |
| Trichloroethylene | 1.34 (15.0) | 2.00 (47.0) | 1.49 (3.13) |
| Tetrachloroethylene | 2.60 (27.0) | 5.60 (250) | 2.15 (9.26) |
| Styrene | 0.67 (11.0) | 1.80 (53.5) | 2.69 (4.86) |
| *m,p*-Dichlorobenzene | 0.80 (13.0) | 2.80 (915) | 3.50 (70.4) |
| Ethylbenzene | 3.20 (20.0) | 6.10 (320) | 1.91 (16.0) |
| *o*-Xylene | 3.00 (27.0) | 4.98 (46.0) | 1.66 (1.70) |
| *m,p*-Xylene | 9.90 (70.0) | 15.50 (120) | 1.57 (1.71) |

*Source*: Adapted from Wallace et al. (1986) with permission.
[a]Outdoor heading corresponds to overnight outdoor air in TEAM nomenclature.
[b]Indoor heading corresponds to overnight personal air in TEAM nomenclature. Summary
statistics presented include a small number of personal exposures not in indoor environments.
[c]Ratio of indoor median to outdoor median (ratio of indoor maximum to outdoor
maximum).
[d]Median (maximum).

EPA's research on total human exposure, Ott et al. (1986) acknowledged these
major contributions of the TEAM studies: (a) Variability of two to three orders of
magnitude in exposures is found over small geographic regions, suggesting a need
to reconsider epidemiologic approaches that assume homogeneous exposures
across broad areas; (b) personal and indoor exposures consistently exceed outdoor
concentrations; (c) although inhalation is the prime exposure route to many VOCs,
ingestion by drinking water can be a major route of exposure to chloroform and
other species; and (d) breath samples are a reliable biologic marker for VOC
exposure and correlate well with personal exposures.

### SUMMARY

The majority of daily activity is spent in indoor settings, and therefore, on a time-
weighted basis, indoor exposures may dominate the total exposure of most individuals when concentrations experienced in other microenvironments are of comparable magnitude. An understanding of the personal exposures in the indoor
setting is essential and will continue to be an important focus in air pollution
epidemiology and public health planning. This chapter has reviewed the basic
concepts of human exposure assessment and has presented some of the methodologic considerations. These approaches to the estimation of actual personal
exposures offer encouraging prospects for improvement of our understanding of
the relationship between air pollutant exposures and health effects and the potential
for intervention to reduce those exposures.

# REFERENCES

Akland, G. G., et al. 1985. Measuring human exposure to carbon monoxide in Washington, D.C., and Denver, Colorado, during the winter of 1982–1983. *Environ. Sci. Technol.* 19:911–18.

Annest, J. L. 1983. Trends in blood lead levels of the United States population. In *Lead Versus Health.* Ed. M. Rutter and R. R. Jones, 33–58. New York: John Wiley & Sons.

Billick, I. H. 1983. Sources of lead in the environment. In *Lead Versus Health.* Ed. M. Rutter and R. R. Jones, 59–77. New York: John Wiley & Sons.

Coburn, R. F.; Forster, R. E.; and Kane, P. B. 1965. Considerations of the physiology and variables that determine blood carboxyhemoglobin concentrations in man. *J. Clin. Invest.* 44:1899–1910.

Contant, C. F., et al. 1987. The estimation of personal exposures to air pollutants for a community-based study of health effects in asthmatics: Exposure model. *J. Air Pollut. Control Assoc.* 37:587–94.

Duan, N. 1982. Models for human exposure to air pollution. *Environ. Int.* 8:305–9.

Fugas, M. 1986. Assessment of true human exposures to air pollution. *Environ. Int.* 12:363–67.

Harlos, D. P., et al. 1987. Relating indoor $NO_2$ levels to infant personal exposures. *Atmos. Environ.* 21:369–76.

Joumard, R., et al. 1981. Mathematical models of the uptake of carbon monoxide on hemoglobin at low carbon monoxide levels. *Environ. Health Perspect.* 41:277–89.

Lambert, W. E. 1990. Cardiac response to carbon monoxide in the community setting. Ph.D. diss., University of California, Irvine.

Lambert, W. E.; Colome, S. D.; and Wojciechowski, S. L. 1988. Application of end-expired breath sampling to estimate carboxyhemoglobin levels in community air pollution exposure assessments. *Atmos. Environ.* 22:2171–81.

Michelson, W. 1985. Measuring macroenvironment and behavior: The time budget and time geography. In *Methods in Environmental and Behavioral Research.* Ed. R. B. Bechtel, R. W. Marans, and W. Michelson, 216–43. New York: Van Nostrand Reinhold.

Ott, W. R. 1985. Total human exposure. *Environ. Sci. Technol.* 19:880–86.

Ott, W. R., 1988. Validation of the simulation of human activity and pollution exposure (SHAPE) model using paired days from the Denver, Colorado, carbon monoxide field study. *Atmos. Environ.* 22:2101–13.

Ott, W. R., et al. 1986. The Environmental Protection Agency's program on total human exposure. *Environ. Int.* 12:475–94.

Ozkaynak, H., et al. 1986. Bias due to misclassification of personal exposures in epidemiologic studies of indoor and outdoor air pollution. *Environ. Int.* 12:389–93.

Quackenboss, J. J., et al. 1986. Personal exposure to nitrogen dioxide: Relationship to indoor/outdoor air quality and activity patterns. *Environ. Sci. Technol.* 20:775–83.

Robinson, J. P. 1988. Time-diary research and human exposure assessment: Some methodological considerations. *Atmos. Environ.* 22:2085–92.

Ryan, P. B., et al. 1987. Nitrogen dioxide exposure assessment in greater Boston: Evaluation of personal monitoring. *Fourth international conference on indoor air quality and climate.* August, West Berlin.

Ryan, P. B., et al. 1988a. The Boston residential $NO_2$ characterization study, I: A preliminary evaluation of the survey methodology. *J. Air Pollut. Control Assoc.* 38:22–27.

Ryan, P. B., et al. 1988b. The Boston residential $NO_2$ characterization study, II: Survey methodology and population concentration estimates. *Atmos. Environ.* 22:2115–25.

Ryan, P. B., et al. 1989. Nitrogen dioxide exposure studies, I: The Boston personal monitoring studies. Presented at EPA/AWMA symposium on total exposure assessment methodology. 27–30 November, Las Vegas.

Ryan, P. B.; Spengler, J. D.; and Letz, R. 1986. Estimating personal exposures to $NO_2$. *Environ. Int.* 12:394–400.

Schlesinger, R. B. 1988. Biological disposition of airborne particles: Basic principles and application to vehicular emissions. In *Air Pollution, the Automobile, and Public Health*. Ed. A. Y. Watson, R. B. Bates, and D. Kennedy, 239–98. Washington, D.C.: National Academy Press.

Sexton, K., and Ryan, P. B. 1988. Assessment of human exposure to air pollution: Methods, measurements, and models. In *Air Pollution, the Automobile, and Public Health*. Ed. A. Y. Watson, R. B. Bates, and D. Kennedy, 207–38. Washington, D.C.: National Academy Press.

Shy, C. M.; Kleinbaum, D. G.; and Morgenstern, H. 1978. The effect of misclassification of exposure status in epidemiological studies of air pollution health effects. *Bull. N.Y. Acad. Med.* 54:1155–65.

Spengler, J. D., et al. 1985. Personal exposures to respirable particulates and implications for air pollution epidemiology. *Environ. Sci. Technol.* 19:700–707.

Spengler, J. D., et al. 1989. An overview of the Los Angeles and Boston $NO_2$ personal monitoring studies. Presented at EPA/AWMA symposium on total exposure assessment methodology. 27–30 November, Las Vegas.

Spengler, J. D., et al. Forthcoming. Human exposure to nitrogen dioxide in the Los Angeles Basin: Study design and results. *Journal of the Air and Waste Management Association*.

Spengler, J. D., and Soczek, M. L. 1984. Evidence for improved air quality and the need for personal exposure research. *Environ. Sci. Technol.* 18:268A–80.

Stock, T. H., et al. 1985. The estimation of personal exposures to air pollutants for a community-based study of health effects in asthmatics: Design and results of air monitoring. *J. Air Pollut. Control Assoc.* 35:1266–73.

U.S. Department of Health and Human Services. 1986. *The health consequences of involuntary smoking. A report of the surgeon general*. Rockville, Md.: U.S. Government Printing Office. DHHS, PHS Publication no. (CDC) 87-8398.

Wallace, L. A. 1987. *The total exposure assessment methodology (TEAM) study: Summary and analysis*. Vol. 1. Washington, D.C.: Office of Research and Development, U.S. Environmental Protection Agency. Publication no. EPA/600/6-87/002a.

Wallace, L. A., and Ott, W. R. 1982. Personal monitors: A state-of-the-art survey. *J. Air Pollut. Control Assoc.* 32:601–10.

Wallace, L. A., et al. 1986. Total exposure assessment methodology (TEAM) study: Personal exposures, indoor-outdoor relationships, and breath levels of volatile organic compounds in New Jersey. *Environ. Int.* 12:369–87.

Wallace, L., et al. 1988. Comparison of breath CO, CO exposure, and Coburn model predictions in the U.S. EPA Washington, D.C.-Denver CO study. *Atmos. Environ.* 22:2183–93.

World Health Organization. 1982. Estimating human exposure to air pollutants. Geneva, Switzerland: WHO. WHO Offset Publication no. 69.

# II. HEALTH EFFECTS

# 6

# ENVIRONMENTAL TOBACCO SMOKE

Jonathan M. Samet, M. D., M.S., William S. Cain, Ph.D.,
Brian P. Leaderer, Ph.D., M.P.H.

Extensive toxicologic, experimental, and epidemiologic data, largely collected since the 1950s, have established that active cigarette smoking is the major preventable cause of morbidity and mortality in the United States (U.S. Department of Health, Education, and Welfare [DHEW] 1979; U.S. Department of Health and Human Services [DHHS] 1989). More recently, involuntary exposure to tobacco smoke has been investigated as a risk factor for disease and also found to be a cause of preventable morbidity and mortality in nonsmokers. The 1986 report of the surgeon general on smoking and health (U.S. DHHS 1986) and a report by the National Research Council (NRC 1986a), also published in 1986, comprehensively reviewed the data on involuntary exposure to tobacco smoke; both reports concluded that involuntary smoking was a cause of disease in nonsmokers.

This chapter will summarize the converging evidence on the health effects of involuntary exposure to tobacco smoke. To date, research on involuntary smoking has focused on respiratory effects although recent investigations have examined associations with diverse conditions including nonrespiratory cancers, ischemic heart disease, age at menopause, sudden infant death syndrome, and birth weight (Table 6.1).

## EXPOSURE TO ENVIRONMENTAL TOBACCO SMOKE

### CHARACTERISTICS OF ENVIRONMENTAL TOBACCO SMOKE

Nonsmokers inhale environmental tobacco smoke (ETS), the combination of the sidestream smoke that is released from the cigarette's burning end with the mainstream smoke exhaled by the active smoker (First 1985). The inhalation of ETS is generally referred to as *passive smoking* or *involuntary smoking*. The exposures of involuntary and active smoking differ quantitatively and, to some

Table 6.1  Established and Potential Health
Effects of Involuntary Exposure
to Tobacco Smoke

Established
    Increased lower respiratory infections in children
    Increased respiratory symptoms in children
    Reduced lung growth in children
    Increased lung cancer risk in nonsmokers
    Irritation of the eyes, nose, throat, and lower res-
        piratory tract
Potential
    Increased respiratory symptoms in adults
    Reduced lung function in adults
    Increased risk for asthma
    Exacerbation of asthma
    Increased risk for cardiovascular disease
    Increased risk for nonrespiratory cancers
    Earlier age at menopause
    Increased risk for sudden infant death
    Reduced birth weight

extent, qualitatively (NRC 1981, 1986a; Sterling and Kobayashi 1982; U.S. DHHS 1984, 1986). Because of the lower temperature in the burning cone of the smoldering cigarette, most partial pyrolysis products are enriched in sidestream as compared with mainstream smoke. Consequently, sidestream smoke has higher concentrations of some toxic and carcinogenic substances than mainstream smoke does; however, dilution by room air markedly reduces the concentrations inhaled by the involuntary smoker in comparison with those inhaled by the active smoker. Nevertheless, involuntary smoking is accompanied by exposure to many of the toxic agents generated by tobacco combustion (NRC 1981, 1986a; Sterling and Kobayashi 1982; U.S. DHHS 1984, 1986).

ENVIRONMENTAL TOBACCO SMOKE CONCENTRATIONS
    Tobacco smoke is a complex mixture of gases and particles which contains myriad chemical species (U.S. DHEW 1979; U.S. DHHS 1984). Not surprisingly, tobacco smoking in indoor environments increases levels of respirable particles, nicotine, polycyclic aromatic hydrocarbons, carbon monoxide (CO), acrolein, nitrogen dioxide ($NO_2$), and many other substances (Table 6.2). The extent of the increase in concentration varies with the number of smokers, the intensity of smoking, the ventilation rate of the indoor space, and the use of air cleaning devices. Several components of cigarette smoke have been measured in indoor environments as markers of the contribution of tobacco combustion to indoor air pollution. Particles have been measured most often because both sidestream and mainstream smoke contain high concentrations of particles in the respirable size range (NRC 1986a; U.S. DHHS 1986). Particles are a nonspecific marker of tobacco smoke contamination, however, because numerous sources other than

Table 6.2    Selected Studies of Tobacco Smoke Component Concentrations
in Various Environments

| Referenced | Location | Component | Mean Concentration |
|---|---|---|---|
| Badre et al. (1978) | Room, 18 smokers | Acrolein | $0.19$ mg/m$^3$ |
| Badre et al. (1978) | Room, 18 smokers | Benzene | $0.11$ mg/m$^3$ |
| Wallace (1987) | New Jersey homes, smokers | Benzene | 16 $\mu$g/m$^3$, overnight |
| | New Jersey homes, nonsmokers | Benzene | 8.4 $\mu$g/m$^3$, overnight |
| Chappell and Parker (1977) | Office | CO | 2.5 ppm, 2- to 3-min samples |
| Chappell and Parker (1977) | Nightclub | CO | 13.0 ppm, 2- to 3-min samples |
| Hinds and First (1975) | Restaurant | Nicotine | 5.2 $\mu$g/m$^3$, 2.5-h samples |
| Hinds and First (1975) | Train | Nicotine | 6.3 $\mu$g/m$^3$, 2.5-h samples |
| Muramatsu et al. (1984) | Cafeteria | Nicotine | 26.4 $\mu$g/m$^3$ |
| Weber and Fischer (1980) | Office | NO$_2$ | 24 ppb |
| Repace and Lowrey (1980) | Cocktail party | Particles | 351 $\mu$g/m$^3$, 15-min sample |
| | Bowling alley | Particles | 202 $\mu$g/m$^3$, 20-min sample |
| | Bar | Particles | 334 $\mu$g/m$^3$, 26-min sample |
| Spengler et al. (1981) | Residence, $\geq 2$ smokers | Particles | 70 $\mu$g/m$^3$, 24-h sample |
| | Residence, 1 smoker | Particles | 37 $\mu$g/m$^3$, 24-h sample |
| Henderson et al. (1989) | Residence, cigarette smoking | Nicotine | 3.4 $\mu$g/m$^3$, 14-h sample |
| | Residence, no cigarette smoking | Nicotine | 0.3 $\mu$g/m$^3$, 14-h sample |

tobacco combustion add particles to indoor air. Studies of levels of ETS components have been conducted largely in public buildings; fewer studies have been conducted in the home and office environments (NRC 1986a; U.S. DHHS 1986).

The contribution of various environments to personal exposure to tobacco smoke varies with the time-activity pattern, the distribution of time spent in different locations. Time-activity patterns may heavily weight exposures in particular environments for certain groups of individuals. For example, exposure in the home predominates for infants who do not attend day-care (Harlos et al. 1987). For adults residing with nonsmokers, the workplace may be the principal location at which exposure takes place.

The contribution of smoking in the home to indoor air pollution has been demonstrated by studies using personal monitoring and monitoring of homes for respirable particles. Spengler et al. (1981) monitored homes in six U.S. cities for respirable particle concentrations over several years and found that a smoker of one pack of cigarettes daily contributed about 20 $\mu$g/m$^3$ to twenty-four-hour indoor particle concentrations. In homes with two or more heavy smokers, this study showed that the old twenty-four-hour national ambient air quality standard of 260 $\mu$g/m$^3$ for total suspended particulates could be exceeded. Because cigarettes are not smoked uniformly over the day, higher peak concentrations must occur when cigarettes are actually smoked. Spengler et al. (1985) measured the personal exposures to respirable particles sustained by nonsmoking adults in two rural Tennessee communities. The mean twenty-four-hour exposures were substantially higher for those exposed to smoke at home, 64 $\mu g/m^3$ for those exposed versus 36 $\mu g/m^3$ for those not exposed.

In several recent studies, small numbers of homes have been monitored for nicotine. In a study of ETS exposure of day-care children, average nicotine concentration during the time that the ETS-exposed children were at home was 3.7 $\mu g/m^3$; in homes without smoking, the average was 0.3 $\mu g/m^3$ (Henderson et al. 1989). Coultas, et al. (1990) measured twenty-four-hour nicotine and respirable particle concentrations in ten homes on alternate days for a week and then on five more days during alternate weeks. The mean levels were comparable to those in the study of Henderson et al. (1989), but some twenty-four-hour values were as high as 20 $\mu g/m^3$. Nicotine and respirable particle concentrations varied widely in the homes.

The total exposure assessment methodology (TEAM) study, conducted by the U.S. Environmental Protection Agency, provided extensive data on concentrations of twenty volatile organic compounds in a sample of homes in several communities (Wallace 1987). Indoor monitoring showed increased concentrations of benzene, xylenes, ethylbenzene, and styrene in homes with smokers compared with homes without smokers.

More extensive information is available on levels of environmental tobacco smoke in public buildings of various types (Table 6.2). Monitoring in locations where smoking may be intense, such as bars and restaurants, has generally shown elevations of particles and other markers of smoke pollution where smoking is taking place (NRC 1986a; U.S. DHHS 1986). For example, Repace and Lowrey (1980) used a piezobalance to sample aerosols in restaurants, bars, and other locations. In the places sampled, respirable particulate levels ranged up to 700 $\mu g/m^3$, and the levels varied with the intensity of smoking. Similar data have been reported for the office environment, although the information is more limited (NRC 1986a; U.S. DHHS 1986).

Transportation environments may also be affected by cigarette smoking. Contamination of air in trains, buses, automobiles, airplanes, and submarines has been documented (NRC 1986a; U.S. DHHS 1986). A recent NRC report (NRC 1986b) on air quality in airliners summarized studies of tobacco smoke pollutants in commercial aircraft. In one study, during a single flight, the $NO_2$ concentration varied with the number of passengers with a lighted cigarette. In another study, respirable particles in the smoking section were measured at concentrations fivefold or greater than in the nonsmoking section. Peaks as high as 1,000 $\mu g/m^3$ were measured in the smoking section. Mattson and colleagues (1989) used personal exposure monitors to assess nicotine exposures of passengers and flight attendants. All persons were exposed to nicotine, even if seated in the nonsmoking portion of the cabin. Exposures were much greater in the smoking than in the nonsmoking section and were also greater on aircraft with recirculated air.

Biologic markers of tobacco smoke exposure can be used to describe the prevalence and the dosimetry of involuntary smoking and to validate questionnaire-based measures of exposure. In both active and involuntary smokers, the detection of smoke components or their metabolites in body fluids or alveolar air provides evidence of exposure to tobacco smoke, and levels of these markers can be used to gauge the intensity of exposure. The risks of involuntary smoking have also been estimated by comparing levels of biologic markers in active and involuntary smokers.

At present, the most sensitive and specific markers for tobacco smoke exposure are nicotine and its major metabolite, cotinine (Jarvis and Russell 1984; NRC 1986a; U.S. DHHS 1988). Neither nicotine nor cotinine is present in body fluids in the absence of exposure to tobacco smoke. Because the circulating half-life of nicotine is generally shorter than two hours (Rosenberg et al. 1980), nicotine concentrations in body fluids reflect more recent exposures. In contrast, cotinine has a half-life in the blood or plasma of active smokers which ranges from less than ten hours to about forty hours (Kyerematen et al. 1982; Benowitz et al. 1983; U.S. DHHS 1988); hence, cotinine levels provide information about more chronic exposure to tobacco smoke in both active and involuntary smokers. Whether cotinine has the same half-life in plasma, saliva, and urine is presently controversial, as is the choice of the optimal body fluid for measuring cotinine for research purposes (Jarvis et al. 1988; Wall et al. 1988; Coultas and Samet 1990; Haley, Spekovic, and Hoffmann 1989). Thiocyanate concentration in body fluids, concentration of CO in expired air, and carboxyhemoglobin level distinguish active smokers from nonsmokers but are not as sensitive and specific as cotinine for assessing involuntary exposure to tobacco smoke (Hoffman et al. 1984a, 1984b; Jarvis and Russell 1984).

Cotinine levels have been measured in adult nonsmokers and in children (Table 6.3). In the studies of adult nonsmokers, exposures at home, in the workplace, and in other settings determined cotinine concentrations in urine and saliva. The cotinine levels in involuntary smokers ranged from less than 1 percent to about 8 percent of cotinine levels measured in active smokers. Smoking by parents was the predominant determinant of the cotinine levels in their children. For example, Greenberg et al. (1984) found significantly higher concentrations of cotinine in the urine and saliva of infants exposed to cigarette smoke in their homes in comparison with unexposed controls. Urinary cotinine levels in the infants increased with the number of cigarettes smoked during the previous twenty-four hours by the mother. In a study of schoolchildren in England, salivary cotinine levels rose with the number of smoking parents in the home (Jarvis et al. 1985).

The results of studies on biologic markers have important implications for research on involuntary smoking and add to the biologic plausibility of associations between involuntary smoking and disease documented in epidemiologic studies. The data on marker levels provide ample evidence that involuntary exposure leads to absorption, circulation, and excretion of tobacco smoke compo-

Table 6.3   Selected Studies of Cotinine Levels in Nonsmokers

| Population | Findings |
|---|---|
| 100 adult patients attending clinics in London (Jarvis et al. 1984) | Cotinine levels parallel self-reported exposure. In non-smoking, mean = 1.5 ng/ml in saliva; in active smokers, mean = 309.9 ng/ml. |
| 151 adult males attending a clinic in London and 70 subjects from Oxford (Wald et al. 1984; Wald and Ritchie 1984) | Urinary cotinine level increased with reported duration of smoke exposure. In nonexposed nonsmokers, median level = 2.0 ng/ml; exposed nonsmokers, median = 6.0 ng/ml; active cigarette smokers, median = 1,645 ng/ml. Smoking by wife increased cotinine concentrations threefold in nonsmoking men. |
| 51 infants attending clinics in North Carolina (Greenberg et al. 1984) | In nonexposed, median urinary level = 4 ng/mg creatinine; exposed, median = 351 ng/mg creatinine. Salivary creatinine levels higher in exposed. |
| 472 nonsmoking adults in Japan (Matsukura et al. 1984) | Exposure at home and at work independently increased urinary cotinine level. In nonsmokers, median = 680 ng/mg creatinine; active smokers, median = 8,570 ng/mg creatinine. |
| 569 schoolchildren, age 11–16 years, in Bristol, England (Jarvis et al. 1985) | Salivary cotinine level increased with the number of smoking parents. If neither parent smoked, median = 0.20 ng/ml; if both smoked, median = 2.70 ng/ml. |
| 38 children, age 3–15 months, attending a child center in North Carolina (Pattishall et al. 1985) | Serum cotinine level increased with the number of smokers in the home. In children without household exposure, mean = 1.0 ng/ml; exposed, mean = 4.1 ng/ml. |
| 839 children and adults in a population sample in New Mexico (Coultas et al. 1987) | Salivary cotinine level increased with the number of smokers in the home. If no smokers in the home, median level was zero. If one or more smokers, median was greater than zero and increased with the number of smokers |
| 260 adult municipal workers in Dallas, Texas (Haley et al. 1989) | Urinary cotinine level about 2.5 times greater for persons living with smokers. Somewhat greater levels for those exposed at work. |

nents. The studies of biologic markers also confirm the high prevalence of involuntary smoking, as ascertained by questionnaire (Coultas et al. 1987). The observed correlations between reported exposures and levels of markers suggest that questionnaire methods for assessing recent exposure have some validity.

Comparisons of levels of biologic markers in smokers and nonsmokers have been made in order to estimate the relative intensities of active and involuntary smoking. However, proportionality cannot be assumed between the ratio of the levels of markers in passive and active smokers and the relative doses of other tobacco smoke components. Nonetheless, several investigators have attempted to characterize involuntary smoking in terms of active smoking. For example, Foliart and colleagues (Foliart, Benowitz, and Becker 1983) measured urinary excretion of nicotine in flight attendants during an eight-hour flight and estimated that the average exposure was 0.12–0.25 mg of nicotine. Russell, West, and Jarvis (1985) compared nicotine levels in nonsmokers exposed to tobacco smoke with levels achieved following infusion of known doses of nicotine. On the basis of this comparison the investigators estimated that the average rate of nicotine absorption was 0.23 mg/h in a smoky tavern, 0.36 mg/h in an unventilated smoke-filled room, and 0.014 mg/h from average daily exposure. In active smokers the first cigarette of the day resulted in absorption of 1.4 mg of nicotine.

## HEALTH EFFECTS OF INVOLUNTARY SMOKING

### LOWER RESPIRATORY TRACT ILLNESSES IN CHILDHOOD

Epidemiologic investigations have linked involuntary smoking in children to increased occurrence of lower respiratory tract illness during infancy and childhood; presumably these illnesses are infectious in etiology and do not represent a direct response of the lung to toxic components of ETS. Investigations conducted throughout the world have demonstrated an increased risk of lower respiratory tract illness in infants with smoking parents (Table 6.4). These studies indicate a significantly increased frequency of bronchitis and pneumonia during the first year of life of children with smoking parents. Although the health outcome measures varied somewhat among the studies, the relative risks associated with involuntary smoking were similar, and dose-response relationships with the extent of parental smoking were demonstrable. Although most of the studies have shown that maternal smoking rather than paternal smoking underlies the increased risk, a recent study from China shows that paternal smoking alone can increase the incidence of lower respiratory illness (Yue Chen, Wanxian, and Shunzhang 1986). In these studies (Table 6.4), an effect of passive smoking has not been readily identified after the first year of life. The strength of the effect of passive smoking during the first year of life may reflect higher exposures consequent to the time-activity patterns of young infants, which place them in close proximity to cigarettes smoked by their mothers.

For school-age children, parental smoking also increases the occurrence of chest illnesses. For example, in a survey of 4,071 Pennsylvania children ages five to fourteen years, the proportion of children having a chest illness of three days or more during the past year rose from 8.8 to 11.8 to 13.6 percent with none, one, and two smoking parents, respectively (Schenker, Samet, and Speizer 1983). The findings in other large surveys have been similar (Ware et al. 1984; Somerville, Rona, and Chinn 1988).

### RESPIRATORY SYMPTOMS AND ILLNESSES IN CHILDREN

Data from numerous surveys demonstrate a greater frequency of the most common respiratory symptoms, cough, phlegm, and wheeze in the children of smokers (U.S. DHHS 1986). In these studies the subjects have generally been schoolchildren, and the effects of parental smoking have been examined. Thus, the less

Table 6.4  Early Childhood Respiratory Illnesses and Involuntary Smoking

| Study Population | Study Design | Effect of Involuntary Smoking | Comments |
|---|---|---|---|
| 10,672 births in Israel, 1967–68 (Harlap and Davies 1974) | Antenatal maternal smoking history, monitoring of admissions during first year of life | Significant increase in hospitalization for pneumonia and bronchitis; $RR^a$ = 1.4 | Dose-response relationship present; maternal smoking only |
| 2,205 births in England, 1963–65 (Leeder et al. 1976) | Prospective cohort with annual questionnaire | Significant increase in bronchitis or pneumonia in first year of life; RR = 1.7 if one parent smoked, RR = 2.6 if both smoked | Sex of smoking parent not examined |
| 12,068 births in Finland, 1966 (Rantakallio 1978) | Prospective cohort with follow-up of hospitalizations, physician visits, and mortality | Significant increase of hospitalization for respiratory diseases during first 5 years, RR = 1.7 | Effect largest during first year; maternal smoking only and measured during pregnancy |
| 1,265 births in New Zealand, 1977 (Fergusson and Horwood 1985) | Prospective cohort with diaries, physician, and hospital record review | Significant increase in bronchitis or pneumonia during the first year of life; RR = 2.0, if mother smoked; dose-response present in first | No effect of paternal smoking; effect of maternal smoking equivocal in second year, absent in third |
| 1,565 infants in Scotland, 1980 (Ogston, Florey, and Walker 1985, 1987) | Prospective cohort with record review and interview at one year of age | Significant increase in report of a respiratory illness during the first year of life; RR = 1.54 if either parent smoked | Incidence lowest for group with mother alone smoking |
| 130 children with RS virus infection in infancy, England (Pullan and Hey 1982) | Case-control with 111 controls, performed 10 years after index illness | Significant effect of maternal smoking at time of illness; RR = 3.2 | Effect of paternal smoking also present |
| 29 children hospitalized with respiratory syncytial virus infection before age 2 years, and 58 controls, New York (Hall et al. 1984) | Case-control study with controls hospitalized for nonrespiratory condition | Significant effect of smoking in the household; odds ratio = 4.8 | Smoking by specific parents not considered |

$^a$RR = relative risk. Calculated from published data if not provided by the authors.

prominent effects of passive smoking, in comparison with the studies of lower respiratory illness in infants, may reflect lower exposures to ETS by older children who spend less time with their parents.

Recent results from several large studies provide convincing evidence that involuntary exposure to tobacco smoke/increases the occurrence of cough and phlegm in the children of smokers although earlier data from smaller studies had been ambiguous (Table 6.5). In a study of ten thousand schoolchildren in six U.S. communities, smoking by parents increased the frequency of persistent cough in their children by about 30 percent (Ware et al. 1984). The effect of parental smoking derived primarily from smoking by the mother. Charlton (1984) conducted a survey on cigarette smoking which included 15,709 English children, ages eight to nineteen years. In the nonsmoking children, the prevalence of frequent cough was significantly higher if either the father or the mother smoked. In another large study in the United Kingdom, parental smoking was associated with day or night cough in children aged five to eleven years (Somerville, Rona, and Chinn 1988).

For the symptom of chronic wheeze, the preponderance of the evidence also indicates an excess associated with involuntary smoking (Table 6.5). In a survey of 650 schoolchildren in Boston, persistent wheezing was the most frequent symptom (Weiss et al. 1980); the prevalence of persistent wheezing increased significantly as the number of smoking parents increased. In the large study of children in six U.S. communities, the prevalence of persistent wheezing during the previous year was significantly increased if the mother smoked (Ware et al. 1984). In English children aged five to eleven years, parental smoking was associated with a

Table 6.5   Prevalence of Respiratory Symptoms in Selected Investigations
of Children, by Number of Smoking Parents

| Subjects | Respiratory Symptoms | Prevalence (per 100) by Number of Smoking Parents | | |
|---|---|---|---|---|
| | | 0 | 1 | 2 |
| 2,426 children, aged 6–14, England (Colley 1974) | Chronic cough | 15.6 | 17.2 | 22.2 |
| 3,105 nonsmoking children, aged 12–13, England (Bland et al. 1978) | Cough during the day or at night | 16.4 | 19.0 | 23.5 |
| 650 children, aged 5–9, Massachusetts (Weiss et al. 1980) | Chronic cough and phlegm | 1.7 | 2.7 | 3.4 |
| | Persistent wheeze | 1.8 | 6.8 | 11.8 |
| 4,071 children, aged 5–14, Pennsylvania (Schenker, Samet, and Speizer 1983) | Chronic cough | 6.3 | 7.0 | 8.3 |
| | Chronic phlegm | 4.1 | 4.8 | 4.0 |
| | Persistent wheeze | 7.2 | 7.7 | 5.4 |
| 8,528 children, aged 5–9, six U.S. cities (Ware et al. 1984) | Chronic cough | 7.7 | 8.4 | 10.6 |
| | Persistent wheeze | 9.9 | 11.0 | 13.1 |
| 1,733 nonsmoking children, aged 8–10, England (Charlton 1984) | Frequent cough (boys) | 35 | 42 | 48 |
| | Frequent cough (girls) | 32 | 40 | 52 |

*Source*: abstracted from U.S. DHHS (1986, Table 4, pp. 360–62) and from Charlton (1984).

more frequent report of persistent wheezing (Somerville, Rona, and Chinn 1988). The odds ratio for exposure to twenty cigarettes per day at home was 1.6 (95 percent confidence interval 1.2–2.2) compared with no exposure. McConnochie and Roghmann (1986) assessed predictors of wheeze in a retrospective study of children who had mild bronchiolitis in infancy and of control children. At a mean age of 8.3 years, current exposure to tobacco smoke increased the risk of wheezing (relative risk = 1.9). Parental smoking predicted the occurrence of wheezing at age five years in a study of children at risk for atopy (Cogswell, Mitchell and Alexander 1987). Passive smoking has not been significantly associated with wheezing in all studies, however (Leeder et al. 1976; Schenker, Samet, and Speizer 1983; Tashkin et al. 1984).

Although involuntary exposure to tobacco smoke is associated with the symptom of wheeze, evidence for association of involuntary smoking with childhood asthma is conflicting. Exposure to ETS might cause asthma as a long-term consequence of the increased occurrence of lower respiratory infection in early childhood or through other mechanisms (Samet, Tager, and Speizer 1983; Tager 1988). Gortmacker et al. (1982) collected data from two U.S. population samples. The relative risk for asthma associated with maternal smoking was 1.5 in a midwestern urbanized county and 1.8 in a more rural eastern county. In a longitudinal study of children in Tecumseh, Michigan, parental smoking increased the prevalence of asthma at the first examination and was associated with a doubling of the risk for developing asthma during a fifteen-year follow-up period (Burchfiel 1984). A case-control study in the United Kingdom also showed increased risk for asthma in association with exposure to ETS at home (Kershaw 1987). In contrast, in a longitudinal study in New Zealand, parental smoking habits were not found to affect the incidence of asthma during the first six years of life (Horwood, Fergusson, and Shannon 1985). In another longitudinal study of more than two thousand children in Harrow, England, parental smoking was not a significant predictor of the development of asthma during a five-year follow-up period (Leeder et al. 1976). Some cross-sectional studies have also not demonstrated a relationship between parental smoking and asthma (Schenker, Samet, and Speizer 1983; Tashkin et al. 1984; Somerville, Rona, and Chinn 1988). The inconsistencies among these investigations cannot be readily explained.

Although involuntary exposure to tobacco smoke has not been established as a cause of asthma, recent evidence indicates that involuntary smoking worsens the status of those with asthma. Murray and Morrison (1986) evaluated ninety-four asthmatic children of ages seven to seventeen years. Level of lung function, symptom frequency, and responsiveness to inhaled histamine were adversely affected by maternal smoking. In a study of twenty-one asthmatics, ages six to twenty-one years, O'Connor and colleagues (1987) also found that maternal smoking increased the level of airways responsiveness. Male nine-year-old Italian schoolchildren had greater bronchial responsiveness if their parents smoked; the association with smoking was strongest for children with asthma (Martinez et al. 1988). The increased level of airways responsiveness associated with maternal smoking would be expected to increase the clinical severity of asthma. In this regard, exposure to smoking in the home has been shown to increase the number of emergency room visits made by asthmatic children (Evans et al. 1987).

Recent studies have also shown that children exposed to cigarette smoke in their homes are at increased risk for middle ear disease. Both acute otitis media (Pukander et al. 1985) and persistent middle ear effusions (Kraemer et al. 1983; Black 1985; Iversen et al. 1985; Strachan, Jarvis, and Feyerabend 1989) have been associated with involuntary smoking.

LUNG FUNCTION IN CHILDREN

On the basis of the primarily cross-sectional data available at the time, the 1984 report of the surgeon general (U.S. DHHS 1984) concluded that the children of smoking parents in comparison with those of nonsmokers had small reductions of lung function, but the long-term consequences of these changes were regarded as unknown. In the two years between the 1984 and the 1986 reports, sufficient longitudinal evidence accumulated to support the conclusion in the 1986 report (U.S DHHS 1986) that involuntary smoking reduces the rate of lung function growth during childhood. New cross-sectional studies have continued to confirm the evidence reviewed in the 1984 report of the surgeon general (Burchfiel 1984; Tashkin et al. 1984; Tsimoyianis et al. 1987), although not all studies have shown adverse effects of involuntary smoking on the lung function of children (Hosein and Corey 1984; Lebowitz, Knudson, and Burrows 1984).

The effects of involuntary smoking on lung growth have been demonstrated in three separate longitudinal studies. Based on cross-sectional data from children in East Boston, Massachusetts, Tager and co-workers (1979) reported in 1979 that the level of $FEF_{25-75}$, a spirometric flow rate sensitive to subtle effects on airways and parenchymal function, declined with increasing number of smoking parents in the household. In 1983, this investigative group reported the results obtained on follow-up of these children over a seven-year period (Tager et al. 1983). Using a multivariate technique, the investigators showed that both maternal smoking and active smoking by the child reduced the growth rate of the one-second forced expiratory volume ($FEV_1$). Lifelong exposure of a child to a smoking mother was estimated to reduce growth of the $FEV_1$ by 10.7, 9.5, and 7.0 percent after one, two, and five years of follow-up, respectively.

Recent longitudinal data from the study in six U.S. cities also showed reduced growth of the $FEV_1$ in children whose mothers smoked cigarettes (Berkey et al. 1986). The growth rate of the $FEV_1$ from ages six through ten years was calculated for 7,834 white children. From ages six through ten years, the findings of a statistical analysis were that $FEV_1$ growth rate is reduced by 0.17 percent per pack of cigarettes smoked daily by the mother. This effect was somewhat smaller than that reported by Tager et al. (1983), although if extrapolated to age twenty years, a cumulative effect of 2.8 percent is predicted.

Burchfiel and co-workers (Burchfiel 1984; Burchfiel et al. 1986) examined the effects of parental smoking on fifteen-year lung function change in subjects in the Tecumseh study, who had been enrolled at ages ten through nineteen years. In the female subjects who remained nonsmokers across the follow-up period, parental smoking did not affect lung function change. In nonsmoking males, parental smoking reduced the growth of the $FEV_1$, forced vital capacity (FVC), and maximum flow rate at 50 percent of FVC ($V_{max50}$) although the sample size was limited, and the effects were not statistically significant. For the $FEV_1$ in males, the analysis estimated 7.4 percent and 9.4 percent reductions in fifteen-year growth associated with one or two smoking parents, respectively.

RESPIRATORY SYMPTOMS AND ILLNESSES IN ADULTS

Only a few cross-sectional investigations provide information on the association between respiratory symptoms in nonsmokers and involuntary exposure to tobacco smoke. These studies have only considered exposure to a smoking spouse and have not evaluated sources of exposure outside the home. Consistent evidence of an effect of passive smoking on respiratory symptoms in adults has not been found (Lebowitz and Burrows 1976; Schilling et al. 1977; Comstock et al. 1981; Schenker, Samet and Speizer 1982; Kauffmann et al. 1989).

Neither epidemiologic nor experimental studies have established the role of ETS in exacerbating asthma in adults. The acute responses of asthmatics to ETS have been assessed by exposing persons with asthma to tobacco smoke in a chamber. This experimental approach cannot be readily controlled because of the impossibility of blinding subjects as to exposure to ETS. However, suggestibility does not appear to underlie physiologic responses of asthmatics to ETS (Urch et al. 1988). Of three studies involving exposure of unselected asthmatics to ETS, only one showed a definite adverse effect (Shephard et al. 1979; Dahms, Bolin, and Slavin 1981; Wiedemann et al. 1986). Stankus et al. (1988) recruited twenty-one asthmatics who reported exacerbation with exposure to ETS. With challenge in an exposure chamber, seven of the subjects experienced a more than 20 percent decline in $FEV_1$.

LUNG FUNCTION IN ADULTS

With regard to involuntary smoking and lung function in adults, exposure to passive smoking has been associated with reduction of the $FEF_{25-75}$ in cross-sectional investigations. White and Froeb (1980) compared spirometric test results in middle-aged nonsmokers with at least twenty years of involuntary smoking in the workplace with the results in an unexposed control group of nonsmokers. The mean $FEF_{25-75}$ of the exposed group was significantly reduced, by 15 percent of predicted value in women and by 13 percent in men. This investigation has been intensely criticized with regard to the spirometric test procedures, the determination and classification of exposures, and the handling of former smokers in the analyses.

A subsequently reported investigation in France examined the effect of marriage to a smoker in more than 7,800 adults in seven cities (Kauffmann, Tessier, and Oriol 1983). The study included 849 male and 826 female nonsmokers exposed to tobacco smoking by their spouses' smoking. At more than age forty years, the $FEF_{25-75}$ was reduced in nonsmoking men and women with a spouse who smoked. The investigators interpreted this finding as representing a cumulative adverse effect of marriage to a smoker. In a subsequent report, the original findings in the French women were confirmed, but a parallel analysis in a large population of U.S. women did not show effects of involuntary smoking on lung function (Kauffmann et al. 1989).

The results of an investigation of 163 nonsmoking women in The Netherlands also suggested adverse effects of tobacco smoke exposure in the home on lung function (Brunekreef et al. 1985; Remijn et al. 1985). Cross-sectional analysis of spirometric data collected in 1982 demonstrated adverse effects of tobacco smoke exposure in the home, but in a sample of the women, domestic exposure to tobacco smoke was not associated with longitudinal decline of lung function during the period 1965 to 1982.

Svendsen and co-workers (1987) assessed the effects of spouse smoking on 1,400 nonsmoking male participants in the Multiple Risk Factor Intervention Trial (MRFIT). The subjects were aged thirty-five to fifty-seven years at enrollment and were at high risk for mortality from coronary artery disease. At the baseline visit, the maximum $FEV_1$ was approximately 100 milliliters lower for the men married to a smoker.

Masi and colleagues (1988) evaluated the lung function of 293 young adults using spirometry and measurement of the diffusing capacity and lung volumes. The results varied with gender. In men, reduction of the maximal mid-expiratory flow rate was associated with maternal smoking and exposure to ETS during childhood. In women, reduction of the diffusing capacity was associated with exposure to ETS at work.

Other studies have not shown chronic effects of involuntary exposure to tobacco smoke in adult nonsmokers. In two cross-sectional studies, marriage to a smoker was not significantly associated with reduction of ventilatory function (Schilling et al. 1977; Comstock et al. 1981). Jones and co-workers (Jones et al. 1983) conducted a case-control study of twenty- to thirty-nine-year-old nonsmoking women in the longitudinal study in Tecumseh. Subjects from the highest and lowest quartiles of the lung function distribution had comparable exposure to smokers in the home. In a study conducted in Germany, the effects of involuntary and active smoking were examined in a population of 1,351 white-collar workers (Kentner, Triebig, and Weltle 1984). Self-reported exposure to ETS at home and at work was not associated with reduction of spirometric measures of lung function.

A conclusion cannot yet be reached on the effects of ETS exposure on lung function in adults. However, further research is warranted because of widespread exposure in workplaces and homes.

LUNG CANCER

In 1981, reports were published from Japan (Hirayama 1981) and from Greece (Trichopoulos et al. 1981) that indicated increased lung cancer risk in nonsmoking women married to cigarette smokers. Subsequently, this controversial association has been examined in investigations conducted in the United States, Scotland, Japan, Hong Kong, Sweden, and China. The association of involuntary smoking with lung cancer derives biologic plausibility from the presence of carcinogens in sidestream smoke and the lack of a documented threshold dose for respiratory carcinogenesis in active smokers (U.S. DHHS 1982).

Time trends of lung cancer mortality in nonsmokers have been examined with the rationale that temporally increasing exposure to ETS should be paralleled by increasing mortality rates (Enstrom 1979; Garfinkel 1981). These data provide only indirect evidence on the lung cancer risk associated with involuntary exposure to tobacco smoke. Epidemiologists have tested directly the association between lung cancer and involuntary smoking utilizing conventional designs: the case-control and cohort studies. In a case-control study, the exposures of nonsmoking persons with lung cancer to ETS are compared with those of an appropriate control group. In a cohort study, the occurrence of lung cancer over time in nonsmokers is assessed in relationship to involuntary tobacco smoke exposure. The results of both study designs may be affected by inaccurate assessment of exposure to ETS, by inaccurate information on personal smoking habits that leads to classification of smokers as nonsmokers, and by the misdiagnosis of a cancer of another site as a primary cancer of the lung.

Methodologic investigations suggest that accurate information can be obtained by interview in an epidemiologic study on the smoking habits of a spouse (i.e., never or ever smoker) (Pron et al. 1988; Coultas, Peake, and Samet 1989; Cummings et al. 1989). However, information concerning quantitative aspects of the spouse's smoking is reported with less accuracy. Misclassification of current or former smokers as never smokers may introduce a positive bias because of the concordance of spouse smoking habits (Lee 1988). The extent to which this bias explains the numerous reports of association between spouse smoking and lung cancer is controversial (Wald et al. 1986; Lee 1988).

The evidence from the case-control and the cohort studies does not uniformly indicate increased lung cancer risk in persons exposed to ETS, but most of the studies indicate increased risk in nonsmokers married to smokers (Table 6.6). Hirayama's (1981) early report was based on a prospective cohort study of 91,540 nonsmoking women in Japan. Standardized mortality ratios for lung cancer increased significantly with the amount smoked by the husbands. The findings could not be explained by confounding factors and were unchanged when follow-up of the study group was extended (Hirayama 1984). Based on the same cohort, Hirayama has also reported significantly elevated standardized mortality ratios for lung cancer of 2.1 and 2.3 in nonsmoking men with wives smoking one to nineteen cigarettes and twenty or more cigarettes daily, respectively (Hirayama 1984).

In 1981, Trichopoulos et al. (1981) also reported increased lung cancer risk in nonsmoking women married to cigarette smokers. These investigators conducted a case-control study in Athens, Greece, which included cases with a diagnosis other than adenocarcinoma or bronchioloalveolar carcinoma and controls selected

Table 6.6   Cohort and Case-Control Studies of Passive Exposure
to Tobacco Smoke and Lung Cancer

| Study | Findings | Comments |
|---|---|---|
| Prospective cohort study in Japan of 91,540 nonsmoking females, 1966–81 (Hirayama 1981) | Age-occupation-adjusted SMRs,[a] by husband smoking: Nonsmokers = 1.00 Exsmokers = 1.36 Current smokers <20/day = 1.45 >20/day = 1.91 | Trend statistically significant; all histologies |
| Prospective cohort study in the U.S. of 176,139 nonsmoking females, 1960–72 (Garfinkel 1981) | Age-adjusted SMRs, by husband smoking: Nonsmokers = 1.00 Current smokers <20/day = 1.27 >20/day = 1.10 | All histologies; effect of husband smoking not significant |
| Prospective cohort study in Scotland of 8,128 males and females, 1972–82 (Gillis et al. 1984) | Age-adjusted mortality ratios for domestic exposure: Males = 3.25 Females = 1.00 | Preliminary, small numbers of cases |
| Case-control study in Greece of 40 nonsmoking female cases, 149 controls, 1978–80 (Trichopoulos et al. 1981; Trichopoulos, Kalandidi, and Sparros 1983) | Odds ratios by husband smoking: Nonsmokers = 1.0 Exsmokers = 1.8 Current smokers <20/day = 2.4 >20/day = 3.4 | Trend statistically significant; histologies other than adenocarcinoma and bronchioloalveolar carcinoma |
| Case-control study in Hong Kong of 84 female cases and 139 controls, 1976–77 (Chan et al. 1979; Chan and Fung 1982) | Crude odds ratio of 0.75 associated with smoking spouse | All histologies; two reports are inconsistent on the exposure variable |
| Case-control study in the U.S. with 22 female and 8 male nonsmoking cases, 133 female and 180 male controls (Correa et al. 1983) | Odds ratios by spouse smoking: Nonsmokers = 1.00 <40 pack years = 1.48 >41 pack years = 3.11 | Significant increase for >41 pack years; bronchioloalveolar carcinoma excluded |
| Case-control study in the U.S. 25 male and 53 female nonsmoking cases with matched controls, 1971–80 (Kabat and Wynder 1984) | Odds ratio not significantly increased for current exposure at home: Males = 1.26 Females = 0.92 | All histologies; findings negative for spouse smoking variable as well |
| Case-control study in Hong Kong with 88 nonsmoking female cases, 1981–82 (Koo, Ho, and Saw 1984; Koo, Ho, and Lee 1985) | Odds ratio of 1.24 ($p > .40$) for combined home and workplace exposure; no association with cumulative hours of exposure | All histologies |
| Case-control study in the U.S. with 31 nonsmoking and 189 smoking female cases (Wu et al. 1985) | No significant effects of exposure from parents, spouse, or workplace in smokers and nonsmokers | Adenocarcinoma and squamous cell carcinoma only |
| Case-control study in the U.S. with 134 nonsmoking female cases (Wu et al. 1985) | Nonsignificant odds ratio of 1.22 if husband smoked; significantly increased odds ratio of 2.11 if husband smoked 20 | All histologies; careful exclusion of smokers from the case group |

(*continued*)

Table 6.6 (*Continued*)

| Study | Findings | Comments |
|---|---|---|
| | or more cigarettes daily at home; significant trend with number of cigarettes smoked at home by the husband | |
| Case-control study in England with 15 male and 32 female nonsmoking cases, and 30 male and 66 female nonsmoking controls (Lee, Chamberlain, and Alderson 1986) | Overall odds ratio for spouse smoking of 1.1 | Hospital-based study |
| Case-control study in Japan with 19 male and 94 female nonsmoking cases, and 110 male and 270 female nonsmoking controls (Akiba, Kato, and Blot 1986) | For females, odds ratio of 1.5 if husband smoked; for males, odds ratio of 1.8 if wife smoked | Clinical or radiologic diagnosis for 43%; all histologies |
| Case-control study in Louisiana, Texas, and New Jersey with 99 nonsmoking cases and 736 controls (Dalager et al. 1986) | Adjusted odds ratio for marriage to a smoking spouse was 1.5 | Nearly 100% histologic confirmation; all histologies |
| Case-control study in New Mexico with 28 nonsmoking cases and 292 nonsmoking controls (Humble, Samet, and Pathak 1987) | Adjusted odds ratio for marriage to a smoking spouse was 3.2; no effect in active smokers | All histologies other than bronchiolo-alveolar carcinoma |
| Case-control study in Sweden with 77 nonsmoking cases, two matched control series (Pershagen, Hrubec, and Svensson 1987) | Odds ratio for marriage to a smoker was 3.3 for squamous and small cell carcinomas | No effect of exposure for other types; study based within a cohort |
| Case-control study in Colorado with 102 adenocarcinoma cases, 50 males and 52 females, and 131 controls (Brownson et al. 1987) | No effect in entire group; in nonsmoking women, odds ratio of 1.7 for exposure $\geq 4$ h/day | Passive smoking effect not significant in nonsmoking women but only 19 such cases included |
| Case-control study in Hong Kong with 199 never smoking female cases and 335 controls (Lam et al. 1987) | Overall odds ratio = 1.7, significantly increased for marriage to a smoker; odds ratio = 2.1 for adenocarcinoma | All histologies; no evidence for exposure response |
| Case-control study in Shanghai with 246 nonsmoking female cases and 375 controls (Gao et al. 1987) | Overall odds ratio = 0.9 for ever living with a smoker; risk increased with duration of living with a smoking husband | All histologies, but majority adenocarcinoma; no effect of childhood exposure |
| Case-control study in Japan with 90 nonsmoking female cases and 163 controls (Shimizu et al. 1988) | Odds ratio for husband's smoking was 1.1; no effect of exposure at work | All histologies; increased risk from other household members' smoking |
| Case-control study in Japan with 28 smoking female cases and | Overall odds ratio = 2.3 for marriage to a smoker | Risk increased with the number of |

(*continued*)

Table 6.6    (*Continued*)

| Study | Findings | Comments |
|---|---|---|
| 62 controls (Inoue and Hirayama 1988) Case-control study in Tianjin China with 54 nonsmoking female cases and 93 controls (Geng et al. 1987) | Overall odds ratio = 2.2 for marriage to a smoker | cigarettes smoked by the husband All histologies |

[a]Standardized mortality ratio.

at a hospital for orthopedic disorders. The positive findings reported in 1981 were unchanged with expansion of the study population (Trichopoulos, Kalandidi, and Sparrows, 1983).

The results of other subsequently reported case-control studies have also demonstrated statistically significant associations between involuntary smoking and lung cancer (Table 6.6). The findings from the more recent reports greatly strengthen the evidence from the earlier studies. Several of the newer studies included relatively large numbers of nonsmokers (Garfinkel, Auerbach, and Joubert 1985; Akiba, Kato, and Blot 1986; Dalager et al. 1986; Gao et al. 1987; Lam et al. 1987). Furthermore, in most of these studies, involuntary smoking was assessed in greater detail than in the earlier reports so that exposure-response relationships could be examined more fully.

The results of two other investigations have also been interpreted as showing an increased lung cancer risk associated with passive smoking although both have methodologic limitations. In Germany, Knoth, Bohn, and Schmidt (1983) described a series of fifty-nine female lung cancer cases of which thirty-nine were in nonsmokers. Based on census data, these investigators projected that a much greater than expected proportion of these nonsmokers had lived in households with smokers. This report did not include an appropriate comparison series, however. Gillis et al. (1984) described the preliminary results of a cohort study of 16,171 males and females in western Scotland; domestic exposure to tobacco smoke increased the lung cancer risk for nonsmoking men but not for women. The report was based on only sixteen cases of lung cancer in nonsmokers, however.

The results of some investigations indicate lesser or no effects of exposure to ETS (Table 6.6). In these studies, however, confidence limits for the relative risks associated with marriage to a smoker are wide and overlap with the confidence limits in the studies with significant results (NRC 1986a). Two separate case-control studies in Hong Kong, where lung cancer incidence rates in females are particularly high, did not indicate excess risk from passive smoking (Chan et al. 1979; Chan and Fung 1982; Koo, Ho, and Saw 1984; Koo, Ho, and Lee 1985; Koo et al. 1987). In the more recent of the two studies, the questionnaire comprehensively assessed cumulative exposure from home and workplace sources (Koo, Ho, and Saw 1984; Koo, Ho, and Lee 1985; Koo et al. 1987). A subsequent study in

Hong Kong did find a significant association of spouse smoking and lung cancer risk (Lam et al. 1987). Lee and co-workers (Lee, Chamberlain, and Alderson 1986) reported a hospital-based case-control study in England. Although the investigators considered that their findings indicated little or no effect of involuntary smoking, the case series was small. Another recent hospital-based case-control study, conducted in Japan, also did not show an association between lung cancer risk and spouse smoking (Shimizu et al. 1988).

The results of the American Cancer Society's prospective cohort study of mortality in 176,139 nonsmoking women have also been construed by many as not showing an association between involuntary smoking and lung cancer (Garfinkel 1981). However, the standardized mortality ratios for the nonsmoking women with husbands who smoked were greater than unity, but not significantly greater. Recent and preliminary results from a nationwide case-control study also did not demonstrate increased lung cancer risk from domestic exposure to tobacco smoke (Kabat and Wynder 1984). In another case-control study that was performed in Los Angeles, Wu et al. (1985) did not find significantly increased risk for adenocarcinoma associated with involuntary smoking in smoking and nonsmoking women. These investigators estimated exposure from parental smoking, spouse smoking, and workplace sources. The relative risk for lung cancer was slightly, but not significantly, increased by exposure from spouse smoking and from smoking by co-workers.

The current extent of the data on involuntary smoking and lung cancer contrasts with the more extensive literature cited in the 1964 surgeon general's report, which characterized active cigarette smoking as a cause of lung cancer (U.S. Public Health Service [PHS] 1964). The variability of the data on involuntary smoking also contrasts with that on active smoking. However, most of the studies on involuntary smoking and lung cancer have small numbers of cases, and confidence intervals for the effect of involuntary smoking in the various studies would overlap. Variation in the results of the studies may also reflect random and nonrandom errors in the classification of exposure to ETS. In fact, assessment of exposure relevant to lung cancer appears more difficult than for other health effects of involuntary smoking. The relevant exposures may begin at birth and occur under a wide variety of circumstances. Thus, some inconsistency among the studies would be anticipated in the face of the relatively small study populations and the difficulties of estimating exposure.

In spite of the variable epidemiologic evidence, ETS has been characterized as a cause of lung cancer. The International Agency for Research on Cancer of the World Health Organization (IARC 1986) has concluded that "passive smoking gives rise to some risk of cancer." In its monograph on tobacco smoking, the agency supported this conclusion on the basis of the characteristics of sidestream and mainstream smoke, the absorption of tobacco smoke materials during involuntary smoking, and the nature of dose-response relationships for carcinogenesis.

The NRC (NRC 1986a) and the U.S. surgeon general (U.S. DHHS 1986) have also concluded that involuntary smoking increases the incidence of lung cancer in nonsmokers. In reaching this conclusion, the NRC (NRC 1986a) cited the biologic plausibility of the association between exposure to ETS and lung cancer and the supporting epidemiologic evidence. Based on a pooled analysis of the epidemiologic data which adjusted for bias, the report concluded that the best estimate for the excess risk of lung cancer in nonsmokers married to smokers was 25 percent. The 1986 report of the surgeon general (U.S. DHHS 1986) characterized involuntary smoking as a cause of lung cancer in nonsmokers. This conclusion was based on the extensive information already available on the carcinogenicity of active smoking, on the qualitative similarities between ETS and mainstream smoke, and on the epidemiologic data on involuntary smoking.

The extent of the lung cancer hazard associated with involuntary smoking in the United States remains uncertain, however (U.S. DHHS 1986; Weiss 1986). The epidemiologic studies provide varying and imprecise measures of risk, and exposures have not been characterized for large and representative population samples. Risk estimation procedures have been used to describe the lung cancer risk associated with involuntary smoking, but assumptions and simplifications must be made in order to use this method. For example, Repace and Lowrey (1985) calculated that approximately 5,000 lung cancer deaths occur annually in U.S. nonsmokers as a result of involuntary smoking. Wells (1988) attributed 3,000 lung cancer deaths annually in the United States to involuntary smoking.

OTHER CANCERS
Several recent reports have suggested that exposure to ETS may increase the risk of cancer at sites other than the lung. One study found that in children, maternal exposure to environmental tobacco smoke during pregnancy was associated with increased risk of brain tumors (Preston-Martin et al. 1982), and in another study paternal but not maternal smoking increased the risk of childhood rhabdomyosarcoma (Grufferman et al. 1982). Such effects might arise from smoking-induced changes in germ cells of the parents or through transplacental exposure rather than as a direct effect of smoke inhalation (Everson 1980; Grufferman et al. 1983).

In adults, involuntary smoking has been linked to a generally increased risk of malignancy and to excess risk at specific sites. Miller (1984) interviewed surviving relatives of 537 deceased nonsmoking women in western Pennsylvania concerning the smoking habits of their husbands. A significantly increased risk of cancer death (odds ratio = 1.94, $p < .05$) was found in women who were married to smokers and also not employed outside the homes. The large number of potential subjects who were not interviewed and the possibility of information bias detract from this report.

Sandler and colleagues (Sandler, Everson, and Wilcox 1985, Sandler et al. 1985; Sandler, Wilcox, and Everson 1985) conducted a case-control study on the effects of exposures to ETS during childhood and adulthood on the risk of cancer. The 518 cases included cancers of all types other than basal cell cancer of the skin; the cases and the matched controls were between the ages of fifteen and fifty-nine years. For all sites combined, significantly increased risk was found for parental smoking (crude odds ratio = 1.6) and for marriage to a smoking spouse (crude odds ratio = 1.5); the effects of these two exposures were independent (Sandler, Wilcox, and Everson 1985). Significant associations were also found for some individual sites: for childhood exposure (Sandler et al. 1985), maternal and paternal smoking increased the risk of hematopoietic malignancy, and for adulthood exposure (Sandler, Everson, and Wilcox 1985), spouse's smoking increased the risk for cancers of the female breast, female genital system, and the endocrine system. These findings are primarily hypothesis generating and require replication. In a case-control study, such as reported by Sandler et al. (1985), biased information on exposure to environmental tobacco smoke is of particular concern. Hirayama (1984) has reported significantly increased mortality from nasal sinus cancers and from brain tumors in nonsmoking women married to smokers in the Japanese cohort. In a case-control study of bladder cancer, involuntary smoke exposure at home and at work did not increase risk (Kabat, Dieck, and Wynder 1986). Cervical cancer, which has been linked to active smoking, was associated with duration of involuntary smoking in a case-control study in Utah (Slattery et al. 1989).

These associations of involuntary smoking with cancer at diverse nonrespiratory sites cannot be supported readily with arguments for biologic plausibility. Increased risks at some of the sites, for example, cancer of the nasal sinus and female breast cancer, have not been observed in active smokers (U.S. DHHS 1982). In fact, the IARC has concluded that effects would not be produced in passive smokers which would not be produced to a larger extent in active smokers (IARC 1986).

CARDIOVASCULAR DISEASE

Although extensive data establish active cigarette smoking as a causal risk factor for cardiovascular diseases (U.S. DHHS 1983), few studies have examined involuntary smoking as a risk factor for these diseases. In the cohort of nonsmoking Japanese women, Hirayama (1983) found a small, statistically significant increased risk of death from ischemic heart disease associated with the husband's smoking. Garland et al. (1985) prospectively determined mortality from ischemic heart disease in nonsmoking older women residing in southern California. After adjustment for established risk factors, marriage to a smoking spouse was associated with a relative risk of 2.7 ($p < .10$). Gillis et al. (1984) assessed the baseline prevalence of cardiovascular symptoms and major electrocardiographic abnormalities in a population sample residing in Scotland and then determined cause-specific mortality for up to ten years of follow-up. In a preliminary report, involuntary smoking was not associated with the prevalence of cardiovascular symptoms at baseline or with cardiovascular mortality on follow-up. A case-control study in England did not show increased risk for ischemic heart disease or for stroke in nonsmokers married to smokers (Lee, Chamberlain, and Alderson 1986).

The effect of involuntary smoking was assessed among the nonsmoking male participants in the MRFIT; these men had been selected to be in the upper 10–15 percent of risk for mortality from coronary artery disease, based on a score from the Framingham study (Svendsen et al. 1987). In comparison with men married to nonsmokers, never smokers with smoking wives had increased risk for coronary heart disease (relative risk = 2.11, 95 percent confidence interval 0.69–6.46), fatal or nonfatal coronary heart disease event (relative risk = 1.48, 95 percent confidence interval 0.89–2.47), and death from any cause (relative risk = 1.96, 95 percent confidence interval 0.93–4.11). These relative risks changed little when former smokers were included in the analysis or with adjustment for other risk factors for coronary heart disease.

Helsing and colleagues (1988) reported on the heart disease mortality of non-smokers enrolled in a cohort study in Washington County, Maryland. In comparison with persons married to nonsmokers, both men and women married to smokers had a significantly increased risk of dying from heart disease ($RR$ = 1.3 for males and 1.2 for females).

The effects of involuntary exposure to tobacco smoke on athletic performance, which largely depends on cardiovascular responses, have also been examined. Such effects derive plausibility from the composition of ETS, which contains agents that might affect level of lung function and oxygen delivery by the cardiovascular system. Irritation of the upper and lower respiratory tracts following acute exposure might also adversely affect performance when exercise requires high minute ventilation.

Of the many toxic agents in ETS, CO and nicotine are candidates to influence performance adversely because of their cardiovascular effects (Schievebein and Richter 1984). CO interferes with oxygen transport by avidly binding to hemoglobin to form carboxyhemoglobin and by shifting the oxyhemoglobin dissociation curve to the left. Nicotine releases epinephrine and norepinephrine and elevates pulse rate, blood pressure, and oxygen demand. Although these effects of CO and nicotine might impair performance, exposures to ETS are generally at concentrations below which physiologic effects would be expected to occur (Schievebein and Richter 1984; U.S. DHHS 1986).

In two studies, healthy nonsmoking subjects were exposed to tobacco smoke and their performance subsequently assessed (Pimm, Silverman, and Shephard 1978; McMurray, Hicks, and Thompson 1985). In both studies, attempts were made to blind the subjects as to whether clean air or smoke-contaminated air was inhaled. Given the unmistakable odor and other characteristics of cigarette smoke, it seems unlikely that these studies were truly blinded, and their findings must be interpreted with this constraint.

Pimm, Silverman, and Shephard (1978) exposed ten males and ten females to levels of cigarette smoke described as characteristic of "levels typically encountered in public buildings." The subjects were exposed in a chamber and subsequently underwent a progressive exercise test. Maximal oxygen uptake was not significantly affected, and a consistent pattern of adverse effects on lung function was not found. The subjects did have symptomatic responses to the exposure.

In the study conducted by McMurray, Hicks, and Thompson (1985), air or cigarette smoke was inhaled by eight female subjects through a mouthpiece, and submaximal and maximal exercise performance were assessed. The inhalation of cigarette smoke led to a reduction of maximal oxygen uptake and a reduction of time to exhaustion. Effects on the respiratory exchange ratio (R), maximal blood lactate, and ratings of perceived exertion were also found during the maximal testing. Adverse effects of smoke exposure were also suggested by the submaximal testing.

TOTAL MORTALITY

Several cohort studies provide information on involuntary smoking and mortality from all causes. In the Scottish cohort study, total mortality was increased for women living with a smoker but not for men (Gillis et al. 1984). As described previously, total mortality was also increased among nonsmoking participants in MRFIT who lived with smokers (Svendsen et al. 1987). In contrast, mortality was not increased for nonsmoking female subjects in a study in Amsterdam (Vandenbroucke et al. 1984). Neither the study in Scotland nor the study in Amsterdam controlled for other factors that influence total mortality. In the cohort study in Washington County, all-cause mortality rates were significantly increased for men ($RR = 1.17$) and for women ($RR = 1.15$) after adjustment for housing quality, schooling, and marital status (Sandler et al. 1989).

## ODOR AND IRRITATION

Tobacco smoke contains numerous irritants, including particulate material and gases (U.S. DHHS 1986). Both questionnaire surveys and laboratory studies involving exposure to ETS have shown annoyance and irritation of the eyes and upper and lower airways from involuntary smoking. In several surveys of nonsmokers, complaints about tobacco smoke at work and in public places were common (U.S. DHHS 1986); about 50 percent of respondents complained about tobacco smoke at work, and a majority was disturbed by tobacco smoke in restaurants. The experimental studies show that the rate of eye blinking is increased by ETS, as are complaints of nose and throat irritation (U.S. DHHS 1986). In the study of passive smoking on commercial airline flights reported by Mattson and colleagues (1989), changes in nose and eye symptoms were associated with nicotine exposure. The odor and irritation associated with ETS merit special consideration because a high proportion of nonsmokers are annoyed by exposure to ETS, and control of the concentrations in indoor air poses difficult problems in the management of heating, ventilating, and air-conditioning systems.

EXPERIMENTAL STUDIES

Experimental exposure of volunteer subjects has provided convincing evidence of the irritant effects of exposure to ETS. Studies reviewed in the 1986 report of the surgeon general (U.S. DHHS 1986) documented eye irritation through both objective measurements of blink rates and of stability of the precorneal tear film and subjective reports. Symptoms of nose and throat irritation were also associated with ETS exposure. More recent experimental studies have provided further data concerning the odor and annoyance associated with ETS exposure.

The usual experimental setting to assess the effects of indoor contaminants on the senses is exposure in a climate-controlled environmental chamber with relatively inert surfaces, for example, aluminum or stainless steel, and variable ventilation. To investigate occupancy odor, human beings occupy the chamber for a given time. Judges of the odor of interest either enter the chamber briefly or place their faces into a box fed with the atmosphere of the chamber and may thus be considered to visit the space. The odor judgment may comprise a mark on an annotated rating scale (e.g., *no odor* to *overpowering odor*) or the choice of a matching odor intensity, generally using a device called an *olfactometer,* which delivers the vapor of a standard odorant, such as *n*-butyl alcohol (1-butanol), at various concentrations.

Many modern investigations also obtain judgments of acceptability in order to "calibrate" intensity judgments. Acceptability judgments address the question: How many people object to any given level of odor (or irritation)? The answer depends upon individual differences in olfactory sensitivity and upon aesthetic criteria. Whereas we can expect average intensity judgments to remain constant through the decades for any fixed stimulus, we can expect acceptability judgments to shift with prevailing standards.

Figure 6.1 shows the relationship between ventilation rate and occupant satisfaction in a recent study conducted in a climate chamber with from four to twelve occupants (Cain et al. 1983). Visitors made judgments of air circulated through an outside sampling box and were therefore naïve to the conditions of occupancy. The scale refers to the concentration of 1-butanol matched to the occupancy odor present after one hour of occupancy. Both odor level and dissatisfaction decreased with increases in ventilation rate.

The ventilation standard of the American Society of Heating, Refrigerating, and Air-Conditioning Engineers (ASHRAE) (1989) recommends a maximum of 20 percent dissatisfaction among visitors to a space. By this criterion, the data from the investigation imply the need for 17 cubic feet per minute (cfm) per occupant (Figure 6.1). The ASHRAE standard suggests 15 cfm or more per occupant for most spaces, for example, 15 cfm for classrooms, libraries, auditoriums, and dormitories; 20 cfm for offices, conference rooms, dining rooms, and lobbies; 25 cfm for discotheques and beauty shops; 30 cfm for bars and casinos; and 60 cfm for smoking lounges. Thus, the ASHRAE standard specifies sufficient air to control odor associated with the occupants of a space.

When cigarettes were smoked in the climate chamber, odor level increased markedly (Figure 6.2). Figure 6.2 shows ETS odor for various conditions of smoking: intermittent (four cigarettes per hour) or continuous (eight and sixteen cigarettes per hour). The intensity of the odor increased with the number of cigarettes smoked and declined with increasing ventilation. As shown in Figure 6.3, the degree of dissatisfaction mirrored the higher odor level. Based on the rule of 20 percent maximum dissatisfaction, the ventilation rate required per cigarette

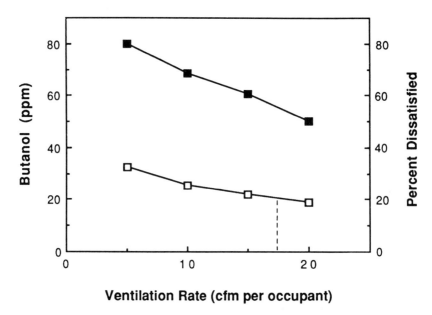

Figure 6.1. Relation between level of occupancy odor (indicated by concentration of 1-butanol matched to the odor [*filled squares*]) and ventilation rate per occupant when four to twelve persons occupied a climate chamber for an hour. Judgments of odor were made by visitors who sampled the air of the chamber at a remote sampling box. Also shown is the frequency of dissatisfaction expressed by the visitors in response to the question, "Is the air acceptable or unacceptable (*unfilled squares*)?" The *dashed line* shows the ventilation rate that led to 20 percent dissatisfaction. *Source:* Reprinted with permission from *Atmospheric Environment* 17, Cain W. S. et al., Ventilation requirements in buildings—I. Control of occupancy odor and tobacco smoke odor. Copyright 1983, Pergamon Press PLC.

during active smoking exceeded 4,000 ft$^3$. In order to convert ventilation per cigarette into ventilation rate per person for typical conditions of occupancy in a "smoking-permitted" space, we assumed that 10 percent of the occupants would be smoking at any given time. The resulting requirement for ventilation was 53 cfm, more than three times that for nonsmoking occupancy.

The higher ventilation rate for smoking calculated from these data does not appear to represent a special aversion to the odor of cigarettes on the part of the judges. The judges, one-third of whom were smokers and two-thirds of whom were not, seemed to base their dissatisfaction strictly on odor intensity. Degree of dissatisfaction varied with odor intensity in the same way for both occupancy odor and tobacco smoke odor (Figure 6.4); stronger odors yielded greater dissatisfaction regardless of the source of odor.

The adequacy of the ASHRAE standard can be evaluated using these experimental data. The standard recommends 60 cfm per occupant in a smoking lounge, where presumably most or all occupants may be smoking. If 100 percent rather than 10 percent of the occupants smoke simultaneously, then the ventilation rate would need to exceed an unachievable 500 cfm per occupant. If 50 percent smoke

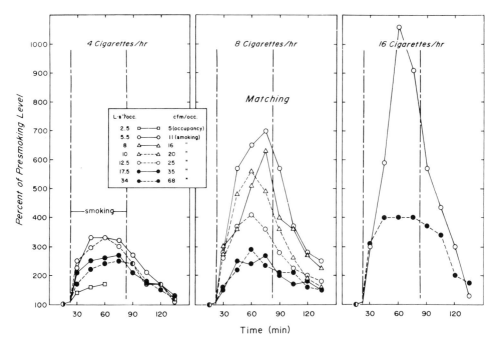

Figure 6.2. Intensity of ETS odor perceived by visitors to the sampling box during and after intermittent (four cigarettes per hour) or continuous (eight to sixteen cigarettes per hour) smoking in the climate chamber. Results are expressed relative to level of butanol matched to odor during presmoking occupancy. The *open squares* in the *left panel* show a function for nonsmoking occupancy for comparison. *Ventilation rate per occupant under smoking conditions* refers to smokers, who were the only occupants in the chamber. *Source:* Reprinted with permission from *Atmospheric Environment* 17, Cain W. S. et al., Ventilation requirements in buildings—I. Control of occupancy odor and tobacco smoke odor. Copyright 1983, Pergamon Press PLC.

simultaneously, perhaps a more realistic scenario, then the rate would need to exceed a still unachievable 250 cfm per occupant. The maximum achievable rate for typical design occupancy in a mechanically ventilated space will usually equal about 60 cfm per occupant, although a generous allotment of space per person can increase that value.

The smoker, however, seems less concerned about the odor of ETS than the nonsmoker. Smokers as a group seem satisfied with about one-quarter of the ventilation air needed by a group containing a typical proportion of smokers and nonsmokers. Hence, a rate of 60 cfm per occupant in smoking areas may almost meet the customary ASHRAE criterion of a maximum of 20 percent dissatisfaction for a group of smokers. The data from the investigation suggest that under typical conditions of smoking occupancy (10 percent smoking at any given time), nonsmokers would need over 100 cfm per occupant to hold dissatisfaction at only 20 percent. We do not know whether the difference between smokers and nonsmokers reflects olfactory sensitivity to ETS or other criteria.

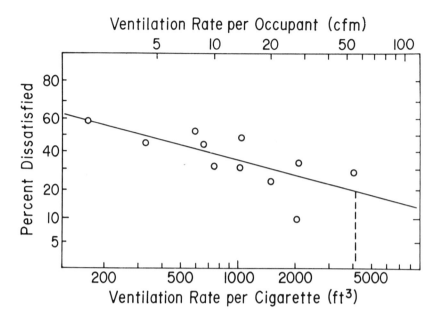

Figure 6.3. Percent dissatisfaction among visitors versus ventilation during the last 15 minutes of smoking in the experiments shown in Figure 6.2. The ventilation rate per cigarette is based on 7.5-minute smoking time per cigarette. The ventilation rate per occupant is adjusted to typical conditions of smoking occupancy in which 10 percent of occupants will be smoking at any given time. *Source:* Reprinted with permission from *Atmospheric Environment* 17, Cain W. S. et al., Ventilation requirements in buildings—I. Control of occupancy odor and tobacco smoke odor. Copyright 1983, Pergamon Press PLC.

Clausen and co-workers (1986b) found similar differences in tolerance of ETS odor between smokers and nonsmokers. For any given level of odor (expressed as concentration of butanol), nonsmokers expressed much more dissatisfaction than smokers. For both groups, odor intensity and dissatisfaction were associated, but the relationship was steeper for nonsmokers. At the point at which 20 percent of the smokers expressed dissatisfaction, almost half of nonsmokers were dissatisfied with the air quality.

In a laboratory situation in which other sources of combustion can be eliminated, CO can serve as an index of the level of ETS. Clausen related dissatisfaction to concentration of CO in ETS as well as to matched level of butanol; in the experiment, odor intensity and the increment in CO concentration due to smoking were strongly correlated. The concentration at which 20 percent of the nonsmokers expressed dissatisfaction fell about eight times below that at which 20 percent of the smokers expressed dissatisfaction.

As ETS enters the atmosphere, its many chemical constituents react both chemically and physically with each other and with surrounding materials. Nevertheless, the odor of ETS behaves over short time periods as though ETS were a stable contaminant. After the source has been removed, ETS odor decays in a manner

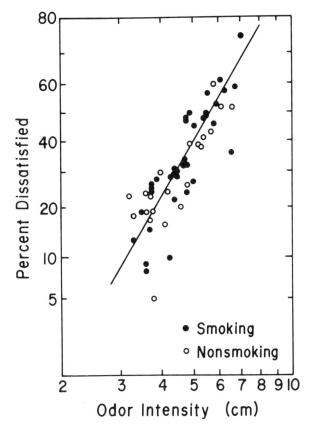

Figure 6.4. Percent dissatisfaction versus odor intensity (graphic rating) during smoking and nonsmoking odors. *Source:* Reprinted with permission from *Atmospheric Environment* 17, Cain W. S. et al., Ventilation requirements in buildings—I. Control of occupancy odor and tobacco smoke odor. Copyright 1983, Pergamon Press PLC.

entirely predictable from ventilation rate (Clausen et al. 1985). In this respect, it differs from occupancy odor, which has a half-life of 55 minutes, presumably dictated by slow oxidation of chemical constituents into less odorous products (Clausen et al. 1986a).

Standards for ventilation have focused on the reactions of the visitor to a space, rather than those of the occupant, on the assumption that the visitor will be more sensitive to, and hence more critical of, the contaminant than the person who has adapted to it. On the other hand, a focus on the visitor may not adequately address irritation, which is an important time-dependent sensory response of the occupant. Whereas air containing an irritant may initially be only slightly irritating, it may become intolerably so over time.

Figure 6.5 illustrates the time course of eye irritation experienced by occupants

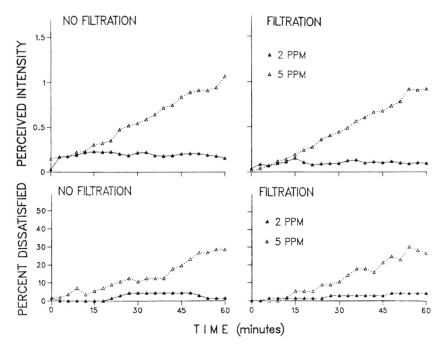

Figure 6.5. Perceived magnitude of eye irritation and degree of dissatisfaction expressed by occupants exposed to ETS for an hour. Concentrations of CO were held constant throughout the exposures and indicate severity of exposure. *Filtration* refers to elimination of particles via electrostatic precipitation. Filtration had little effect on irritation. *Source:* Reprinted with permission from *Atmospheric Environment* 21, Cain W. S. et al., Environmental tobacco smoke: Sensory reactions of occupants. Copyright 1987, Pergamon Press PLC.

exposed to ETS at constant concentrations of 2 or 5 ppm of CO, used as an index of ETS concentration (Cain et al. 1987). The lower concentration led to slight, although statistically significant, irritation above the presmoking baseline. The higher concentration led to irritation that increased over time in sensory magnitude and caused an increasing degree of dissatisfaction. Whereas essentially none of the occupants found the irritation objectionable at first, by the end of an hour about 30 percent were irritated. In an extension of this study, Clausen, Mäller, and Fanger (1987) found that a level of 20 percent dissatisfaction would occur at a concentration of 3.8 ppm of CO. A comparison with the odor judgments of visitors suggests that only smokers would find such a level tolerable by the "20 percent rule." Clausen, Mäller, and Fanger (1987) estimated that the ventilation rate necessary to control irritation of occupants to a dissatisfaction level of 20 percent would equal only one-tenth of that needed to control odor perceived by visitors to the same level of dissatisfaction.

Although Clausen and co-workers did not argue in favor of lowering ventilation to meet only the dissatisfaction of occupants, others have suggested this approach

(Winneke et al. 1984). Cain and co-workers (1987) cautioned against handling irritation and odor in the same fashion. The appropriateness of applying the 20 percent rule to dissatisfaction based on irritation alone, as it is applied to dissatisfaction based on odor alone, has been questioned. Whereas odor may be interpretable narrowly on grounds of comfort, irritation would seem interpretable on grounds of health.

CONTROL

The standards of ASHRAE mandate specific levels of ventilation to provide occupant satisfaction with indoor air quality. The experimental studies reviewed above provide insights concerning the level of ventilation needed to achieve satisfaction for nonsmokers and for smokers in the presence of ETS. In actual indoor environments, when ventilation fails to eliminate the contaminant entirely, the physical interaction of ETS with surfaces may increase the need for ventilation. Because the liquid aerosol of ETS, known in the aggregate as *tar,* adsorbs strongly to walls, fabrics, and so on, it becomes a source of odor as components volatilize to the air. The background odor of the emitted products carries its own demands for ventilation, predictable in part from the typical amount of smoking in a space (Clausen et al. 1986b).

Obviously, ETS can be readily controlled by eliminating smoking from indoor environments or its impact lessened by limiting smoking to specific areas. Air cleaning offers another approach.

Although the odor of ETS can be postulated to come from its vapor phase and the irritation from its particulate phase, recent investigations that have employed electrostatic air cleaning have shown clearly that the gas phase accounts for most of the odor and irritation (Hugod 1984; Weber 1984). Comparison of the right and left sides of Figure 6.5 shows that elimination of the particulate phase had only a trivial effect on the eye irritation caused by ETS at 2 and 5 ppm carbon monoxide (Cain et al. 1987). The findings were similar for judgments of odor and of nose and throat irritation. Clausen, Mäller, and Fanger (1987) confirmed these results. In finding that particles played essentially no role in odor, both investigations also confirmed Clausen and colleagues' (1985) earlier experiments with visitors. Particle filtration holds no promise for immediate elimination of the discomfort of exposure to ETS. The major advantage of such air cleaning derives from reduction of haze and collection of tar that would otherwise adsorb elsewhere in the space.

Although both the odor and irritation of ETS come from the vapor phase, the chemical constituents responsible for these two effects may be different. Undoubtedly, the odor comes from a very large number of constituents. The sense of smell responds to almost all airborne organic materials present in sufficient concentration (Cain 1988). For one substance, however, a "sufficient concentration" may fall a millionfold below that of another. Furthermore, individual constituents may combine perceptually in mixtures in complicated, nonlinear ways.

Many single compounds can cause irritation at the concentrations present in ETS, which represents a complex mixture with numerous components capable of causing odor and irritation. Little is known about the effects upon perception of the combination of ETS irritants although it is known that odor and irritation interact (Cain and Murphy 1980). Irritation can suppress the perception of odor and vice versa (Cain, See, and Tosun 1986). Insofar as irritation may have a less complex origin than odor, it may offer easier opportunities for control through filtration. As yet, however, experiments on ETS have told more about what fails to cause irritation than about what causes it (Weber, Jermini, and Grandjean 1976; Weber-Tschopp, Fischer, and Grandjean 1977; Weber-Tschopp et al. 1977; Hugod, Hawkins, and Astrup 1978).

The complexity of ETS more or less assures that almost any means of air cleaning will eliminate part of it even though no simple procedure will eliminate all of it. Through the use of air washing that presumably eliminated some water-soluble constituents of ETS, Clausen, Mäller, and Fanger (1987) achieved some reduction in level of dissatisfaction although not in the perceived intensity of ETS. The results offered little encouragement for using air washing alone but showed that the odor character of ETS can play some role in the degree of acceptance.

A combination of particulate air cleaning and vapor phase cleaning via adsorption on activated carbon or via chemisorption on oxidant-impregnated alumina can likely control both the irritation and odor of ETS to some degree. Unfortunately, standards for assessing the efficacy of vapor phase filtration media have not been developed. The installation of such media occurs more commonly in special environments, for example, libraries and computer facilities, under expert guidance than in spaces designed for general occupancy. In the overwhelming majority of cases, attempts to control ETS rely on ventilation (dilution). As shown by the experimental studies, however, ventilation has limitations.

## SUMMARY

The effects of active smoking and the toxicology of cigarette smoking have been examined comprehensively. The periodic reports of the U.S. surgeon general and other summary reports have considered the extensive evidence on active smoking; these reports have provided definitive conclusions concerning the adverse effects of active smoking, which have prompted public policies and scientific research directed at prevention and cessation of smoking.

Although the evidence on involuntary smoking is not as extensive as that on active smoking, health risks of involuntary smoking have been identified. The 1986 report of the U.S. surgeon general (U.S. DHHS 1986) and the 1986 report of the NRC (NRC 1986a) both concluded that involuntary exposure to tobacco smoke increases respiratory infections in children, increases the prevalence of respiratory symptoms in children, reduces the rate of functional growth as the lung matures, and causes lung cancer in nonsmokers. Involuntary smoking may also adversely affect asthmatics, and annoyance and irritation are well documented. These adverse effects of involuntary exposure to tobacco smoke have provided a strong rationale for policies directed at reducing and eliminating exposure of nonsmokers to ETS (U.S. DHHS 1986). Complete protection of nonsmokers in public locations and the workplace may require the banning of smoking since the 1986 report of the surgeon general (U.S. DHHS 1986) concluded that "the simple separation of smokers and nonsmokers within the same air space may reduce, but does not eliminate, the exposure of nonsmokers to environmental tobacco smoke."

## REFERENCES

Akiba, S.; Kato, H.; and Blot, W. J. 1986. Passive smoking and lung cancer among Japanese women. *Cancer Res.* 46:4804–7.

American Society of Heating, Refrigerating, and Air-Conditioning Engineers. 1989. ASHRAE *Standard 62-1989: Ventilation for acceptable indoor air quality.* Atlanta, Ga.: ASHRAE.

Badre, R., et al. 1978. Pollution atmospherique par la fumée de tabac. *Ann. Pharm. Fr.* 36:443–52.

Benowitz, N. L., et al. 1983. Cotinine disposition and effects. *Clin. Pharmacol. Ther.* 34:604–11.

Berkey, C. S., et al. 1986. Indoor air pollution and pulmonary function growth in preadolescent children. *Am. J. Epidemiol.* 123:250–60.

Black, N. 1985. The aetiology of glue ear: A case-control study. *Int. J. Pediatr. Otorhinolaryngol.* 9:121–33.

Bland, M., et al. 1978. Effect of children's and parents' smoking on respiratory symptoms. *Arch. Dis. Child.* 53:100–105.

Brownson, R. C., et al. 1987. Risk factors for adenocarcinoma of the lung. *Am. J. Epidemiol.* 125:25–34.

Brunekreef, B., et al. 1985. Indoor air pollution and its effect on pulmonary function of adult nonsmoking women, III: Passive smoking and pulmonary function. *Int. J. Epidemiol.* 14:227–30.

Burchfiel, C. M., III. 1984. Passive smoking, respiratory symptoms, lung function and initiation of smoking in Tecumseh, Michigan. Ph.D. diss., University of Michigan, Ann Arbor.

Burchfiel, C. M., et al. 1986. Passive smoking in childhood: Respiratory conditions and pulmonary function in Tecumseh, Michigan. *Am. Rev. Respir. Dis.* 133:966–73.

Cain, W. S. 1988. Olfaction. In *Stevens' handbook of experimental psychology, Vol. 1: Perception and motivation,* rev. ed. Ed. R. C. Atkinson, et al., 409–59. New York: John Wiley & Sons.

Cain, W. S., and Murphy, C. L. 1980. Interaction between chemoreceptive modalities of odour and irritation. *Nature* 284:255–57.

Cain, W. S.; See, L. C.; and Tosun, T. 1986. Irritation and odor from formaldehyde: Chamber studies. In *IAQ '86: Managing indoor air for health and energy conservation,* 126–37. Atlanta, Ga.: ASHRAE.

Cain, W. S., et al. 1983. Ventilation requirements in buildings, I: Control of occupancy odor and tobacco smoke odor. *Atmos. Environ.* 17:1183–97.

Cain, W. S., et al. 1987. Environmental tobacco smoke: Sensory reactions of occupants. *Atmos. Environ.* 21:347–53.

Chan, W. C., and Fung, S. C. 1982. Lung cancer in nonsmokers in Hong Kong. In *Cancer campaign*, Vol. 6: *Cancer epidemiology*. Ed. E. Grundman, 199–202. Stuttgart: Gustav Fischer Verlag.

Chan, W. C., et al. 1979. Bronchial cancer in Hong Kong 1976–1977. *Br. J. Cancer* 39:182–92.

Chappell, S. B., and Parker, R. J. 1977. Smoking and carbon monoxide levels in enclosed public places in New Brunswick. *Can. J. Public Health,* 68:159–61.

Charlton, A. 1984. Children's coughs related to parental smoking. *Br. Med. J.* 288:1647–49.

Clausen, G. H. 1986. Tobaksrog: Lugtgener og ventilationsbehov. Ph.D. diss., Technical University of Denmark, Copenhagen.

Clausen, G. H.; Møller, S. B.; and Fanger, P. O. 1987. The impact of air washing on environmental tobacco smoke odor. In *Indoor air '87, Volume 2*. Ed. B. Seifert, et al., 47–51. Berlin: Institute for Water, Soil, and Air Hygiene.

Clausen, G. H., et al. 1985. The influence of aging, particle filtration and humidity on tobacco smoke odor. In *Clima 2000, Vol. 4: Indoor climate*. Ed. P.O. Fanger, 345–49. Copenhagen: VVS Kongres-VVS Messe.

Clausen, G. H., et al. 1986a. Stability of body odor in enclosed spaces. *Environ. Int.* 12:201–5.

Clausen, G. H., et al. 1986b. Background odor caused by previous tobacco smoking. In *IAQ '86: Managing indoor air for health and energy conservation, 119–25*. Atlanta: ASHRAE.

*Cogswell, J. J.; Mitchell, E. B.; and Alexander, J. 1987. Parental smoking, breast feeding, and respiratory infection in development of allergic diseases. Arch. Dis. Child. 62:338–44.*

Colley, J. R. 1974. Respiratory symptoms in children and parental cigarette smoking and phlegm production. *Br. Med. J.* 2:201–4.

Comstock, G. W., et al. 1981. Respiratory effects of household exposures to tobacco smoke and gas cooking. *Am. Rev. Respir. Dis.* 124:143–48.

Correa, P., et al. 1983. Passive smoking and lung cancer. *Lancet* 2:595–97.

Coultas, D. B., and Samet, J. M. 1990. Comparability of salivary and urinary cotinine determination for assessment of exposure to environmental tobacco smoke. Submitted for publication.

Coultas, D. B., et al. 1990. Variability of measures of exposure to environmental tobacco smoke in the home. *Am. Rev. Respir. Dis.* 142:602–6.

Coultas, D. B., et al. 1987. Salivary cotinine levels and involuntary tobacco smoke exposure in children and adults in New Mexico. *Am. Rev. Respir. Dis.* 136:305–9.

Coultas, D. B., et al. 1988. Variability of measures of exposure to environmental tobacco smoke in the home. Air Pollution Control Association, International specialty conference on combustion processes and the quality of the indoor environment.

Cummings, K. M., et al. 1989. Measurement of lifetime exposure to passive smoke. *Am. J. Epidemiol.* 130:122–32.

Dahms, T. E.; Bolin, J. F.; and Slavin, R. G. 1981. Passive smoking: Effect on bronchial asthma. *Chest* 80:530–34.

Dalager, N. A., et al. 1986. The relation of passive smoking to lung cancer. *Cancer Res.* 46:4808–11.

Enstrom, J. E. 1979. Rising lung cancer mortality among nonsmokers. *J. Natl. Cancer Inst.* 62:755–60.

Evans, D., et al. 1987. The impact of passive smoking on emergency room visits of urban children with asthma. *Am. Rev. Respir. Dis.* 135:567–72.

Everson, R. B. 1980. Individuals transplacentally exposed to maternal smoking may be at increased cancer risk in adult life. *Lancet* 2:123–27.

Fergusson, D. M., and Horwood, L. J. 1985. Parental smoking and respiratory illness during early childhood: A six-year longitudinal study. *Pediatr. Pulmonol.* 1:99–106.

First, M. W. 1985. Constituents of sidestream and mainstream tobacco smoke and markers to quantify exposure to them. In *Indoor air and human health*. Ed. R. B. Gammage and S. V. Kaye, 195–203. Chelsea, Mich.: Lewis Publishers.

Foliart, D.; Benowitz, N. L.; and Becker, C. E. 1983. Passive absorption of nicotine in flight attendants (letter). *N. Engl. J. Med.* 308:1105.

Gao, Y. T., et al. 1987. Lung cancer among Chinese women. *Int. J. Cancer* 40:604–9.

Garfinkel, L. 1981. Time trends in lung cancer mortality among nonsmokers and a note on passive smoking. *J. Natl. Cancer Inst.* 66:1061–66.

Garfinkel, L.; Auerbach, O.; and Joubert, L. 1985. Involuntary smoking and lung cancer: A case-control study. *J. Natl. Cancer Inst.* 75:463–69.

Garland, C., et al. 1985. Effects of passive smoking on ischemic heart disease mortality of nonsmokers. *Am. J. Epidemiol.* 121:645–50.

Geng, G. Y., et al. 1987. On the relationship between smoking and female lung cancer. In *Smoking and health 1987*. Ed. M. Aoki, S. Hisamichi, and S. Tominaga, 483–86. Amsterdam: Excerpta Medica.

Gillis, C. R., et al. 1984. The effect of environmental tobacco smoke in two urban communities in the west of Scotland. *Eur. J. Respir. Dis.* 65(Suppl. 133):121–26.

Gortmacker, S. L., et al. 1982. Parental smoking and the risk of childhood asthma. *Am. J. Public Health* 72:574–79.

Greenberg, R. A., et al. 1984. Measuring the exposure of infants to tobacco smoke: Nicotine and cotinine in urine and saliva. *N. Engl. J. Med.* 310:1075–78.

Grufferman, S., et al. 1982. Environmental factors in the etiology of rhabdomyosarcoma in childhood. *J. Natl. Cancer Inst.* 68:107–13.

Grufferman, S., et al. 1983. Parents' cigarette smoking and childhood cancer. *Med. Hypotheses* 12:17–20.

Haley, N. J.; Sepkovic, D.; and Hoffman, D. 1989. Elimination of cotinine from body fluids: Disposition in smokers and nonsmokers. *Am. J. Public Health* 79:1046–48.

Haley, N. J., et al. 1989. Biochemical validation of self-reported exposure to environmental tobacco smoke. *Environ. Res.* 49:127–35.

Hall, C. B., et al. 1984. Long-term prospective study in children after respiratory syncytial virus infection. *J. Pediatr.* 105:358–64.

Harlap, S., and Davies, A. M. 1974. Infant admissions to hospital and maternal smoking. *Lancet* 1:529–32.

Harlos, D. P., et al. 1987. Relating indoor $NO_2$ levels to infant personal exposures. *Atmos. Environ.* 21:369–78.

Helsing, K. J., et al. 1988. Heart disease mortality in nonsmokers living with smokers. *Am. J. Epidemiol.* 127:915–22.

Henderson, F. W., et al. 1989. Home air nicotine levels and urinary cotinine excretion in preschool children. *Am. Rev. Respir. Dis.* 140:197–201.

Hinds, W. C., and First, M. W. 1975. Concentrations of nicotine and tobacco smoke in public places. *N. Engl. J. Med.* 292:844–45.

Hirayama, T. 1981. Nonsmoking wives of heavy smokers have a higher risk of lung cancer: A study from Japan. *Br. Med. J.* 282:183–85.

Hirayama, T. 1983. Passive smoking and lung cancer, nasal sinus cancer, brain tumor and ischemic heart disease. In *Proceedings of the Fifth World Conference on Smoking and Health, Vol. 1*. Ed. W. F. Forbes, R. C. Frecker, and D. Nostbakken, 137–41. Ottawa: Canadian Council on Smoking and Health.

Hirayama, T. 1984. Cancer mortality in nonsmoking women with smoking husbands based on a large-scale cohort study in Japan. *Prev. Med.* 13:680–90.

Hoffman, D., et al. 1984a. Indoor air pollution by tobacco smoke: Model studies on the uptake by nonsmokers. In *Indoor air, Vol. 2: Radon, passive smoking, particulates and housing epidemiology*. Ed. B. Berglund, T. Lindvall, and J. Sundell, 313–18. Stockholm: Swedish Council for Building Research.

Hoffman, D., et al. 1984b. Tobacco sidestream smoke: Uptake by nonsmokers. *Prev. Med.* 13:608–17.

Horwood, L. J.; Fergusson, D. M.; and Shannon, F. T. 1985. Social and familial factors in the development of early childhood asthma. *Pediatrics* 75:859–68.

Hosein, R., and Corey, P. 1984. Multivariate analyses of nine indoor factors on $FEV_1$ of Caucasian children. *Am. Rev. Respir. Dis.* 129(suppl.):140 (abstr.).

Hugod, C. 1984. Indoor air pollution with smoke constituents: An experimental investigation. *Prev. Med.* 13:582–88.

Hugod, C.; Hawkins, L. H.; and Astrup, P. 1978. Exposure of passive smokers to tobacco smoke constituents. *Int. Arch. Occup. Environ. Health* 42:21–29.

Humble, C. G.; Samet, J. M.; and Pathak, D. R. 1987. Marriage to a smoker and lung cancer risk in New Mexico. *Am. J. Public Health* 77:598–602.

Inoue, R., and Hirayama, T. 1988. Passive smoking and lung cancer in women. In *Smoking and health 1987*. Ed. M. Aoki, S. Hisamichi, and S. Tominaga, 283–85. Amsterdam: Excerpta Medica.

International Agency for Research on Cancer. 1986. IARC monographs on the evaluation of the carcinogenic risk of chemicals to humans: Tobacco smoking, Vol. 38. Lyon, France: World Health Organization, IARC.

Iversen, M., et al. 1985. Middle ear effusion in children and the indoor environment: An epidemiological study. *Arch. Environ. Health* 40:74–79.

Jarvis, M. J., and Russell, M. A. 1984. Measurement and estimation of smoke dosage to nonsmokers from environmental tobacco smoke. *Eur. J. Respir. Dis.* 65(Suppl. 133):68–75.

Jarvis, M. J., et al. 1984. Biochemical markers of smoke absorption and self-reported exposure to passive smoking. *J. Epidemiol. Community Health* 38:335–39.

Jarvis, M. J., et al. 1985. Passive exposure to tobacco smoke: Saliva cotinine concentrations in a representative population sample of nonsmoking school children. *Br. Med. J.* 291:927–29.

Jarvis, M. J., et al. 1988. Elimination of cotinine from body fluids: Implications for noninvasive measurement of tobacco smoke exposure. *Am. J. Public Health* 78:696–98.

Jones, J. R., et al. 1983. Effects of cooking fuels on lung function in nonsmoking women. *Arch. Environ. Health.* 38:219–22.

Kabat, G. C., and Wynder, E. L. 1984. Lung cancer in nonsmokers. *Cancer* 53:1214–21.

Kabat, G. C.; Dieck, G. S.; and Wynder, E. L. 1986. Bladder cancer in nonsmokers. *Cancer* 2:362–67.

Kauffmann, F.; Tessier, J. S.; and Oriol, P. 1983. Adult passive smoking in the home environment: A risk factor for chronic airflow limitation. *Am. J. Epidemiol.* 117:269–80.

Kauffmann, F., et al. 1989. Respiratory symptoms and lung function in relation to passive smoking: A comparative study of American and French women. *Int. J. Epidemiol.* 18:334–44.

Kentner, M.; Triebig, G.; and Weltle, D. 1984. The influence of passive smoking on pulmonary function: A study of 1,351 office workers. *Prev. Med.* 13:656–69.

Kershaw, C. R. 1987. Passive smoking, potential atopy and asthma in the first five years. *J. R. Soc. Med.* 80:683–88.

Knoth, A.; Bohn, H.; and Schmidt, F. 1983. Passivrauchen als lung enkrebsursache bei nichtraucherinnen. *Med. Klin.* 2:66–69.

Koo, L. C.; Ho, J. H.; and Lee, N. 1985. An analysis of some risk factors for lung cancer in Hong Kong. *Int. J. Cancer* 35:149–55.

Koo, L. C.; Ho, J. H.; and Saw, D. 1984. Is passive smoking an added risk factor for lung cancer in Chinese women? *J. Exp. Clin. Cancer Res.* 3:277–83.

Koo, L. C., et al. 1987. Measurements of passive smoking and estimates of lung cancer risk among nonsmoking Chinese females. *Int. J. Cancer* 39:162–69.

Kraemer, J. M., et al. 1983. Risk factors for persistent middle-ear effusions: Otitis media, catarrh, cigarette exposure, and atopy. *JAMA* 249:1022–25.

Kyerematen, G. A., et al. 1982. Smoking-induced changes in nicotine disposition: Application of a new HPLC assay for nicotine and its metabolites. *Clin. Pharmacol. Ther.* 32:769–80.

Lam, T. H., et al. 1987. Smoking, passive smoking and histological types in lung cancer in Hong Kong Chinese women. *Br. J. Cancer* 56:673–78.

Lebowitz, M. D., and Burrows, B. 1976. Respiratory symptoms related to smoking habits of family adults. *Chest* 69:48–50.

Lebowitz, M. D.; Knudson, R. J.; and Burrows, B. 1984. Family aggregation of pulmonary function measurements. *Am. Rev. Respir. Dis.* 129:8–11.

Lee, P. N. 1988. *Misclassification of smoking habits and passive smoking.* Heidelberg: Springer-Verlag.

Lee, P. N.; Chamberlain, J.; and Alderson, M. R. 1986. Relationship of passive smoking to risk of lung cancer and other smoking-associated diseases. *Br. J. Cancer* 54:97–105.

Leeder, S. R., et al. 1976. Influence of family factors on the incidence of lower respiratory illness during the first year of life. *Br. J. Prev. Soc. Med.* 30:203–12.

Martinez, F. D., et al. 1988. Parental smoking enhances bronchial responsiveness in nine-year-old children. *Am. Rev. Respir. Dis.* 138:518–23.

Masi, M. A., et al. 1988. Environmental exposure to tobacco smoke and lung function in young adults. *Am. Rev. Respir. Dis.* 138:296–99.

Matsukura, S., et al. 1984. Effects of environmental tobacco smoke on urinary cotinine excretion in nonsmokers: Evidence for passive smoking. *N. Engl. J. Med.* 311:828–32.

Mattson, M. E., et al. 1989. Passive smoking on commercial airline flights. *JAMA* 261:867–72.

McConnochie, K. M., and Roghmann, K. J. 1986. Breast feeding and maternal smoking as predictors of wheezing in children age 6 to 10 years. *Pediatr. Pulmonol.* 2:260–68.

McMurray, R. G.; Hicks, L. L.; and Thompson, D. L. 1985. The effects of passive inhalation of cigarette smoke on exercise performance. *Eur. J. Appl. Physiol.* 54:196–200.

Miller, G. H. 1984. Cancer, passive smoking and nonemployed and employed wives. *West. J. Med.* 140:632–35.

Muramatsu, M., et al. 1984. Estimation of personal exposure to tobacco smoke with a newly developed nicotine personal monitor. *Environ. Res.* 35:218–27.

Murray, A. B., and Morrison, B. J. 1986. The effect of cigarette smoke from the mother on bronchial responsiveness and severity of symptoms in children with asthma. *J. Allergy Clin. Immunol.* 77:575–81.

National Research Council (committee on indoor pollutants). 1981. *Indoor pollutants.* Washington, D.C.: National Academy Press.

National Research Council (committee on passive smoking). 1986a. *Environmental tobacco smoke: measuring exposures and assessing health effects.* Washington, D.C.: National Academy Press.

National Research Council (committee on airliner cabin air quality). 1986b. *The airliner cabin environment: Air quality and safety.* Washington, D.C.: National Academy Press.

O'Connor, G. T., et al. 1987. The effect of passive smoking on pulmonary function and nonspecific bronchial responsiveness in a population-based sample of children and young adults. *Am. Rev. Respir. Dis.* 135:800–804.

Ogston, S. A.; Florey, C. V.; and Walker, C. H. M. 1985. The Tayside infant morbidity and mortality study: Effect on health of using gas for cooking. *Br. Med. J.* 290:957–60.

Ogston, S. A.; Florey, C. V.; and Walker, C. H. M. 1987. Association of infant alimentary and respiratory illness with parental smoking and other environmental factors. *J. Epidemiol. Community Health* 41:21–25.

Pattishall, E. N., et al. 1985. Serum cotinine as a measure of tobacco smoke exposure in children. *Am. J. Dis. Child.* 139:1101–4.

Pershagen, G.; Hrubec, Z.; and Svensson, C. 1987. Passive smoking and lung cancer in Swedish women. *Am. J. Epidemiol.* 125:17–24.

Pimm, P. E., Silverman, F., and Shephard, R. J. 1978. Physiological effects of acute passive exposure to cigarette smoke. *Arch. Environ. Health* 33:201–13.

Preston-Martin, S., et al. 1982. *N*-Nitroso compounds and childhood brain tumors: A case-control study. *Cancer Res.* 42:5240–45.

Pron, G. E., et al. 1988. The reliability of passive smoking histories reported in a case-control study of lung cancer. *Am. J. Epidemiol.* 127:267–73.

Pukander, J., et al. 1985. Risk factors affecting the occurrence of acute otitis media among 2–3-year-old urban children. *Acta Otolaryngol.* 100:260–65.

Pullan, C. R., and Hey, C. N. 1982. Wheezing, asthma, and pulmonary dysfunction 10 years after infection with respiratory syncytial virus in infancy. *Br. Med. J.* 284:1665–69.

Rantakallio, P. 1978. Relationship of maternal smoking to morbidity and mortality of the child up to the age of five. *Acta Paediatr. Scand.* 67:621–31.

Remijn, B., et al. 1985. Indoor air pollution and its effect on pulmonary function of adult nonsmoking women, I: Exposure estimates for nitrogen dioxide and passive smoking. *Int. J. Epidemiol.* 14:215–20.

Repace, J. L., and Lowrey, A. H. 1980. Indoor air pollution, tobacco smoke, and public health. *Science* 208:464–72.

Repace, J. L., and Lowrey, A. H. 1985. A quantitative estimate of nonsmokers' lung cancer risk from passive smoking. *Environ. Int.* 11:3–22.

Rosenberg, J., et al. 1980. Disposition kinetics and effects of intravenous nicotine. *Clin. Pharmacol. Ther.* 28:517–22.

Russell, M. A.; West, R. J.; and Jarvis, M. J. 1985. Intravenous nicotine simulation of passive smoking to estimate dosage to exposed nonsmokers. *Br. J. Addict.* 80:201–6.

Samet, J. M.; Tager, I. B.; and Speizer, F. E. 1983. The relationship between respiratory illness in childhood and chronic air-flow obstruction in adulthood. *Am. Rev. Respir. Dis.* 127:508–23.

Sandler, D. P., Everson, R. B., and Wilcox, A. J. 1985. Passive smoking in adulthood and cancer risk. *Am. J. Epidemiol.* 121:37–48.

Sandler, D. P.; Wilcox, A. J.; and Everson, R. B. 1985. Cumulative effects of lifetime passive smoking on cancer risk. *Lancet* 1:312–15.

Sandler, D. P., et al. 1985. Cancer risk in adulthood from early life exposure to parents' smoking. *Am. J. Public Health* 74:487–92.

Sandler, D. P., et al. 1989. Deaths from all causes in non-smokers who lived with smokers. *Am. J. Public Health* 79:163–67.

Schenker, M. B.; Samet, J. M.; and Speizer, F. E. 1982. Effect of cigarette tar content and smoking habits on respiratory symptoms in women. *Am. Rev. Respir. Dis.* 125:684–90.

Schenker, M. B.; Samet, J. M.; and Speizer, F. E. 1983. Risk factors for childhood respiratory disease: The effect of host factors and home environmental exposures. *Am. Rev. Respir. Dis.* 128:1038–43.

Schievebein, H., and Richter, F. 1984. The influence of passive smoking on the cardiovascular system. *Prev. Med.* 13:626–44.

Schilling, R. S., et al. 1977. Lung function, respiratory disease, and smoking in families. *Am. J. Epidemiol.* 106:274–83.

Shephard, R. J., et al. 1979. Effect of cigarette smoke on the eyes and airway. *Int. Arch. Occup. Environ. Health* 135–44.

Shimizu, H., et al. 1988. A case-control study of lung cancer in nonsmoking women. *Tohoku J. Exp. Med.* 154:389–97.

Slattery, M. L., et al. 1989. Cigarette smoking and exposure to passive smoke are risk factors for cervical cancer. *JAMA* 261:1593–98.

Somerville, S. M.; Rona, R. J.; and Chinn, S. 1988. Passive smoking and respiratory conditions in primary school children. *J. Epidemiol. Community Health* 42:105–10.

Spengler, J. D., et al. 1981. Long-term measurements of respirable sulfates and particles inside and outside homes. *Atmos. Environ.* 15:23–30.

Spengler, J. D., et al. 1985. Personal exposures to respirable particulates and implications for air pollution epidemiology. *Environ. Sci. Technol.* 19:700–707.

Stankus, R. P., et al. 1988. Cigarette smoke-sensitive asthma: Challenge studies. *J. Allergy Clin. Immunol.* 82:331–38.

Sterling, T. D., and Kobayashi, D. 1982. Indoor byproduct levels of tobacco smoke: A critical review of the literature. *J. Air Pollut. Control Assoc.* 32:250–59.

Strachan, D. P.; Jarvis, M. J.; and Feyerabend, C. 1989. Passive smoking, salivary cotinine concentrations, and middle ear effusion in 7-year-old children. *Br. Med. J.* 298:1549–52.

Svendsen, K. H., et al. 1987. Effects of passive smoking in the multiple risk factor intervention trial. *Am. J. Epidemiol.* 126:783–95.

Tager, I. B. 1988. Passive smoking-bronchial responsiveness and atopy (editorial). *Am. Rev. Respir. Dis.* 138:507–9.

Tager, I. B., et al. 1979. Effect of parental cigarette smoking on the pulmonary function of children. *Am. J. Epidemiol.* 110:15–26.

Tager, I. B., et al. 1983. Longitudinal study of the effects of maternal smoking on pulmonary function in children. *N. Engl. J. Med.* 309:699–703.

Tashkin, D. P., et al. 1984. The UCLA population studies of chronic obstructive respiratory disease, VII: Relationship between parental smoking and children's lung function. *Am. Rev. Respir. Dis.* 129:891–97.

Trichopoulos, D.; Kalandidi, A.; and Sparros, L. 1983. Lung cancer and passive smoking: Conclusion of Greek study (letter). *Lancet* 2:677–78.

Trichopoulos, D., et al. 1981. Lung cancer and passive smoking. *Int. J. Cancer* 27:1–4.

Tsimoyianis, G. V., et al. 1987. Reduction in pulmonary function and increased frequency of cough associated with passive smoking in teenage athletes. *Pediatrics* 80:32–36.

U.S. Department of Health, Education, and Welfare. 1979. *Smoking and health. A report of the surgeon general.* Washington, D.C.: U.S. Government Printing Office. DHEW Publication no. (PHS) 79-50066.

U.S. Department of Health and Human Services. 1982. *The health consequences of smoking: Cancer. A report of the surgeon general.* Washington, D.C.: U.S. Government Printing Office. DHHS Publication no. (PHS) 82-50179.

U.S. Department of Health and Human Services. 1983. *The health consequences of smoking: Cardiovascular disease. A report of the surgeon general.* Washington, D.C.: U.S. Government Printing Office. DHHS Publication no. (PHS) 84-50204.

U.S. Department of Health and Human Services. 1984. *The health consequences of smoking: Chronic obstructive lung disease. A report of the surgeon general.* Washington, D.C.: Government Printing Office. DHHS Publication no. (PHS) 84-50205.

U.S. Department of Health and Human Services. 1986. *The health consequences of involuntary smoking. A report of the surgeon general.* Washington, D.C.: U.S. Government Printing Office. DHHS, PHS Publication no. (CDC) 87-8398.

U.S. Department of Health and Human Services. 1988. *The health consequences of smoking: Nicotine addiction. A report of the surgeon general.* Washington, D.C.: U.S. Government Printing Office. DHHS Publication no. (CDC) 88-8406.

U.S. Department of Health and Human Services. 1989. *Reducing the health consequences of smoking: 25 years of progress. A report of the surgeon general.* Washington, D.C.: U.S. Government Printing Office. DHHS Publication no. (CDC) 89-8411.

U.S. Public Health Service. 1964. *Smoking and health. Report of the advisory committee to the surgeon general of the Public Health Service.* Washington, D.C.: U.S. Government Printing Office. PHS Publication no. 1103.

Urch, R. B., et al. 1988. Does suggestibility modify acute reactions to passive cigarette smoke exposure? *Environ. Res.* 47:34–47.

Vandenbroucke, J. P., et al. 1984. Active and passive smoking in married couples: Results of 25-year follow up. *Br. Med. J.* 288:1801–2.

Wald, N., and Ritchie, C. 1984. Validation of studies on lung cancer in nonsmokers married to smokers (letter). *Lancet* 1:1067.

Wald, N. J., et al. 1984. Urinary cotinine as marker of breathing other people's tobacco smoke (letter). *Lancet* 1:230–31.

Wald, N. J., et al. 1986. Does breathing other people's smoke cause lung cancer? *Br. Med. J.* 293:1217–22.

Wall, M. A., et al. 1988. Cotinine in the serum, saliva and urine of nonsmokers, passive smokers, and active smokers. *Am. J. Public Health* 78:699–701.

Wallace, L. A. 1987. *The total exposure assessment methodology (TEAM) study: Summary and analysis,* Vol. 1. Washington, D.C.: Office of Research and Development, U.S.

Environmental Protection Agency. Publication no. EPA/600/6-87/002a.

Ware, J. H., et al. 1984. Passive smoking, gas cooking, and respiratory health of children living in six cities. *Am. Rev. Respir. Dis.* 129:366–74.

Weber, A. 1984. Annoyance and irritation by passive smoking. *Prev. Med.* 13:618–25.

Weber, A., and Fischer, T. 1980. Passive smoking at work. *Int. Arch. Occup. Environ. Health* 47:209–21.

Weber, A.; Jermini, C.; and Grandjean, E. 1976. Irritating effects on man of air pollution due to cigarette smoke. *Am. J. Public Health* 66:672–76.

Weber-Tschopp, A.; Fischer, T.; and Grandjean, E. 1977. Reizwirkungen des Formaldehyds (HCHO) auf den Menschen. (Irritating effects of formaldehyde on men.) *Int. Arch. Occup. Environ. Health* 39:207–18.

Weber-Tschopp, A., et al. 1977. Experimentelle Reizwirkungen von Akrolein auf den Menschen. (Experimentally induced irritating effects of acrolein on men.) *Arch. Occup. Environ. Health* 40:117–30.

Weiss, S. T. 1986. Passive smoking and lung cancer: What is the risk? (editorial). *Am. Rev. Respir. Dis.* 133:1–3.

Weiss, S. T., et al. 1980. Persistent wheeze: Its relation to respiratory illness, cigarette smoking, and level of pulmonary function in a population sample of children. *Am. Rev. Respir. Dis.* 122:697–707.

Wells, A. J. 1988. An estimate of adult mortality in the United States from passive smoking. *Environ. Int.* 14:249–65.

White, J. R., and Froeb, H. F. 1980. Small airways dysfunction in nonsmokers chronically exposed to tobacco smoke. *N. Engl. J. Med.* 302:720–23.

Wiedemann, H. P., et al. 1986. Acute effects of passive smoking on lung function and airway reactivity in asthmatic subjects. *Chest* 89:180–85.

Winneke, G., et al. 1984. Patterns and determinants of reaction to tobacco smoke in an experimental exposure setting. In *Indoor air.* Ed. B. Berglund, T. Lindvall, and J. Sundell, Vol. 2, 351–56. Stockholm: Swedish Council for Building Research.

Wu, A. H., et al. 1985. Smoking and other risk factors for lung cancer in women. *J. Natl. Cancer Inst.* 4:747–51.

Yue Chen, B. M.; Wanxian, L. I.; and Shunzhang, Y. 1986. Influence of passive smoking on admissions for respiratory illness in early childhood. *Br. Med. J.* 293:303–6.

# 7

# NITROGEN
# DIOXIDE

Jonathan M. Samet, M.D., M.S.

Nitrogen dioxide ($NO_2$) causes lung damage at high concentrations (Lowry and Schuman 1956; National Research Council [NRC] 1976), but effects at levels currently encountered in outdoor and indoor air have been difficult to characterize. Early epidemiologic studies focused on the health effects of ambient $NO_2$ (Shy et al. 1978). Few investigations directed at $NO_2$ exposure from ambient sources have involved populations exposed primarily to $NO_2$ (NRC 1976). More often, the $NO_2$ has been a component of a complex pollutant mixture, and the effects of exposure could not be attributed to $NO_2$ alone. Studies of occupationally exposed individuals have the same potential limitation. Thus, the evidence from studies of persons exposed to $NO_2$ in outdoor air or in the workplace cannot be extended to the indoor environment.

Studies conducted during the 1970s in the laboratory and in homes showed that indoor combustion sources were adding $NO_2$ and nitric oxide (NO) to indoor air and that indoor concentrations often exceeded outdoor concentrations in many homes (NRC 1981). The predominant role of indoor sources in determining personal exposure to nitrogen oxides was quickly recognized. Consequently, more recent epidemiologic studies have emphasized sources and effects of indoor $NO_2$ concentrations.

Combustion processes generate NO and, to a lesser extent, $NO_2$ (NRC 1976). Nitric oxide, however, is converted to $NO_2$, the nitrogen oxide of principal concern with regard to health in indoor environments. Combustion processes may also produce other potentially toxic derivatives of the nitrogen oxides such as nitric acid and nitrates, but the extent of these compounds in indoor air and their effects on health have not been addressed.

$NO_2$ is an oxidant gas that is soluble in tissues. Dosimetric studies show that most inhaled $NO_2$ is retained in the lungs and deposited primarily in the large and small airways, with little deposition in the alveoli (Goldstein et al. 1980; Miller et al. 1982). Because of its degree of tissue solubility, $NO_2$ reacts not only with the alveolar epithelium, but also with the interstitium and endothelium of the pulmonary capillaries (Mustafa and Tierney 1978). Inhaled $NO_2$ is thought to combine with water in the lung to form nitric ($HNO_3$) and nitrous ($HNO_2$) acids (Goldstein et al. 1980; Overton and Miller 1988), although substantial uncertainty remains concerning the tissue reactions to $NO_2$ (Morrow 1984).

Oxidant injury has been postulated to be the principal mechanism through which $NO_2$ damages the lung (Mustafa and Tierney 1978). At high concentrations, $NO_2$ causes extensive lung injury in animals and in humans (NRC 1976). Fatal pulmonary edema and bronchopneumonia have been reported at extremely high concentrations; lower concentrations are associated with bronchitis, bronchiolitis, and pneumonia (NRC 1976; Morrow 1984).

Experimental evidence indicates that $NO_2$ exposure adversely affects lung defense mechanisms (Gardner 1984; Morrow 1984). Lung defense mechanisms against inhaled particles and gases include aerodynamic filtration, mucociliary clearance, particle transport and detoxification by alveolar macrophages, and local and systemic immunity. In experimental models, $NO_2$ reduces the efficacy of several of these lung defense mechanisms; effects on mucociliary clearance, the alveolar macrophage, and the immune system have been demonstrated (NRC 1976; Dawson and Schenker 1979; Gardner 1984; Morrow 1984; Pennington 1988). The results of some experimental models, however, have not implied adverse effects of $NO_2$ on lung defenses (Lefkowitz, McGrath, and Lefkowitz 1986; Mochitate et al. 1986).

In animal experiments involving challenge with respiratory pathogens, exposure to $NO_2$ reduces clearance of infecting organisms and increases the mortality of the experimental animals (Dawson and Schenker 1979; Jakab 1980; Morrow 1984; Pennington 1988). In these infectivity models, the pathogens have most often been bacteria although viruses have also been used. The viral exposure studies have generally, but not uniformly, suggested an adverse effect of $NO_2$ on the outcome of infection (Buckley and Loosli 1969; Henry et al. 1970; Fenters et al. 1973; NRC 1976; Pennington 1988). Adverse effects have generally been demonstrated at concentrations an order of magnitude greater than generally found in indoor environments. Investigators at the U.S. Environmental Protection Agency have conducted a series of experiments to assess the consequences of various exposure patterns. These studies indicate that for short-term exposures, concentration has a greater effect on susceptibility than duration (Gardner et al. 1982), and the adverse effects of short-term spikes of exposure may be biologically significant (Miller et al. 1987). The studies with spikes of exposure may parallel the general pattern of human exposure to $NO_2$ from indoor sources, as short-term peak exposures can result from appliances used during cooking or space heating.

*EXPOSURE*

In the home environment, the principal combustion sources of $NO_2$ include gas stoves, gas water heaters, and space heaters. Central gas furnaces are vented to the outside and release little $NO_2$ into a home unless the venting system is malfunctioning. Automobile exhaust containing $NO_2$ may enter a home from an attached garage, and tobacco smoking also produces $NO_2$. The air of commercial buildings may be contaminated with $NO_2$ from entrained exhaust and from tobacco combustion. In locations with higher concentrations of $NO_2$ in ambient air, the entry of outdoor air into indoor environments elevates indoor concentrations further.

Combustion of gas during cooking and the burning of pilot lights releases NO, $NO_2$, carbon monoxide (CO), carbon dioxide ($CO_2$), and water (NRC 1981). On average, normal use of an unvented gas cooking range adds 25 parts per billion (ppb) $NO_2$ to the background concentration in a home (Spengler et al. 1983). The distributions of $NO_2$ levels in homes with gas and electric cooking ranges are distinct but overlap to some extent (Figure 7.1). The increase is greater during cold weather when the air exchange rate is usually reduced. Use of a gas stove or oven for space heating, a common practice in some cities in cold climates, results in particularly high concentrations of $NO_2$ (Sterling, Dimich, and Kobayashi 1981). During cooking with a gas range, peak levels in the kitchen may reach 200–400 ppb (Spengler and Sexton 1983), and measured personal exposures to $NO_2$ are therefore higher for persons living in homes with gas stoves than for persons living in homes with electric stoves (Quackenboss et al. 1982; Yocom 1982; Spengler et al. 1983).

Exposure to $NO_2$ from gas cooking stoves and ovens is widespread. About 50 percent of homes in the United States have gas cooking appliances; in some urban areas, such as Los Angeles, more than 90 percent of homes are equipped with gas appliances (U.S. Bureau of the Census 1983). The potential importance for health of indoor exposure to $NO_2$ is underscored by a comparison of the federal standard set for ambient air, 50 ppb annual average, with the levels measured in homes with gas cooking appliances. For example, Spengler and co-workers (Spengler et al. 1983) measured $NO_2$ in 137 homes in Portage, Wisconsin, a rural community with extremely low ambient levels of $NO_2$. The annual mean levels in the kitchens exceeded the present national ambient air quality standard in 10 percent of the homes with gas stoves. Sexton and co-workers (Sexton, Letz, and Spengler 1983) used data generated by personal, indoor, and outdoor monitoring to develop a computer model for personal and indoor exposure. The model was applied to residents of six U.S. cities. Although none of the cities experienced $NO_2$ concentrations in outdoor air above the federal standard (50 ppb), the model predicted that more than 25 percent of the residents of homes with gas ranges would have annual personal exposures above the level of the standard if ambient $NO_2$ con-

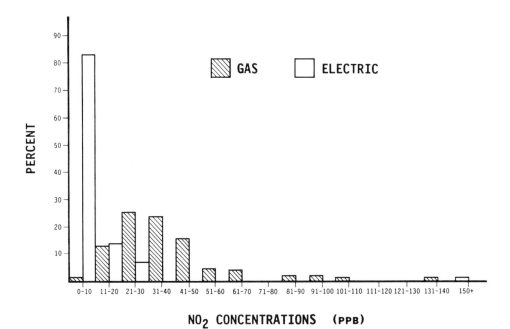

Figure 7.1. Two-week integrated $NO_2$ concentrations in the activity room in homes in Albuquerque, New Mexico. *Source:* Marbury et al. (1988), reprinted with permission.

centrations averaged 30 ppb. Furthermore, persons in a kitchen during cooking with a gas stove may receive short-term exposures at concentrations substantially above the annual standard for ambient air.

The use of space heaters, which produce heat by combustion, may also increase the level of exposure to $NO_2$. Gas-fired space heaters that are not vented to the outside emit NO, $NO_2$, and CO (NRC 1981). Unvented kerosene space heaters, increasingly popular for home heating since the energy crises of the 1970s, produce $NO_2$, CO, and sulfur dioxide ($SO_2$) (Leaderer 1982; Traynor et al. 1985). In a study of Connecticut homes, the presence of a kerosene space heater and the pattern of its use were strong determinants of $NO_2$ concentrations measured during the winter (Leaderer et al. 1987). In fourteen homes in the South with unvented gas space heaters, $NO_2$ concentrations exceeded the ambient standard of 50 ppb in eleven of the fourteen homes during a four-day monitoring period (McCarthy, Yarmac, and Yocom 1987).

### HEALTH EFFECTS

To date, studies on the health effects of exposure to $NO_2$ in indoor air have only addressed exposure in the home environment. Most of these studies have focused on respiratory symptoms and illnesses and on the level of pulmonary function.

Experimental investigations support the choice of these outcome measures; $NO_2$ may damage the lung directly through its oxidant properties or indirectly by increasing susceptibility to respiratory infections (NRC 1976; Jakab 1980).

Data on the health effects of $NO_2$ concentrations likely to be encountered by the general population are derived from experimental and epidemiologic studies. The results of some human exposure studies imply that levels comparable to those measured in homes may increase the level of airways reactivity in some asthmatics, but the results of other studies are inconsistent (Orehek et al. 1976; Bauer et al. 1984; Morrow 1984; Bromberg 1988). Although experimental studies are useful for describing effects of acute exposures in specific populations, they cannot address the issue of chronic effects from chronic lower level exposures. Numerous epidemiologic investigations that provide evidence on the health effects of $NO_2$ in indoor environments have now been carried out.

The majority of these investigations are cross-sectional surveys of school-children (Tables 7.1 and 7.2). The investigators generally assessed current symptom status and retrospective illness histories, as obtained by parent-completed questionnaire, and pulmonary function. Although $NO_2$ levels were measured in several of the investigations (Florey et al. 1979; Melia et al. 1982; Fischer et al. 1985), exposure was most often assessed by simple questions concerning type of fuel used for cooking. Consistent evidence of excess respiratory symptoms and illnesses in children exposed to gas stoves has not been demonstrated (Table 7.1).

Early reports from two cross-sectional surveys of schoolchildren in Great Britain indicated that children from homes with gas stoves had a higher prevalence of respiratory symptoms than children from homes with electric stoves (Melia et al. 1977; Melia, Florey, and Chinn 1979). When one of the survey groups was followed longitudinally, however, the relative risks associated with gas stove use became highly variable and tended to decrease as the children grew older (Melia, Florey, and Chinn 1979). These same British investigators surveyed a third group of 808 schoolchildren and measured $NO_2$ concentrations in the homes of a small sample ($N = 80$ or 103). The prevalence of respiratory symptoms was higher in children from homes in which gas was used for cooking and increased with higher bedroom $NO_2$ concentrations although both effects were of borderline statistical significance (Florey et al. 1979). A similar association between measured $NO_2$ and respiratory symptoms was not replicated, however, when these same investigators subsequently studied another sample of 183 children (Melia et al. 1982). Two prospective studies of infants in Great Britain also failed to demonstrate an association between the use of gas for cooking and respiratory illness (Melia et al. 1983; Ogston, Florey, and Walker 1985).

Data on children from the United States are similarly inconsistent. Two large cross-sectional studies, one involving the Harvard Six-Cities study (Speizer et al. 1980a, 1980b) and the other involving schoolchildren in Iowa (Ekwo et al. 1983), have demonstrated that reports of serious respiratory illness before age two (Speizer et al. 1980a, 1980b) and hospitalization for respiratory illness before age two (Ekwo et al. 1983) were more common among children from homes with gas

Table 7.1    Effects of Gas Cooking on Respiatory Illnesses and Symptoms in Children

| Study Population | Outcome Measure | Results |
|---|---|---|
| *British Studies* | | |
| 5,758 children, aged 6–11 years, England and Scotland (Melia et al. 1977) | Major respiratory symptoms and diseases individually and as a single composite variable describing the presence of any one of six symptoms or diseases | Significant associations with gas cooking of selected symptoms and diseases, and of a composite variable |
| 2,408 children, 42% of original 5,758 in above study (Melia, Florey, and Chinn 1979) | Single composite variable as described above | Relative risk for composite variable generally exceeded 1.0; risk varied and decreased with age |
| 4,827 children, ages 5–11 years, England and Scotland (Melia, Florey, and Chinn 1979) | Single composite variable as described above | Significant effect of gas stoves on composite variable in urban areas only |
| 808 children, aged 6–7 years, United Kingdom (Florey et al. 1979) | Single composite variable as described above | Borderline significant association between composite variable and gas stoves; increased prevalence as bedroom $NO_2$ levels increased in a sample with measurements ($N = 80$) |
| 191 children, aged 5–6 years, England (Melia et al. 1982) | Single composite variable as described above | No significant association between bedroom $NO_2$ levels and prevalence of composite variable |
| 390 infants, aged 0–1 years, England (Melia et al. 1983) | Respiratory illnesses and symptoms requiring physician visits, assessed prospectively | No association between gas stove use and respiratory illnesses and symptoms |
| 1,565 infants, aged 0–1 years, England (Ogston, Florey, and Walker 1985) | Respiratory illnesses and hospitalizations assessed prospectively to 1 year | No significant association between illness or hospitalizations and use of gas for cooking |
| *Ohio Studies* | | |
| 441 upper-middle-class families including 898 children under age 16 (Keller et al. 1979a) | Incidence of acute respiratory illness, determined by biweekly telephone calls | Respiratory illness incidence similar in homes using gas and electric stoves |
| 120 families from first study, including 176 children under age 12 (Keller et al. 1979b) | Incidence of acute respiratory illness, determined by biweekly telephone calls and validated by home visits | Respiratory illness incidence similar in homes using gas and electric stoves |
| *Harvard Six-Cities Study* | | |
| 8,120 children, aged 6–10 years, six U.S. cities (Speizer et al. 1980a, | History of physician-diagnosed bronchitis or serious respiratory illness | Significant association between current use of gas stove and history of res- |

(*continued*)

Table 7.1  (*Continued*)

| Study Population | Outcome Measure | Results |
|---|---|---|
| 1980b) | before age 2 or respira-tory illness in last year | piratory illness before age 2; odds ratio = 1.23 |
| 10,106 children, aged 6–10 years, six U.S. cities; expansion of above study (Ware et al. 1984) | Same as above | Odds ratio for history of respiratory illness before age 2 decreased to 1.2; $p = .07$) |
| 6,273 children, six U.S. cities, 1983–86 sample (Dockery et al. 1987) | Same as above, and chronic cough and per-sistent wheeze | No significant associations; odds ratio for respiratory illness before age 2 years was 1.09; 95% CI[a] 0.89, 1.33 |
| *Other Studies* | | |
| 676 children, third and fourth grades, Arizona (Dodge 1982) | Prevalence of asthma, wheeze, sputum, cough as determined by parent-completed questionnaire | Significant association be-tween use of gas stove and prevalence of cough; prevalence rate ratio = 1.97 |
| 4,071 children, aged 5–14 years, Pennsylvania (Schenker, Samet, and Speizer 1983) | Major respiratory illnesses and symptoms as deter-mined by parent-completed questionnaire | No significant association between use of gas stove and any symptom or ill-ness variable |
| 1,138 children, aged 6–12 years, Iowa (Ekwo et al. 1983) | Major respiratory symp-toms and illnesses as de-termined by parent-completed questionnaire | Significant association be-tween current gas stove use and hospitalization for respiratory illness be-fore age 2; odds ratio = 2.4 |
| 121 children, aged 0–13 years, Connecticut (Ber-wick et al. 1984) | Number of days of illness | Number of days of illness associated with average hours of space heater use |
| 231 children, aged 6 years, The Netherlands (Hoek et al. 1984) | Comparison of $NO_2$ levels in homes of cases (children with asthma) and controls | $NO_2$ distributions similar in homes of cases and con-trols |

[a]Confidence interval.

stoves. When the original cohort in the Harvard six-cities study was expanded, however, the odds ratio of 1.23 for serious respiratory illness before age two decreased to 1.12 ($p = 0.07$). More recently, the Harvard group enrolled a new sample of preadolescent children ($N = 6,273$) in the same six cities (Dockery et al. 1987). In this new population of children, exposure to a gas stove was not signifi-cantly associated with any respiratory symptoms or doctor-diagnosed chest illness before age two years. In the Iowa study (Ekwo et al. 1983), the effect of exposure to a gas stove varied strongly and inconsistently with parental smoking habits. The effect was absent in homes where one parent smoked, largest where both parents smoked, and intermediate where neither smoked. This pattern of interaction can-not be readily interpreted biologically. Schenker and colleagues (Schenker, Samet, and Speizer 1983) found no association between the type of cooking stove and

Table 7.2    Effects of Gas Cooking on Lung Function in Children

| Study Population | Lung Function Measure | Results |
|---|---|---|
| 808 children, aged 6–7 years, United Kingdom (Florey et al. 1979) | PEFR, $FEV_{0.75}$, $FEF_{25-75}$ | No association with $NO_2$ levels or presence of gas stove |
| 898 children, aged 0–15 years, from 441 families, Ohio (Keller et al. 1979a) | FVC, $FEV_{0.75}$ | Data on children not presented separately; no association with presence of a gas stove |
| 8,120 children, aged 6–10 years, six U.S. cities (Speizer et al. 1980a, 1980b) | FVC, $FEV_1$ | Overall reduction of 16 and 18 ml, respectively, for $FEV_1$ and FVC in children from homes with gas stoves |
| 16,689 children, aged 6–13 years, seven areas in U.S. (Hasselblad et al. 1981) | $FEV_{0.75}$ | Significant reduction of 19 ml associated with gas stove use in older girls only |
| 676 children, third and fourth grades, Arizona (Dodge 1982) | $FEV_1$ | No effect of gas stoves on pulmonary level or rate of growth |
| 183 children, aged 6–12 years, Iowa (Ekwo et al. 1983) | $FEV_1$, $FEF_{75}$, $FEF_{25-75}$ | No change after isoproterenol challenge in children from homes with gas stoves |
| 9,720 children, aged 6–10 years, six U.S. cities (Ware et al. 1984) | $FEV_1$, FVC | Significant reduction in $FEV_1$, of 0.6% and FVC of 0.7%; not significant after adjustment for parental education |
| 3,175 children, aged 5–14 years, Pennsylvania (Vedal et al. 1984) | FVC, $FEV_{0.75}$, $FEF_{25-75}$, $\dot{V}_{max\ 75}$, $\dot{V}_{max\ 90}$ | No association with use of gas stove |

current respiratory symptoms or previous illness history in a cross-sectional survey of 4,071 schoolchildren in western Pennsylvania.

The relationship between stove type and respiratory illness has also been studied prospectively. Keller and colleagues (Keller et al. 1979a, 1979b), in a study of 1,952 family members of all ages in Ohio, found that respiratory illness incidence did not vary with stove type. More recently, Berwick and co-workers (Berwick et al. 1984) followed 121 children for three months, 59 from homes with kerosene heaters and 62 from homes without such heaters. In a preliminary analysis of their data, they found that hours of heater use, which correlated strongly ($r = .70$) with one-week integrated $NO_2$ measurements, was significantly associated with the occurrence of illness lasting for one or more days.

The data concerned with lung function level in children are similarly inconclusive (Table 7.2). Of the four investigations with large sample sizes (Speizer et al. 1980a; Hasselblad et al. 1981; Vedal et al. 1984; Ware et al. 1984), two have demonstrated small but statistically significant effects of exposure to a gas stove (Speizer et al. 1980a; Hasselblad et al. 1981). In initial cross-sectional analysis of data from the Harvard Six-Cities Study, Speizer and co-workers (Speizer et al. 1980a) demonstrated average reductions, adjusted for parental smoking and socioeconomic status, of 16 and 18 ml in the $FEV_1$ and the FVC, respectively, in children from homes with gas stoves compared with children from homes with electric stoves. On expansion of the cohort, however, the reductions in $FEV_1$ and FVC, although still statistically significant, were 0.6 percent of predicted for the former and 0.7 percent for the latter (Ware et al. 1984). With adjustment for parental education, the effects of exposure to a gas stove were reduced by 30 percent and were no longer statistically significant. Cross-sectional analysis of lung function data collected at the children's second examination did not show significant effects of stove type. With extension of the follow-up interval the investigators assessed determinants of pulmonary function growth and found no effect of gas stove exposure (Berkey et al. 1986).

Hasselblad and colleagues (Hasselblad et al. 1981) analyzed data from the Environmental Protection Agency's Community Health Environmental Surveillance System. They reported that in girls ages nine to thirteen years gas stove exposure decreased $FEV_{0.75}$ by an average of 18 ml after adjustment for parental educational level and smoking status. An effect was not observed in girls ages six to eight years nor in boys ages six to thirteen years.

In another large cross-sectional study, Vedal and colleagues (Vedal et al. 1984) examined the effects of stove type on spirometric volumes and flow rates in a sample of 3,175 children ages five to fourteen years. With adjustment for parental smoking and socioeconomic status, exposure to a gas stove was not significantly associated with reduced lung function level.

The effects of gas stove exposure on lung function level were assessed in five other investigations, but the sample sizes were inadequate for detecting effects of the magnitude found in the larger studies. Keller and co-workers (Keller et al. 1979a) performed spirometry on one occasion in a sample of the subjects in their surveillance study. The data were not reported separately for children, and overall there was no effect of stove type. In one of the cross-sectional surveys conducted in Great Britain, the investigators correlated lung function level with one-week measurements of $NO_2$ in the kitchen and in the children's bedrooms (Florey et al. 1979). With a sample of about four hundred children, significant effects of $NO_2$ were not found. Dodge (1982) and Ekwo and colleagues (Ekwo et al. 1983) did not find effects of stove type on lung function measures in their cross-sectional studies. Hosein and Corey (1984) examined the influence of nine indoor factors on $FEV_1$ in 1,357 nonsmoking white children from three U.S. towns. Their preliminary report indicated that exposure to gas stoves was significantly associated with a 0.148-liter reduction in $FEV_1$ level in boys and a 0.75-liter reduction in girls.

Only a few investigations provide data on acute and chronic effects of $NO_2$ exposure indoors on adults (Table 7.3). Prospective studies of acute respiratory illness occurrence have not demonstrated excesses in residents of homes with gas stoves (Keller et al. 1979a, 1979b; Love et al. 1982). Cigarette smoking and chronic respiratory diseases, potential confounding variables, were not considered in these studies.

Potential chronic effects have also been examined in populations of adults (Table 7.3). Comstock and co-workers (Comstock et al. 1981) reported that gas stove use

Table 7.3  Effects of Gas Cooking on Pulmonary Illness, Symptoms,
and Function of Adults

| Study Population | Outcome Measure | Results |
| --- | --- | --- |
| 441 upper-middle-class families, including 1,054 adults over 15 years, Ohio (Keller et al. 1979a) | Incidence of acute respiratory illness, determined by biweekly telephone calls | Respiratory illness incidence similar in homes using gas and electric stoves |
| 120 families from first study, including 269 adults over 18 years, Ohio (Keller et al. 1979b) | Incidence of acute respiratory illness, determined by biweekly telephone calls and validated by home visit | Respiratory illness incidence similar in homes with gas and electric stoves |
| 1,724 adults, aged >20 years, Maryland (Comstock et al. 1981) | Major chronic respiratory symptoms, $FEV_1$, FVC | Association between gas stove use and increased prevalence of respiratory symptoms, $FEV_1$ <80% predicted, $FEV_1/FVC$ <70%, found in nonsmoking males only |
| 708 adults, aged >20 years; nonsmoking sample of above population (Helsing et al. 1982) | Major chronic respiratory symptoms, $FEV_1$, FVC | Significant association between gas stove use and increased prevalence of chronic cough and phlegm, low $FEV_1/FVC$ |
| 102 nonsmoking women in lowest quartile of $FEV_1$ compared with 103 nonsmoking women in highest quartile, Michigan (Jones et al. 1983) | Comparison of proportions of cases and controls currently using gas stoves | Marginal association between use of gas stove and lower lung function; odds ratio = 1.8, $p$ = .08 |
| 97 nonsmoking adult females, Netherlands (Fischer et al. 1985) | IVC, FEV, FVC, PEF, $MEF_{75}$, $MEF_{25}$, MMEF | Cross-sectional analysis showed an association between current $NO_2$ exposure and decreases in most pulmonary function measures; no association with longitudinal decline in pulmonary function |

was associated with a significantly increased prevalence of certain chronic respiratory symptoms and of ventilatory impairment in nonsmoking men but not in smoking men or in women of either smoking status. A subsequent reanalysis limited to the never and former smokers showed significant increases in chronic cough and phlegm and in the prevalence of low $FEV_1/FVC$ in association with gas stove use in both sexes (Helsing et al. 1982).

In a study of ninety-seven nonsmoking rural women from The Netherlands, personal exposure estimates were created by combining one-week measurements of $NO_2$ with time-activity information (Remijn et al. 1985). The investigators demonstrated a cross-sectional association between lung function level and current $NO_2$ exposure but failed to show an association between retrospectively estimated exposure to $NO_2$ and longitudinal decline in pulmonary function during the antecedent seventeen years (Fischer et al. 1985).

Using a case-control design, Jones and coworkers (Jones et al. 1983) compared cooking fuel exposures of twenty- to thirty-nine-year-old nonsmoking women in the highest and lowest quartiles of the lung function distribution in the Tecumseh community health study, a longitudinal study of health in Tecumseh, Michigan. The odds ratio for the effect of cooking with gas compared with electric appliances on lung function level was 1.82 ($p = .076$).

Lebowitz and colleagues (Lebowitz 1984; Lebowitz et al. 1982, 1985) have evaluated acute effects of gas stove exposure on lung function and symptoms in 229 subjects drawn from 117 Tucson households. The families were sampled from a larger study population to include persons with and without asthma, allergies, and airway obstruction. During a two-year period, subjects completed symptom diaries and monitored their peak flow daily. Multivariate analyses indicated adverse effects of gas stoves on symptoms and peak flow rate in asthmatics but not in normal subjects (Lebowitz et al. 1985). However, the magnitude of the effect is difficult to determine from the available publications.

Recently, Kasuga and colleagues (Kasuga 1985) proposed that the urinary hydroxyproline to creatinine ratio is a valid and sensitive indicator of lung damage from environmental pollutants, including tobacco smoke and $NO_2$. Hydroxyproline, an amino acid constituent of collagen, is a product of collagen catabolism; therefore, an increase in its excretion reflects an increase in collagen destruction.

Matsuki and co-workers (Matsuki et al. 1984, 1985) conducted a cross-sectional study of 820 schoolchildren and their 546 mothers during both a summer and a winter period. They measured subjects' twenty-four-hour personal $NO_2$ exposures with filter badges and collected early morning urine samples for evaluation of the hydroxyproline to creatinine ratio. In multiple regression equations, passive smoking status and personal $NO_2$ were independent and significant predictors of this ratio in both schoolchildren and adult women in both seasons. Distance from a main road, as a surrogate for exposure to automobile exhaust, was found to be a stronger predictor of the ratio in summer than in winter in schoolchildren and a predictor only during the summer in adult women. A linear relationship was also found between the value of the ratio and the amount of passive exposure to tobacco smoke. Other studies, however, have not shown relationships of the hydroxyproline to creatinine ratio with either passive exposure to tobacco smoke (Adlkofer, Scherer, and Heller 1984) or with active smoking (Read and Thornton 1985). Although the hydroxyproline to creatinine ratio could serve as a useful biochemical indicator of lung injury by $NO_2$ exposure, further investigations are needed to clarify ambiguities in the available data.

### SUMMARY

Definitive statements concerning the risk of $NO_2$ exposure from cooking with gas stoves and other indoor sources cannot be made at present. Although many studies have examined respiratory illnesses, respiratory symptoms, and lung function in children and adults, their results are not consistent and are not adequate for establishing a causal relationship. Retrospective illness histories may be inaccurate, and their results may be biased by whether the subjects have symptoms or illness at the time of their interview (Samet, Tager, and Speizer 1983). Variations in the characteristics of the study populations and differing end points may partly explain the differences among the studies. Confidence limits have not been uniformly presented in the studies on gas stoves, and the results of many of the smaller studies which have been judged as negative are probably consistent with the larger studies that show small effects.

Unfortunately, $NO_2$ exposures were measured directly in only a few investigations (Florey et al. 1979; Melia et al. 1982; Hoek et al. 1984; Fischer et al. 1985), and in all of these the measurements spanned at most two-week periods. In the other studies, categorical variables, indicating gas or electric stove use, were employed. However, neither limited area measurements nor variables for stove type tightly predict actual personal exposure (Spengler et al. 1983). Thus, the results of all the investigations of the health effects of $NO_2$ exposure from gas stoves are affected by random misclassification. This type of bias reduces the magnitude of the observed association from the value that would be found if the exposure of subjects was estimated correctly (Shy et al. 1978). Ozkaynak and colleagues (Ozkaynak et al. 1984) have shown that misclassification introduced by the use of a categorical variable for stove type may introduce substantial underestimation of the true relative risk values associated with the actual $NO_2$ exposure.

Bias from inadequate control of confounding factors must also be considered in interpreting the foregoing studies (Vedal 1985). Confounding occurs when the effect of one variable on the outcome of interest has not been separated from the effects of other variables. For example, maternal smoking has been associated with reduced lung function level in children. Confounding by maternal smoking could arise in a particular study if mothers of infants living in homes with gas stoves were more likely to smoke. With regard to $NO_2$ exposure from gas stoves and effects on respiratory illnesses and symptoms, and pulmonary function in children, the potential confounding variables include parental smoking, socioeconomic status, and asthma. Active smoking, occupational exposures, and the presence of chronic respiratory diseases should also be considered in adults. Control of these potentially confounding factors has been variable among published studies (Vedal 1985), and in some studies socioeconomic status has been treated as a confounding factor. However, the effect of socioeconomic status represents a summation of the effects of the associated environmental and familial factors, one of which may be gas stove exposure. Thus, control for socioeconomic status may reduce the likelihood of finding an effect of gas stove exposure.

The findings on $NO_2$ exposure and respiratory illnesses indicate that the magnitude of the $NO_2$ effect at concentrations encountered in most U.S. homes is likely to be small. Groups with particularly high exposures, such as the urban poor who heat with ovens and those who heat their homes with unvented kerosene or gas space heaters, have not yet been investigated adequately. The evidence on respiratory symptoms and lung function level in children and adults is also inconclusive. However, because more than half of U.S. homes have gas cooking stoves and childhood respiratory illness is extremely common, even a small effect of gas stoves would assume public health importance. In order to detect associations of the anticipated small magnitude, future investigations should employ direct measurement of exposure rather than surrogate variables. Infants and other potentially susceptible groups seem the most suitable populations for study. Nevertheless, the epidemiologic evidence implies that clinically relevant effects of $NO_2$ from gas stoves are uncommon at the concentrations found in most U.S. homes.

## REFERENCES

Adlkofer, F.; Scherer, G.; and Heller, W. D. 1984. Hydroxyproline excretion in urine of smokers and passive smokers. *Prev. Med.* 13:670–79.

Bauer, M. A., et al. 1984. 0.30 ppm nitrogen dioxide inhalation potentiates exercise-induced bronchospasm in asthmatics. *Am. Rev. Respir. Dis.* 129 (suppl):151 (abstr.).

Berkey, C. S., et al. 1986. Indoor air pollution and pulmonary function growth in preadolescent children. *Am. J. Epidemiol.* 123:250–60.

Berwick, M., et al. 1984. Respiratory illness in children exposed to unvented combustion sources. In *Indoor air, Vol. 2: Radon, passive smoking, particulates and housing epidemiology.* Ed. B. Berglund, T. Lindvall, and J. Sundell, 255–60. Stockhom: Swedish Council for Building Research.

Bromberg, P. A. 1988. Asthma and automotive emissions. In *Air pollution, the automobile and public health.* Ed. A. Y. Watson, R. R. Bates, and D. Kennedy, 465–98. Washington, D.C.: National Academy Press.

Buckley, R. D., and Loosli, C. G. 1969. Effects of nitrogen dioxide inhalation on germ free mouse lung. *Arch. Environ. Health* 18:588–95.

Comstock, G. W., et al. 1981. Respiratory effects of household exposures to tobacco smoke and gas cooking. *Am. Rev. Respir. Dis.* 124:143–48.

Dawson, S. V., and Schenker, M. B. 1979. Health effects of inhalation of ambient concentrations of nitrogen dioxide (editorial). *Am. Rev. Respir. Dis.* 120:281–92.

Dockery, D. W., et al. 1987. Associations of health status with indicators of indoor air pollution from an epidemiologic study in six U.S. cities. In *Indoor air '87, Vol. 2: Environmental tobacco smoke, multicomponent studies, radon, sick buildings, odours and irritants, hyperreactivities and allergies.* Ed. B. Seifert, et al., 203–7. Berlin: Institute for Water, Soil, and Air Hygiene.

Dodge, R. 1982. The effects of indoor pollution on Arizona children. *Arch. Environ. Health* 37:151–55.

Ekwo, E. E., et al. 1983. Relationship of parental smoking and gas cooking to respiratory disease in children. *Chest* 84:662–68.

Fenters, J. D., et al. 1973. Chronic exposure to nitrogen dioxide: Immunologic, physiologic, and pathologic effects in virus-challenged squirrel monkeys. *Arch. Environ. Health* 27:85–89.

Fischer, P., et al. 1985. Indoor air pollution and its effect on pulmonary function of adult non-smoking women, II: Associations between nitrogen dioxide and pulmonary function. *Int. J. Epidemiol.* 14:221–26.

Florey, C. V., et al. 1979. The relation between respiratory illness in primary school-children and the use of gas for cooking, III: Nitrogen dioxide, respiratory illness and lung function. *Int. J. Epidemiol.* 8:347–53.

Gardner, D. E. 1984. Oxidant-induced enhanced sensitivity to infection in animal models and their extrapolations to man. *J. Toxicol. Environ. Health* 13:423–39.

Gardner, D. E., et al. 1982. Non-respiratory function of the lungs: Host defenses against infection. In *Air pollution by nitrogen oxides.* Ed. T. Schneider and L. Grant, 401–15. New York: Elsevier.

Goldstein, E., et al. 1980. Absorption and transport of nitrogen oxides. In *Nitrogen oxides and their effects on health.* Ed. S. D. Lee, 143–60. Ann Arbor, Mich.: Ann Arbor Science.

Hasselblad, V., et al. 1981. Indoor environmental determinants of lung function in children. *Am. Rev. Respir. Dis.* 123:479–85.

Helsing, K. J., et al. 1982. Respiratory effects of household exposure to tobacco smoke and gas cooking on nonsmokers. *Environ. Int.* 8:365–70.

Henry, M. C., et al. 1970. Chronic toxicity of $NO_2$ in squirrel monkeys. *Arch. Environ. Health.* 20:566–70.

Hoek, G., et al. 1984. Indoor $NO_2$ and respiratory symptoms of Rotterdam children. In *Indoor air, Vol. 3: Sensory and hyperreactivity reactions to sick buildings.* Ed. B. Berglund, T. Lindvall, and J. Sundell, 227–32. Stockholm: Swedish Council for Building Research.

Hosein, H. R., and Corey, P. 1984. Multivariate analyses of nine indoor factors on $FEV_1$ of Caucasian children (abstract). *Am. Rev. Respir. Dis.* 129(Suppl.):A140.

Jakab, G. J. 1980. Nitrogen dioxide-induced susceptibility to acute respiratory illness: A perspective. *Bull. N.Y. Acad. Med.* 56:847–56.

Jones, J. R., et al. 1983. Effects of cooking fuels on lung function in nonsmoking women. *Arch. Environ. Health* 38:219–22.

Kasuga, H. 1985. A review of urinary hydroxyproline as a biochemical marker on health effects of smoking and air pollution with nitrogen dioxide. *Tokai J. Exp. Clin. Med.* 10:439–44.

Keller, M. D., et al. 1979a. Respiratory illness in households using gas and electricity for cooking, I: Survey of incidence. *Environ. Res.* 19:495–503.

Keller, M. D., et al. 1979b. Respiratory illness in households using gas and electricity for cooking, II: Symptoms and objective findings. *Environ. Res.* 19:504–15.

Leaderer, B. P. 1982. Air pollutant emissions from kerosene space heaters. *Science* 218:1113–15.

Leaderer, B. P., et al. 1987. Predicting $NO_2$ levels in residences based upon source use: A multivariate model. *Atmos. Environ.* 21:361–68.

Lebowitz, M. D. 1984. The effects of environmental tobacco smoke exposure and gas stoves on daily peak flow rates in asthmatic and nonasthmatic families. *Eur. J. Respir. Dis.* 65(Suppl. 133):90–97.

Lebowitz, M. D., et al. 1982. The adverse health effects of biological aerosols, other aerosols, and indoor microclimate on asthmatics and nonasthmatics. *Environ. Int.* 8:375–80.

Lebowitz, M. D., et al. 1985. Respiratory symptoms and peak-flow associated with indoor and outdoor air pollutants in the Southwest. *J. Air Pollut. Control Assoc.* 35:1154–58.

Lefkowitz, S. S.; McGrath, J. J.; and Lefkowitz, D. L. 1986. Effects of $NO_2$ on immune responses. *J. Toxicol. Environ. Health* 17:241–48.

Love, G. J., et al. 1982. Acute respiratory illness in families exposed to nitrogen dioxide ambient air pollution in Chattanooga, Tennessee. *Arch. Environ. Health* 37:75–80.

Lowry, T., and Schuman, L. M. 1956. "Silo-filler's disease": A syndrome caused by nitrogen dioxide. *JAMA* 162:153–60.

Marbury, M. C., et al. 1988. Indoor residential NO$_2$ concentrations in Albuquerque, New Mexico. *J. Air Pollut. Control Assoc.* 38:392–98.

Matsuki, H., et al. 1984. Personal exposure to NO$_2$ and its health effect with urinary hydroxyproline to creatinine ratio as biochemical indicator. In *Indoor air, Vol. 2: Radon, passive smoking, particulates and housing epidemiology.* Ed. B. Berglund, T. Lindvall, and J. Sundell, 243–48. Stockholm: Swedish Council for Building Research.

Matsuki, H., et al. 1985. A comparative study on the health effects of smoking and indoor air pollution in summer and winter. *Tokai J. Exp. Clin. Med.* 10:427–37.

McCarthy, S. M.; Yarmac, R. F.; and Yocom, J. E. 1987. Indoor nitrogen dioxide exposure: The contribution from unvented gas space heaters. In *Indoor air '87, Vol. 1: Volatile organic compounds, combustion gases, particles and fibres, microbiological agents.* Ed. B. Seifert et al., 478–82. Berlin: Institute for Water, Soil and Air Hygiene.

Melia, R. J.; Florey, C. V.; and Chinn, S. 1979. The relation between respiratory illness in primary schoolchildren and the use of gas for cooking, I: Results from a national survey. *Int. J. Epidemiol.* 8:333–38.

Melia, R. J., et al. 1977. Association between gas cooking and respiratory disease in children. *Br. Med. J.* 2:149–52.

Melia, R. J., et al. 1982. Childhood respiratory illness and the home environment, II: Association between respiratory illness and nitrogen dioxide, temperature and relative humidity. *Int. J. Epidemiol.* 11:164–69.

Melia, R. J., et al. 1983. The relation between respiratory illness in infants and gas cooking in the UK: A preliminary report. *Proceedings of the sixth world congress on air quality, 16–20 August,* 263–69. Paris: International Union of Air Pollution Prevention Associations.

Miller, F. J., et al. 1982. Pulmonary dosimetry of nitrogen dioxide in animals and man. In *Air pollution by nitrogen oxides.* Ed. T. Schneider and L. Grant, 377–86. New York: Elsevier.

Miller, F. J., et al. 1987. Evaluating the toxicity of urban patterns of oxidant gases, II: Effects in mice from chronic exposure to nitrogen dioxide. *J. Toxicol. Environ. Health* 21:99–112.

Mochitate, K., et al. 1986. Activation and increment of alveolar macrophages induced by nitrogen dioxide. *J. Toxicol. Environ. Health* 17:229–39.

Morrow, P. E. 1984. Toxicological data on NO$_2$: An overview. *J. Toxicol. Environ. Health* 13:205–27.

Mustafa, M. G., and Tierney, D. F. 1978. Biochemical and metabolic changes in the lung with oxygen, ozone, and nitrogen dioxide toxicity. *Am. Rev. Respir. Dis.* 118:1061–90.

National Research Council (committee on medical and biologic effects of environmental pollutants, subcommittee on nitrogen oxides). 1976. *Nitrogen oxides.* Washington, D.C.: National Academy of Sciences.

National Research Council (committee on indoor pollutants). 1981. *Indoor pollutants.* Washington, D.C.: National Academy Press.

Ogston, S. A.; Florey, C. V., and Walker, C. H. 1985. The Tayside infant morbidity and mortality study: Effect on health of using gas for cooking. *Br. Med. J.* 290:957–60.

Orehek, J., et al. 1976. Effect of short-term, low level nitrogen dioxide exposure on bronchial sensitivity of asthmatic patients. *J. Clin. Invest.* 57:301–7.

Overton, J. H., and Miller, F. J. 1988. Dosimetry modeling of inhaled toxic reactive gases. In *Air pollution, the automobile and public health.* Ed. A. Y. Watson, R. R. Bates, and D. Kennedy, 367–85. Washington, D.C.: National Academy Press.

Ozkaynak, H., et al. 1984. Bias due to misclassification of personal exposures in epidemiologic studies of indoor and outdoor air pollution. Presented at the Air Pollution Control Association and American Society for Quality Control specialty conferences on quality assurance in air pollution measurements, 14–18 October, Boulder, Colorado.

Pennington, J. E. 1988. Effects of automotive emissions on susceptibility to respiratory infections. In *Air pollution, the automobile and public health.* Ed. A. Y. Watson, R. R. Bates, and D. Kennedy, 499–518. Washington, D.C.: National Academy Press.

Quackenboss, J. J., et al. 1982. Personal monitoring for nitrogen dioxide exposure: Methodological considerations for a community study. *Environ. Int.* 8:249–58.

Read, G. A., and Thornton, R. E. 1985. Preliminary studies of urinary hydroxyproline levels in rodents and in smokers. *Tokai J. Exp. Clin. Med.* 10:445–50.

Remijn, B., et al. 1985. Indoor air pollution and its effect on pulmonary function of adult non-smoking women, I: Exposure estimates for nitrogen dioxide and passive smoking. *Int. J. Epidemiol.* 14:215–20.

Samet, J. M.; Tager, I. B.; and Speizer, F. E. 1983. The relationship between respiratory illness in childhood and chronic airflow obstruction in adulthood. *Am. Rev. Respir. Dis.* 127:508–23.

Schenker, M. B.; Samet, J. M.; and Speizer, F. E. 1983. Risk factors for childhood respiratory disease: The effect of host factors and home environmental exposure. *Am. Rev. Respir. Dis.* 28:1038–43.

Sexton, K.; Letz, R.; and Spengler, J. D. 1983. Estimating human exposures to nitrogen dioxide: An indoor-outdoor modeling approach. *Environ. Res.* 32:151–66.

Shy, C. M., et al. 1978. Health effects of air pollution. *ATS News* 6:1–63.

Speizer, F. E., et al. 1980a. Respiratory disease rates and pulmonary function in children associated with $NO_2$ exposure. *Am. Rev. Respir. Dis.* 121:3–10.

Speizer, F. E., et al. 1980b. Health effects of indoor $NO_2$ exposure: Preliminary results. In *Nitrogen oxides and their effects on health.* Ed. S. D. Lee, 343–59. Ann Arbor, Mich.: Ann Arbor Science Publishers.

Spengler, J. D., and Sexton, K. 1983. Indoor air pollution: A public health perspective. *Science* 221:9–17.

Spengler, J. D., et al. 1983. Nitrogen dioxide inside and outside 137 homes and implications for ambient air quality standards and health effects research. *Environ. Sci. Technol.* 17:164–68.

Sterling, T. D.; Dimich, H.; and Kobayashi, D. 1981. Use of gas ranges for cooking and heating in urban dwellings. *J. Air Pollut. Control Assoc.* 32:162–65.

Traynor, G. W., et al. 1985. Indoor air pollution due to emissions from unvented gas-fired space heaters. *JAPCA* 35:231–37.

U.S. Bureau of the Census. 1983. *1980 Census of housing, Vol. 1: Characteristics of housing units, Ch. B: Detailed housing characteristics, Pt. 1: United States summary.* Washington, D.C.: Government Printing Office. Publication no. HC80-1-B1.

Vedal, S. 1985. Epidemiological studies of childhood illness and pulmonary function associated with gas stove use. In *Indoor air and human health.* Ed. R. B. Gammage and S. V. Kaye, 303–16. Chelsea, Mich.: Lewis Publishers.

Vedal, S., et al. 1984. Risk factors for childhood respiratory disease. *Am. Rev. Respir. Dis.* 130:187–92.

Ware, J. H., et al. 1984. Passive smoking, gas cooking, and respiratory health of children living in six cities. *Am. Rev. Respir. Dis.* 129:366–74.

Yocom, J. 1982. Indoor-outdoor air quality relationships: A critical review. *J. Air Pollut. Control Assoc.* 32:500–520.

# 8

# CARBON
# MONOXIDE

David B. Coultas, M.D.
William E. Lambert, Ph.D.

Carbon monoxide (CO) is a colorless, odorless gas produced by incomplete combustion of carbonaceous fuels such as wood, gasoline, and natural gas (National Research Council [NRC] 1977). Inhalation of CO, because of its marked affinity for hemoglobin, impairs oxygen transport and often manifests as adverse effects in the cardiovascular system and in the central nervous system. The severity of the health effects increases with the level and duration of exposure to CO.

Exposure to CO may be from outdoor and indoor sources with levels of exposure that vary widely from low concentrations with subtle effects to higher levels and acute poisoning. Although only few data are available on the overall public health impact of CO, it is a public health concern because of its many sources. In the United States, CO is a leading cause of death from poisoning (U.S. Department of Health and Human Services [DHHS] 1987), with an estimated 1,800 accidental deaths annually (U.S. Public Health Service [PHS] 1982). Many of these deaths have been associated with extreme exposures in indoor residential settings caused by faulty or improperly vented combustion appliances. The health effects of low-level exposures to CO are also considered an important public health problem because of the large population at risk.

In this chapter we review exposure to CO as an indoor air pollutant. However, since health data based directly on indoor exposures are limited, we have included information from outdoor exposures or experimental exposures which reflects levels of CO that may be found indoors. The pathophysiology of CO is presented in the first section. This is followed by a description of the sources and levels of exposure to CO. Finally, manifestations of CO intoxication and the health effects of exposures to low levels of CO are reviewed.

In its acute toxic action, CO can be conceptualized as an antimetabolite of oxygen. Inhaled CO binds strongly to hemoglobin in the pulmonary capillary bed; the resulting complex is called carboxyhemoglobin (COHb). The rate of absorption of CO is dependent on ventilatory volume, the hemoglobin content of the blood, the rate of diffusion across the alveolar membrane, the mean pulmonary capillary oxygen tension, and COHb levels in the pulmonary capillaries (Coburn, Forster, and Kane 1965). CO binds to hemoglobin with more than two hundred times the affinity of oxygen, thus effectively outcompeting oxygen for available binding sites on the heme groups. The health consequences of this binding are twofold. First, the oxygen-carrying capacity of the blood is directly reduced; and second, CO bound to one heme subunit induces an allosteric change that slows the dissociation of oxygen bound to any of the three other heme sites on the hemoglobin protein (Stryer 1975). Thus, the absolute oxygen-carrying capacity is reduced by displacement, and lower oxygen tensions are required to release oxygen bound to the hemoglobin (Figure 8.1). This leftward shift of the oxyhemoglobin dissociation curve is physiologically significant and explains the hypoxic differential between simple anemia and the equivalent percentage of COHb (Roughton and Darling 1944; Collier 1976).

In addition to the leftward shift of the oxyhemoglobin dissociation curve, several additional mechanisms of toxicity have been postulated. Ultimately, each is based upon competitive binding interactions and includes the binding of CO to heme proteins including myoglobin, cytochrome oxidase, tryptophan deoxygenase, and tryptophan catalase (Coburn 1979). For example, CO bound to myoglobin in the cardiac muscle could impair oxygen delivery to intracellular contractile processes. In the heart, the marked oxygen gradient from coronary blood to myocardial cells and the low tissue and intracellular oxygen tensions may promote significant CO binding even at relatively low blood COHb levels (Wittenberg 1970); however, experimental data are incomplete. The brain and spinal cord, another sensitive organ system, may be affected similarly.

Within the mitochondria, CO bound to cytochrome oxidase can be expected to interfere with electron transport. Flavoprotein prosthetic groups of the cytochrome enzymes contain iron in a porphyrin configuration that resembles hemoglobin. CO bound to cytochrome oxidase, the terminal oxidase in the system, would prevent the phosphorylation of adenosine diphosphate (ADP). Coburn (1979) observed that increased metabolism may reduce intracellular oxygen tensions and thereby promote CO binding although the affinity of CO for cytochrome oxidase is low at typical physiologic oxygen tensions. Although theoretically plausible, the experimental evidence to support this hypothesis remains limited.

It has been postulated that chronic exposure to CO may accelerate atherosclerotic processes by affecting cholesterol uptake in the arterial wall. Results from animal studies and *in vitro* data are conflicting (Astrup, Kjeldsen, and Wanstrup 1970; Theodore, O'Donnell, and Back 1971; Sarma et al. 1975; Armitage, Davies

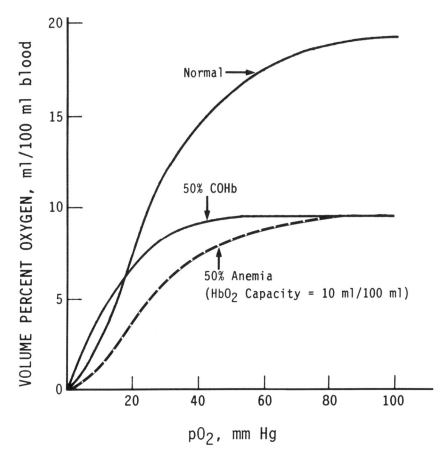

Figure 8.1. Oxyhemoglobin dissociation curves of normal human blood, of blood containing 50 percent COHb, and of blood with a 50 percent normal hemoglobin concentration due to anemia. *Source:* Reprinted from *Carbon Monoxide*, 1977, with permission from the National Academy of Sciences, Washington, D.C. (NRC, 1977).

and Turner 1976). Confident interpretation of this research is hampered by the high CO exposures and high dietary cholesterol employed in the animal studies and the methodologic difficulties in quantifying morphologic changes in the vessel walls. Limited evidence suggests that CO may accelerate clot lysis time (El-Attar and Sairo 1968) and may increase platelet activity and coagulation (Haft 1979). These alterations in the fibrinolytic system imply that CO could potentially increase risk for thromboembolism in the heart or brain.

There are many opportunities for exposure to CO in indoor environments because of the combustion sources placed or used in these settings. Approximately 47 percent of residences in the United States have gas ranges (U.S. Bureau of the Census 1983), a typically unvented source of combustion emissions. Another important unvented source is the kerosene or gas space heater, used in approximately seven percent of U.S. households (Cooper and Alberti 1984). Vented gas appliances, such as furnaces, water heaters, and clothes dryers, can emit CO into the indoor environment if not properly installed or maintained (Wharton et al. 1989). Similarly, improper use of charcoal cookers, wood-burning stoves or fireplaces, and gasoline engines can inject CO and other pollutants into the indoors. Intensive tobacco smoking in indoor locations may also result in CO buildup. The concentrations resulting from these sources are usually far below those that cause acute poisoning; however, the exposures may still be high enough to affect the blood, heart, and nervous systems adversely. In this section, poisonings and high-level exposure situations are discussed followed by presentation of low-level urban exposures in indoor settings.

ACUTE EXPOSURES AND POISONINGS

Investigations into the cause of poisoning accidents provide a *post facto* measure of the CO exposures experienced by the victims. Caplan et al. (1986) reported indoor residential CO concentrations ranging from 100 to 400 ppm. Invariably, evidence of a malfunctioning combustion appliance or tampering and misuse was discovered. Use of a gas range or oven for space heating may result in elevated indoor CO levels (Sterling, Dimich, and Kobayashi 1981) and predict symptomatic CO poisoning (Heckerling et al. 1987).

The U.S. Consumer Product Safety Commission (U.S. CPSC) estimates that 7.6 million unvented gas space heaters are in use in the United States, and directly attributes seventy deaths during 1980 to CO exposures resulting from the use of these heating devices in confined spaces (CPSC 1980). Although no measurements of the CO levels in these accidents were reported, it is known that kerosene space heater emissions are capable of increasing indoor CO concentrations to levels exceeding the eight-hour 9 ppm national primary ambient air quality standard (Cooper and Alberti 1984).

The elevated indoor CO concentrations causing poisonings may be expected to occur more often in the cold seasons when heating sources are in use and homes are kept closed to prevent heat loss. Indeed, CO poisonings in Korean residences were strongly correlated with ambient temperature, a surrogate measure of heating (Kim 1985). Many Korean homes are heated by a traditional system of charcoal briquets placed in pails beneath the flooring of the house. Carbon monoxide concentrations have not been reported for Korean homes. In the United States, poisonings associated with space heating are expected to occur more frequently in the winter. However, summertime poisonings associated with exposures in confined spaces can occur. These poisonings can be caused by the use of gas-fueled campstoves, lamps, and lanterns, radiant heaters, and electric generators in or near tents and recreational vehicles (New Mexico Environmental Improvement Agency 1977; Hopkinson, Pearce, and Oliver 1980). Spengler and Cohen (1985) estimated that CO levels as high as 100 ppm could accumulate in tents during gas campstove use.

LOW-LEVEL URBAN EXPOSURES

Substantial data are available on exposures of urban dwellers to CO in the course of their daily activities. The locations generally making the largest contributions to personal exposure are the auto and residence, but industrial buildings and commercial, institutional, and public buildings are frequent contributors. Early attempts at exposure assessment focused largely on vehicular and occupational exposures, but recent advances in instrumentation for exposure monitoring have facilitated monitoring large numbers of urban residents from population-based samples. Using this type of instrumentation, the U.S. Environmental Protection Agency has conducted studies of personal exposure of five hundred residents of Denver, Colorado, and of Washington, D.C. (Table 8.1) (Akland et al. 1985).

Exposures occurring in automobiles and outdoor settings provide an important reference against which indoor exposures may be compared. In fact, personal monitoring studies indicate that in the total daily exposure profile of urban residents, the highest exposures occur during commuting and when near active internal combustion engines (Akland et al. 1985). In-transit exposures average 5 ppm, and residents of Washington, D.C., and Denver were observed to spend an average of two hours per day in an automobile or bus or on a bicycle. Peak

Table 8.1   Range of Mean Concentrations Observed in Major Urban Environments in the Denver, Colorado, and Washington, D.C., CO Exposure Studies

| Environmental Setting | Mean CO Concentration (ppm) |
| --- | --- |
| Indoor | |
|   Residential | 1.2–1.7 |
|   Public buildings | |
|     Park garages and automobile service facilities | 10.4–18.8 |
|     Stores and service establishments | 2.5–3.0 |
|     Restaurants | 2.1–4.2 |
| Outdoor | |
|   Near active roadways | 2.6–3.8 |
|   Away from roadways, parks | <1.0 |
| In transit | |
|   In vehicle | 3.6–8.0 |
|   Walking or on bicycle | 2.4–4.2 |

*Soruce*: Adapted from Akland et al. (1985), with permission.

exposures of automobile occupants in heavy traffic may attain 50 ppm and average 10–12 ppm (Cortese and Spengler 1976; Flachsbart et al. 1987). Outdoor exposures to CO experienced near roadways and parking areas average 3–4 ppm (Hartwell et al. 1984).

Indoor exposures in residences and public places are generally low (Table 8.1). In the absence of indoor sources, mean indoor CO levels are usually equal to outdoor concentrations. If strong indoor sources are present, however, indoor levels can be severalfold higher than those outside the building. Because CO is an essentially nonreactive gas, removal by ventilation to outside air is the usual route of elimination from the indoor environment. Therefore, in buildings with low ventilation rates, CO may be retained near occupants for extended periods. Residential exposures in Washington, D.C., and Denver during the winter of 1982–83 averaged less than 2 ppm (Hartwell et al. 1984; Johnson 1984; Akland et al. 1985). In Washington, D.C., no significant difference was observed between mean CO levels in residences with an unvented gas stove and in residences with no gas stove when mean levels were integrated over total time spent indoors in the residence (Akland et al. 1985). However, mean personal exposure during cooking activities with a gas stove was higher than those experienced with an electric range and averaged 3 ppm (Hartwell et al. 1984). Similarly, mean hourly CO levels in the kitchens and living rooms of Dutch homes in which unvented gas stoves and infusion water heaters were in use ranged from 1 to 40 ppm, with mean levels of 1–3 ppm (Lebret 1985); however, anecdotal accounts of exposures experienced during the use of gas stoves for space heating describe indoor concentrations ranging from 25 to 50 ppm (Coburn 1979). In general, cigarette smoking contributes little to indoor CO levels (Sterling, Dimich, and Kobayashi 1982; Lebret 1985).

Exposures to CO in public buildings averaged 2–4 ppm in the Washington, D.C., and Denver studies (Akland et al. 1985). Highest mean personal exposures were observed in indoor parking garage locations and averaged 10–18 ppm. Average personal exposures in restaurants averaged 2–4 ppm, and stores and shopping malls averaged 2–3 ppm. Higher indoor levels, averaging 12 ppm and exceeding the eight-hour federal standard of 9 ppm, have been measured in a Honolulu shopping mall with an attached garage (Flachsbart and Brown 1985); this result has important implications for employees and shoppers who spend long periods of time in malls of this architectural design. Some office building settings have been associated with chronically high CO levels. Workers in an underground office located on the same level as an enclosed parking garage experienced mean exposures in the range of 12–22 ppm, with peak exposures to 34 ppm (Wallace 1983). Proper use of garage fans and closure of fire doors leading to the parking garage lowered office concentrations to 5 ppm. Thus, indoor CO levels may accumulate if ventilation systems are operated at low flow rates to reduce energy costs.

Indoor exposures to CO, included under the larger classification of urban exposure, may also be evaluated in terms of the resulting COHb levels. As part of the

1976–80 National Health and Nutrition Examination Survey, more than 8,000 blood samples were analyzed for COHb content and classified according to demographic and personal characteristics (Radford and Drizd 1982). Wintertime mean COHb concentration in never smokers aged twelve to seventy-four years living in urban areas was 1.25 percent. More than 4 percent of nonsmoking adults had levels greater than 2.5 percent; however, the source of exposure could not be identified. Children aged three to eleven years, considered to represent a group not exposed from occupational sources and personal tobacco use, had mean COHb levels of 1.01 percent during the winter months; however, their exposures during transportation may be lower than those of adults. Wintertime COHb levels were substantially higher in the three- to eleven-year-old subgroup than in the adult group; 3.3 percent of the children had a COHb level in excess of 2.5 percent. These results, when extrapolated to the nonsmoking adult population, indicate that 3–4 percent of the population may be exposed during the winter to CO levels exceeding the 9 ppm eight-hour and the 35 ppm one-hour standard assigned to keep COHb levels from rising above 1.5 percent.

Only two studies relate specific indoor exposures with COHb levels. In each study, COHb levels were estimated by measuring CO concentrations in samples of end-expired breath. This methodology is reviewed by Lambert, Colome, and Wojciechowski (1988). In Dutch homes, Verhoeff et al. (1983) observed a small but significant increase in breath CO after occupants used infusion water heaters. Wallace (1983) observed increases in breath CO levels of office workers exposed to motor vehicle exhaust.

## HEALTH EFFECTS OF EXPOSURE

The health effects of CO have been described through clinical observations of patients with CO intoxication and experimental and epidemiologic investigations of persons exposed to low levels of CO. The health effects of CO vary with the level of COHb (Table 8.2) and range from nonspecific symptoms, headache, dizziness, and fatigue, to death (Winter and Miller 1976). CO poisoning, resulting in death, has been recognized since the nineteenth century (Winter and Miller 1976), but the adverse consequences of exposure to low levels of CO have only recently received attention.

Because of the adverse effects of CO on oxygen delivery to tissues, individuals with a need for high oxygen consumption or who have preexisting disorders of oxygen delivery may be highly sensitive to the effects of CO (Table 8.3). These considerations related to oxygen delivery suggest that the developing fetus (Longo 1977), the growing child (Zimmerman and Truxal 1981), and maximally exercising persons may be particularly susceptible to the effects of hypoxia from CO. Other groups that may be unusually sensitive to the adverse consequences of CO include those with chronic hypoxemia, cardiovascular disease, and hemoglobin abnormalities.

Table 8.2    Health Effects Associated with Different
Carboxyhemoglobin Levels

| COHb (%) | Symptoms |
|---|---|
| 10 | No appreciable effect except shortness of breath on vigorous exertion; possible tightness across the forehead; dilatation of cutaneous blood vessels |
| 20 | Shortness of breath on moderate exertion; occasional headache with throbbing in temples |
| 30 | Decided headache; irritable; easily fatigued; judgment disturbed; possible dizziness; dimness of vision |
| 40–50 | Headache; confusion; collapse; fainting on exertion |
| 60–70 | Unconsciousness; intermittent convulsions; respiratory failure; death if exposure is continued for long |
| 80 | Rapidly fatal |

*Source*: Winter and Miller (1976), reprinted with the permission of the American Medical Association.

Table 8.3    Conditions That Potentially
Increase Susceptibility to Adverse
Effects of CO

Fetal development
Children
Chronic hypoxemia
  High altitude
  Chronic lung disease
  Right-to-left shunts
Impaired cardiac output
  Cardiomyopathy
  Valvular heart disease
Vascular disease
  Atherosclerotic heart disease
  Cerebrovascular disease
  Peripheral vascular disease
Hemoglobin abnormalities
  Anemia
  Hemoglobinopathy

CO INTOXICATION

Intoxication from CO may be acute or chronic, depending upon concentration and duration of exposure. Generally, clinically apparent problems with acute exposures appear at COHb levels of 10 percent or greater (Table 8.2). However, the severity of symptoms may not correlate well with COHb levels (Sokal and Kralkowska 1985, Kirkpatrick 1987). Furthermore, because of its nonspecific picture, intoxication may be frequently overlooked (Dolan 1985; Barret, Danel, and Faure 1985).

To determine the frequency of misdiagnosis of CO poisoning, Barret, Danel, and Faure (1985) reviewed records from 340 patients with CO poisoning admitted to a toxicology service in France. Between 1975 and 1977, 30 percent of patients were initially misdiagnosed. The initial diagnoses included food poisoning, neuropsychiatric problems, cardiac disorders, and other intoxications. Food poisoning was the most frequent incorrect diagnosis.

The clinical history and physical examination may suggest the diagnosis of CO intoxication (Table 8.4). However, because the presenting problems of CO poisoning are nonspecific, only a high index of suspicion will result in the correct diagnosis (Hopkinson, Pearce, and Oliver 1980; Heckerling et al. 1987; Kirkpatrick 1987). The history of a potential source of exposure (Heckerling et al. 1987) or the finding of retinal hemorrhages (Kelley and Sophocleus 1978) may provide the first clues to the correct diagnosis. Furthermore, the identification of an index case of CO poisoning should alert the clinician to other potential cases (Wharton et al. 1989).

CO is currently the only air pollutant with a specific and clinically relevant biologic marker, COHb. However, the COHb level may not strongly predict the severity of intoxication, and the duration of exposure may be a better predictor (Sokal and Kralkowska 1985). In a study of thirty-nine patients with CO poisoning, Sokal and Kralkowska (1985) found that the mean duration of exposure was about nine hours among those with clinically severe poisoning, compared with five hours among those with mild to moderate poisoning. There were only slight differences in the COHb levels between the two groups of patients.

CO intoxication, especially with prolonged high levels of COHb, may affect every organ system (Table 8.5). Most complications of CO poisoning are a direct result of tissue hypoxia, and the presence of these complications may provide the first alert to the clinician of possible CO intoxication. For example, an unexplained

---

Table 8.4   Clinical Findings That Suggest
the Possibility of CO Poisoning

History
Exposure to potential source of CO
Nonspecific symptoms (e.g., headache, dizziness,
   fatigue, nausea, vomiting)
Household members or co-workers with similar
   symptoms
Unexplained illness/death among household pets

Physical exam
Retinal hemorrhage
Unexplained coma
Unexplained cardiac arrhythmias

Laboratory
COHb $\geq 10\%^{a}$ in a nonsmoker
Unexplained lactic acidosis

[a]May vary depending upon the chronicity and level of exposure and on the time at which the specimen is drawn in relation to the exposure.

Table 8.5   Complications of CO Poisoning

| Organ System | Complication |
|---|---|
| Cardiac | Myocardial ischemia, arrhythmias, angina |
| Pulmonary | Pulmonary edema, hemorrhage |
| Muscular | Myonecrosis, compartment syndrome |
| Renal | Myglobinuria, acute renal failure |
| Neurologic | Seizure, encephalopathy, cerebral edema |
| Ophthalmologic | Retinal hemorrhage, visual defect |
| Cutaneous | Erythema, listers, bullae |
| Vestibular/auditory | Vertigo, nystagmus, hearing loss, tinnitus |
| Hematologic | Thrombotic thrombocytopenic purpura |
| Fetal | Death, neurologic sequelae |

[a]*Source*: Adapted from Zimmerman and Truxal (1981), with permission.

lactic acidosis strongly suggests CO poisoning (Sokal and Kralkowska 1985).

Although most patients with CO poisoning recover completely, some develop delayed neurologic complications. These problems, which include headache, memory loss, disorientation, hallucinations, apraxia, and aphasia, appear days to weeks after apparent recovery from an acute exposure (Werner et al. 1985). Among patients who develop these delayed neurologic problems, areas of brain necrosis have been demonstrated by magnetic resonance imaging (Horowitz, Kaplan, and Sarpel 1987).

The immediate therapeutic goal in CO poisoning is reversal of the tissue hypoxia (Winter and Miller 1976). As soon as the diagnosis is considered, 100 percent oxygen should be administered. This will increase the dissolved oxygen in plasma and shorten the half-life of COHb. For severe cases, hyperbaric oxygen treatment may be necessary.

LOW-LEVEL EXPOSURE

The health effects of low levels of CO exposure have been examined with two types of investigations: laboratory studies involving short-term exposure, and population studies. The major health outcomes that have been studied include effects on the fetus, on neurobehavioral mechanisms, and on exercise in normal subjects and in patients with coronary artery disease, peripheral vascular disease, and chronic lung disease. For all of these problems we primarily consider information on indoor exposures but include results based on outdoor exposures if indoor data are limited. Similarly, we review relevant data from animal studies only if human data are unavailable.

*Effects on the Fetus*   Because of the adverse consequences of cigarette smoking on the fetus (U.S. Department of Health, Education, and Welfare [DHEW] 1979), researchers have hypothesized that CO may be the component of cigarette smoke which causes the adverse effects (Longo 1977). Animal experiments have been conducted in an attempt to isolate from the other components of tobacco smoke the effects of CO on the fetus (Astrup et al. 1972; Garvey and Longo 1978; Singh and Scott 1984).

In animal experiments, the exposures have been designed to simulate active cigarette smoking rather than exposures to lower levels of CO. Most of the experiments have involved exposures to CO levels of 30–500 ppm, resulting in COHb levels of 4–18 percent (Astrup et al. 1972; Garvey and Longo 1978; Singh and Scott 1984). At the lowest level of 30 ppm, Garvey and Longo (1978) exposed pregnant rats from day 3 to day 20 of gestation, resulting in a mean COHb level of 4.8 percent. The animals were killed, and the percentage of successful pregnancies in the exposed group was 69 percent compared with 100 percent in the unexposed. Other investigators have shown lower birth weight and increased fetal and neonatal mortality at higher levels of exposure (Astrup et al. 1972; Singh and Scott 1984).

For humans, few data are available on fetal and neonatal morbidity and mortality from exposure to CO indoors or outdoors. Alderman, Baron, and Savitz (1987) conducted a case-control study of birth weight and maternal exposure to neighborhood CO during the last three months of gestation. The series included 998 low–birth weight infants (2,500 g or less) and 1,872 normal–birth weight infants from Denver. They used ambient CO levels from stationary monitors to categorize the mother's exposure. For the mothers whose CO exposures were considered most accurate, the odds ratio for having a low–birth weight baby was 1.5 (95 percent confidence interval, 0.7–3.5) for an ambient CO level of 3 ppm or greater compared with lower levels. This finding is limited by the lack of personal smoking histories and personal exposure measurements.

*Neurobehavioral Effects*    To determine the effects of low levels of CO on the central nervous system, investigators have assessed effects in normal volunteers (Table 8.6), including effects on visual perception (Halperin et al. 1959; Hosko 1970; Stewart et al. 1970; Horvath, Dahms, and O'Hanlon 1971; Luria and McKay 1979), on auditory perception (Beard and Wertheim 1967; Wright and Shephard 1978), on manual dexterity (Stewart et al. 1970; McFarland 1973), and on vigilance (Benignus et al. 1977). The results from these investigations have been inconsistent (Benignus et al. 1977; Luria and McKay 1979). Potential reasons for the varied findings include small numbers of subjects and different study designs. Despite the inconsistent results, clinically important neurobehavioral effects in normal subjects are not a major concern with COHb levels below 10–20 percent.

*Effects on Exercise Performance in Normal Subjects*    As in the studies of the neurobehavioral effects of CO, researchers have exposed normal volunteers to CO and then tested its influence on exercise performance (Table 8.7). At COHb levels of 5 percent or less, maximal exercise time and maximal oxygen consumption have generally decreased among healthy subjects compared with preexposure exercise

Table 8.6  Selected Experimental Studies of Normal Human Volunteers on the Neurobehavioral Effects of Exposure to Low Levels of CO

| Reference | Subjects | Exposure | Measure of Effect | Findings |
|---|---|---|---|---|
| Halperin et al. (1959) | 4 males, 16–25 years of age | 100% CO delivered in varying amounts | Discrimination of light intensity | Visual sensitivity was impaired at COHb level of 3.0% and worsened with increasing COHb level |
| Hosko 1970 | 14 males, 24–42 years of age | 0.25–24 h of <1, 25, 50, 100, 200, 500, and 1,000 ppm CO | EEG and visual evoked response (VER) | Changes from baseline found in VER at COHb levels of 20–22% |
| Stewart et al. (1970) | 18 males, 24–42 years of age | 0.5–24 h of <1, 25, 50, 100, 200, 500, and 1,000 ppm CO | Symptoms, VER, visual and auditory tests, tests of reaction time and co-ordination | Exposure to 100 ppm for 8 h resulted in COHb of 11–13% but no impairment of performance; mild headache noted after 4 h of exposure to 200 ppm CO and 1-h exposure to 500 ppm CO; changes in VER occurred at 20% COHb or above; impairment in manual dexterity only at COHb of 28% |
| Luria and McKay (1979) | 12 nonsmokers, 6 smokers, 19–43 years of age | 18 min of 195 ppm CO | Night vision sensitivity, reaction time from visual stimulus, eye movements for letter search, VER | Mean COHb 9% in nonsmokers and COHb level ranged from 10.2 to 13.3% in smokers; no consistent changes in any measures were found |
| Horvath, Dahms, and O'Hanlon (1971) | 10 male non-smokers, 21–32 years of age | 2.25 h of 0, 26, or 111 ppm CO | Tested vigilance by judging light intensities over 1 h | Vigilance impaired at a mean COHb level of 6.6% after breathing 111 ppm CO |

| Reference | Subjects | Exposure | Task | Results |
|---|---|---|---|---|
| Beard and Wertheim (1967) | 18 subjects | Varying times at 0, 50, 100, 175, and 250 ppm CO | Discrimination of time intervals with paired tones | The percentage of correct responses decreased with increased exposure; however, COHb levels unavailable |
| Wright and Shephard (1978) | 3 experiments with 2, 7, and 5 subjects, respectively | Experiment 1: 0, 30, 50, and 75 ppm CO; Experiment 2: Air or CO exposure combined with surrounding office noise or silent conditions; Experiment 3: Air or CO over 10 different days | Discrimination of time interval with paired tones | Experiment 1: the percentage of correct responses decreased with increased exposure and COHb levels of 0.7, 2.0, 3.2, and 4.7%; Experiment 2: No consistent effects of CO with the varied exposure conditions; Experiment 3: Mean COHb 4.9% but no effect of CO observed |
| McFarland (1973) | 27 subjects, 20–50 years of age | Blinded exposure to air or 700 ppm CO for varying times | Psychomotor tasks, dark adaptation and glare recovery, peripheral vision, depth perception, driving performance | Mean COHb levels were $<4$, 6, 11, and 17% decrement in peripheral vision with CO exposure, but no effect on other measures |
| Benignus et al. (1977) | 52 males | 0, 100, and 200 ppm CO | Vigilance task of reporting when 3 consecutive even or odd digits seen among 667 digits | Mean COHb levels were 0.61, 4.6, 12.6%; no effect of CO on vigilance |

Table 8.7  Selected Experimental Studies of Normal Human Volunteers on the Effects of Low Levels of CO on Exercise Performance

| Reference | Subjects/Exercise | Exposure | Mean COHb (%) | Findings |
|---|---|---|---|---|
| Chevalier, Krumholz, and Ross (1966) | 10 nonsmokers, mean age 30 years; bicycle ergometer for 5 min with a mean $\dot{V}o_{2\,max}$ of 1.8 l/min | 2.5–3.5 min of 0.5% CO | $3.95 \pm 1.87$[a] | Oxygen debt and ratio of oxygen debt to total oxygen uptake increased 12.0 and 14%, respectively, compared with no exposure |
| Drinkwater et al. (1974) | 20 normal males, 10 nonsmokers, and 10 smokers; treadmill exercise to exhaustion | Double-blind: Filtered air 50 ppm CO 0.27 ppm PAN[b] CO + PAN | $2.5 \pm 0.30$ | 5% decrement in mean total walking time and 1.9% decrement in $\dot{V}o_{2\,max}$ for nonsmokers with CO exposure but no decrement among smokers |
| Aronow and Cassidy (1975) | 9 males, 1 female, normal nonsmokers, with mean age 50.7; treadmill exercise to exhaustion | Double-blind, 100 ppm CO for 1 h | $3.95 \pm 0.49$ | Mean exercise time decreased 5% |
| Horvath et al. (1975) | 4 healthy males, 24–33 years, 1 pipe smoker; treadmill exercise to exhaustion | Single-blind: Filtered air 75 ppm CO 100 ppm CO delivered by a bolus method or gradual increments on two occasions | 3.18–3.35 4.25–4.30 | Regardless of delivery mode, $\dot{V}o_{2\,max}$ decreased 4.9 and 7.0% at the low and high exposures, respectively |
| Weiser et al. (1978) | 9 male nonsmokers, mean age 24.7 years; treadmill exercise to exhaustion at altitude of 1,610 m | Double-blind: Filtered air CO bolus and rebreathing to achieve 5% COHb | $5.09 \pm 0.11$ | With CO exposure, total exercise time decreased 3.8%, total work decreased 10.0%, and $\dot{V}o_{2\,max}$ decreased 3.5% |
| Horvath et al. (1988) | 11 males and 12 women nonsmokers; exercised to maximal aerobic capacity at simulated altitudes of 55, 1,524, 2,134, and 3,048 m | Double-blind: 0 ppm CO 50 ppm CO 100 ppm CO 150 ppm CO | Not provided | CO and altitude at $\geq 2{,}134$ m decreased $\dot{V}o_{2\,max}$, but COHb did not result in an additional decline at a given altitude |

[a]Calculated COHb level from alveolar gas.
[b]PAN, peroxyacetyl nitrate.

tests. Most exposures have been at sea level, but no additional decrements in exercise performance have been found with CO exposure at higher altitudes (Weiser et al. 1978; Horvath et al. 1988).

*Experimental Studies of Effects on Patients with Cardiovascular and Peripheral Vascular Disease*   Since the early 1970s, numerous investigations studies have been conducted to examine the effects of exposure to low levels of CO on exercise tolerance in patients with vascular disease (Table 8.8). The results of most of these studies have indicated that patients with vascular disease have earlier onset of angina or claudication at COHb levels between about 2 and 5 percent. Although the validity of the investigations conducted by Aronow and his co-workers (1972, 1973, 1974, 1975; Aronow 1981) has been questioned (Budiansky 1983), subsequent investigations have obtained similar results to those reported by Aronow and his co-workers (Table 8.8).

Kleinman and Whittenberger (1989) reported that the exercise tolerance of twenty-four men with reproducible angina was reduced 5.8 percent, and maximal oxygen uptake was decreased 2.2 percent after exposure to 100 ppm for two hours. In a multicenter study (Warren et al. 1989), sixty-three men with reproducible angina and electrocardiographic (ECG) changes indicative of myocardial ischemia were studied at two levels of exposure sufficient to result in COHb levels of 2 and 4 percent. Relative to filtered air, mean time to onset of angina was reduced 4 and 7 percent, respectively. ECG changes preceded angina, and the time to onset of ST segment depression was reduced by 5 and 12 percent, respectively.

*Effects on Patients with Chronic Lung Disease*   The available literature concerning the effects of CO on patients with chronic obstructive lung disease is limited and does not provide definite conclusions (Aronow, Ferlinz, and Glauser 1977; Calverley, Leggett, and Flenley 1981). Calverley, Leggett, and Flenley (1981) studied fifteen patients with severe chronic obstructive pulmonary disease, mean $FEV_1$ of 0.56 liters, and measured the distances walked during a series of twelve-minute walks after breathing air, 2 liters of oxygen, air, and 0.02 percent CO per minute; and 2 liters of oxygen and 0.02 percent CO per minute. The mean increase in COHb was 9.2 percent, which resulted in a mean decrease of 43 m in the walking distance after breathing air and CO. However, since the CO exposures were always last, the decrease in exercise time may have resulted from fatigue.

*Epidemiologic Studies of Effects on Patients with Cardiorespiratory Disease*   Several investigations have been conducted to examine the relationship between ambient CO levels and cardiorespiratory effects (Cohen, Deane, and Goldsmith 1969; Hexter and Goldsmith 1971; Kuller et al. 1975; Kurt, Mogielnicki, and Chandler 1978; Kurt et al. 1979). The health effects that have been examined have ranged from emergency room visits for dyspnea and nontraumatic chest pain to mortality from myocardial infarction. Most of these studies found an association between outdoor measurements of CO and adverse health outcomes.

Table 8.8  Selected Experimental Studies of the Effects of Low Levels of CO Exposure on Patients with Atherosclerotic Heart Disease

| Reference | Subjects/Exposure | Exposure | Mean COHb (%) | Findings |
|---|---|---|---|---|
| Anderson et al. (1973) | 10 males with stable angina, 5 were smokers, mean age 49.9 years, incremental treadmill exercise until onset of angina | Double-blind exposure to room air, 50 or 100 ppm CO for 4 h prior to exercise | 50 ppm = 2.9 ± 0.70, 100 ppm = 4.5 ± 0.80 | Mean time to onset of angina was reduced 15% with exposure to both concentrations of CO; duration of pain was prolonged with 100 ppm CO; ST segment depression appeared earlier and was deeper with CO exposure; no difference between smokers and non-smokers |
| Aronow et al. (1972) | 10 males with angina, 3 were smokers, mean age 48 years; bicycle ergometer exercise until onset of angina | Driven in an open car on Los Angeles freeway for 90 min during traffic; mean CO level in the car was 53 ± 6 ppm. On a second day subjects breathed compressed air during the drive | 5.08 ± 1.19 | Mean exercise time was decreased 75 s after exposure to freeway air, and decreased exercise time persisted for 2 h after the exposure compared with base line or while breathing compressed air |
| Aronow and Isbell (1973) | 10 males with angina, non-smokers; bicycle ergometer exercise until onset of angina | Double-blind exposure to air or 50 ppm CO for 2 hours | 2.68 ± 0.15 | Mean exercise time decreased 37 s with CO exposure compared with air |
| Aronow et al. (1974) | 10 males with intermittent claudication, confirmed angiographically | Double-blind exposure to compressed air or 50 ppm CO for 2 h | 2.8 ± 0.19 | Mean exercise time decreased 30 s with CO exposure compared with air |

| Study | Subjects | Exposure | COHb (%) | Results |
|---|---|---|---|---|
| Aronow (1981) | 15 subjects with stable angina, 14 males, 1 female, nonsmokers; bicycle ergometer exercise until onset of angina | Double-blind exposure to air or 50 ppm CO for 1 h | $2.02 \pm 0.16$ | Mean exercise time was decreased 33 s with CO exposure compared with air |
| Sheps (1985) | 30 subjects with ischemic heart disease, nonsmokers; type of exercise unknown | Double-blind exposure to air or 100 ppm CO on successive days | $4.1 \pm 0.10$ | No effect on time to onset of angina or change in cardiac function with CO exposure |
| Adams et al. (1987) | 30 subjects with ischemic heart disease; type of exercise unknown | Double-blind exposure to air or CO | $5.9 \pm 0.10$ | Mean exercise duration decreased 41 s with CO exposure compared with air; angina only occurred with CO exposure; left ventricular ejection fraction with exercise was less after CO exposure |
| Kleinman and Whittenberger (1989) | 24 males with reproducible angina | Double-blind exposure to filtered air or to 100 ppm CO | $2.9 \pm 0.30$ | Mean exercise time decreased 5.8% and maximal oxygen uptake decreased 2.2% with CO exposure relative to air |
| Warren et al. (1989) | 63 males, ages 35–75 with stable angina; treadmill exercise until onset of angina | Double-blind exposure to air and two levels of CO to achieve COHb of 2.2 and 4.4% | $2.0 \pm 0.10$ $3.9 \pm 0.10$ | 4.2 and 7.1% trimmed mean decrease in time to onset of angina at low and high exposures, respectively; 5.1 and 12.1% trimmed mean decreases in time to development of ischemic ST segment changes |

However, because the ambient measures of exposure used in these studies may not have been representative of personal exposure to CO (Ott and Flachsbart 1982; Akland et al. 1985), these results must be interpreted carefully. Furthermore, exposure misclassification would tend to bias risk estimates downward, making it more difficult to observe an effect.

In contrast to community studies, occupational settings may provide better estimates of exposure to CO. Increased mortality from arteriosclerotic heart disease has been documented in an occupational environment with exposure to elevated levels of CO in an enclosed space (Stern et al. 1988). Among 5,529 New York City bridge and tunnel officers employed between 1952 and 1981, the overall mortality ratio for arteriosclerotic heart disease was 35 percent higher among tunnel workers compared with bridge workers; the former having the higher exposures to CO. The mortality ratio was highest (1.88) for tunnel workers employed for ten or more years. Differences in smoking habits were not sufficient to explain the differences in mortality.

## SUMMARY

Numerous and varied types of observations have documented the adverse health effects of CO. For low levels of CO the effects have largely been studied experimentally with small numbers of subjects. However, these experiments may not provide an accurate description of the free-living environment with variations in exposure, in activity level, and in severity of disease. Nevertheless, the available data demonstrate that levels of COHb greater than 2 percent, which may result from exposure indoors, impair exercise capacity of patients with cardiopulmonary disease and of normal subjects at maximum exercise capacity. Furthermore, CO may exacerbate ischemic symptoms in patients with cardiovascular disease and may contribute to excess mortality. Because nonspecific symptoms result from CO at low or high levels of exposure, a high index of suspicion is necessary to make the diagnosis and to prevent further exposure.

## REFERENCES

Adams, K. F., et al. 1987. Earlier onset of ischemia after exposure to low level carbon monoxide in patients with ischemic heart disease. *J. Am. Coll. Cardiol.* 9:121 (abstr.).

Akland, G. G., et al. 1985. Measuring human exposure to carbon monoxide in Washington, D.C., and Denver, Colorado, during the winter of 1982–83. *Environ. Sci. Technol.* 19:911–18.

Alderman, B. W.; Baron, A. E.; and Savitz, D. A. 1987. Maternal exposure to neighborhood carbon monoxide and risk of low infant birth weight. *Public Health Rep.* 102:410–14.

Anderson, E. W., et al. 1973. Effect of low-level carbon monoxide exposure on onset and duration of angina pectoris: A study in ten patients with ischemic heart disease. *Ann. Intern. Med.* 79:46–50.

Armitage, A. K.; Davies, R. F.; and Turner, D. M. 1976. The effects of carbon monoxide on the development of atherosclerosis in the white carneau pigeon. *Atherosclerosis* 23:333–44.

Aronow, W. S. 1981. Aggravation of angina pectoris by two percent carboxyhemoglobin. *Am. Heart J.* 101:154–57.

Aronow, W. S., and Cassidy, J. 1975. Effect of carbon monoxide on maximal treadmill exercise: A study in normal persons. *Ann. Intern. Med.* 83:496–99.

Aronow, W. S., and Isbell, M. W. 1973. Carbon monoxide effect on exercise-induced angina pectoris. *Ann. Intern. Med.* 79:392–59.

Aronow, W. S.; Ferlinz, J.; and Glauser, F. 1977. Effect of carbon monoxide on exercise performance in chronic obstructive pulmonary disease. *Am. J. Med.* 63:904–8.

Aronow, W. S.; Stemmer, E. A.; and Isbell, M. W. 1974. Effect of carbon monoxide exposure on intermittent claudication. *Circulation* 69:415–17.

Aronow, W. S., et al. 1972. Effect of freeway travel on angina pectoris. *Ann. Intern. Med.* 77:669–76.

Astrup, P.; Kjeldsen, K.; and Wanstrup, J. 1970. Effects of carbon monoxide exposure on the arterial walls. *Ann. N.Y. Acad. Sci.* 174:294–300.

Astrup, P., et al. 1972. Effect of moderate carbon monoxide exposure on fetal development. *Lancet* 2:1220–22.

Barret, L.; Danel, V.; and Faure, J. 1985. Carbon monoxide poisoning: A diagnosis frequently overlooked. *Clin. Toxicol.* 23:309–13.

Beard, R. R., and Wertheim, G. A. 1967. Behavioral impairment associated with small doses of carbon monoxide. *Am. J. Public Health* 57:2012–22.

Benignus, V. A., et al. 1977. Lack of effects of carbon monoxide on human vigilance. *Percept. Mot. Skills* 45:1007–14.

Budiansky, S. 1983. Food and drug data fudged. *Nature* 302:560.

Calverley, P. M. A.; Leggett, R. J. E.; and Flenley, D. C. 1981. Carbon monoxide and exercise tolerance in chronic bronchitis and emphysema. *Br. Med. J.* 283:878–80.

Caplan, Y. H., et al. 1986. Accidental poisonings involving carbon monoxide, heating systems, and confined spaces. *J. Forensic Sci.* 31:117–21.

Chevalier, R. B.; Krumholz, R. A.; and Ross, J. C. 1966. Reaction of non-smokers to carbon monoxide inhalation: Cardio-pulmonary responses at rest and during exercise. *JAMA* 198:1061–64.

Coburn, R. F. 1979. Mechanisms of carbon monoxide toxicity. *Prevent. Med.* 8:310–22.

Coburn, R. F.; Forster, R. E.; and Kane, P. B. 1965. Considerations of the physiological variables that determine blood carboxyhemoglobin concentration in man. *J. Clin. Invest.* 44:1899–1910.

Cohen, S. I.; Deane, M.; and Goldsmith, J. R. 1969. Carbon monoxide and survival from myocardial infarction. *Arch. Environ. Health* 19:510–17.

Collier, C. R. 1976. Oxygen affinity of human blood in the presence of carbon monoxide. *J. Appl. Physiol.* 40:487–90.

Cooper, K. R., and Alberti, R. R. 1984. Effect of kerosene space heater emissions on indoor air quality and pulmonary function. *Am. Rev. Respir. Dis.* 129:629–31.

Cortese, A. D., and Spengler, J. D. 1976. Ability of fixed-monitoring stations to represent carbon monoxide exposure. *J. Air Pollut. Control Assoc.* 26:1144–50.

Dolan, M. C. 1985. Carbon monoxide poisoning. *Can. Med. Assoc. J.* 133:392–99.

Drinkwater, B. L., et al. 1974. Air pollution, exercise, and heat stress. *Arch. Environ. Health* 28:177–81.

El-Attar, O. A., and Sairo, D. M. 1968. Effect of carbon monoxide on the whole fibrinolytic activity. *Industr. Med. Surg.* 37:774–77.

Flachsbart, P. G., and Brown, D. E. 1985. Surveys of personal exposure to vehicle exhaust in Honolulu microenvironments. Honolulu: Department of Urban and Regional Planning.

Flachsbart, P. G., et al. 1987. Carbon monoxide exposures of Washington commuters. *J. Air Pollut. Control Assoc.* 37:135–42.

Garvey, D. J., and Longo, L. D. 1978. Chronic low level maternal carbon monoxide exposure and fetal growth and development. *Biol. Reprod.* 19:8–14.

Haft, J. I. 1979. Role of blood platelets in coronary artery disease. *Am. J. Cardiol.* 43:1197–1206.

Halperin, M. H., et al. 1959. The time course of the effects of carbon monoxide on visual thresholds. *J. Physiol.* 146:583–93.

Hartwell, T. D., et al. 1984. Study of carbon monoxide exposures of residents of Washington, D.C. Paper 84-121.4, presented at the seventy-seventh annual meeting of the Air Pollution Control Association, 24–29 June, San Francisco, Calif.

Heckerling, P. S., et al. 1987. Predictors of occult carbon monoxide poisoning in patients with headache and dizziness. *Ann. Intern. Med.* 107:174–76.

Hexter, C. A., and Goldsmith, J. R. 1971. Carbon monoxide: Association of community air pollution with mortality. *Science* 172:265–67.

Hopkinson, J. M.; Pearce, P. J.; and Oliver, J. S. 1980. Carbon monoxide poisoning mimicking gastroenteritis. *Br. Med. J.* 281:214–15.

Horowitz, A. L.; Kaplan, R.; and Sarpel, G. 1987. Carbon monoxide toxicity: MR imaging in the brain. *Radiology* 162:787–88.

Horvath, S. M.; Dahms, T. E.; and O'Hanlon, J. F. 1971. Carbon monoxide and human vigilance. *Arch. Environ. Health* 23:343–47.

Horvath, S. M., et al. 1975. Maximal aerobic capacity at different levels of carboxyhemoglobin. *J. Appl. Physiol.* 38:300–303.

Horvath, S. M., et al. 1988. Maximal aerobic capacity at several ambient concentrations of carbon monoxide at several altitudes. Presented at the fifth Health Effects Institute annual conference, 17–20 April, Colorado Springs, Colo.

Hosko, J. M. 1970. The effect of carbon monoxide on the visual evoked response in man, and the spontaneous electroencephalogram. *Arch. Environ. Health* 21:174–80.

Johnson, T. R. 1984. A study of personal exposure to carbon monoxide in Denver, Colorado. Paper 84-121.3, presented at the seventy-seventh annual meeting of the Air Pollution Control Association, 24–29 June, San Francisco, Calif.

Kelley, J. S., and Sophocleus, G. J. 1978. Retinal hemorrhages in subacute carbon monoxide poisoning: Exposure in homes with blocked furnace flues. *JAMA* 239:1515–17.

Kim, Y. S. 1985. Seasonal variation in carbon monoxide poisoning in urban Korea. *J. Epidemiol. Community Health* 39:79–81.

Kirkpatrick, J. N. 1987. Occult carbon monoxide poisoning. *West. J. Med.* 146:52–56.

Kleinman, M. T., and Whittenberger, J. L. 1989. Effects of short-term exposure to carbon monoxide in subjects with coronary artery disease. Paper 89-54.4, presented at the eighty-second annual meeting of the Air and Waste Management Association, 25–30 June, Anaheim, Calif.

Kuller, L., et al. 1975. Carbon monoxide and heart attacks. *Arch. Environ. Health* 30:477–82.

Kurt, T. L.; Mogielnicki, R. P.; and Chandler, J. E. 1978. Association of the frequency of acute cardiorespiratory complaints with ambient levels of carbon monoxide. *Chest* 74:10–13.

Kurt, T. L., et al. 1979. Ambient carbon monoxide levels and acute cardiorespiratory complaints: An exploratory study. *Am. J. Public Health* 69:360–63.

Lambert, W. E.; Colome, S. D.; and Wojciechowski, S. L. 1988. Application of end-expired breath sampling to estimate carboxyhemoglobin levels in community air pollution exposure assessments. *Atmos. Environ.* 22:2171–81.

Lebret, E. 1985. *Air pollution in Dutch homes: An exploratory study in environmental epidemiology.* Report R-138, Wageningen Agricultural University, The Netherlands: Department of Environmental and Tropical Health.

Longo, L. D. 1977. The biological effects of carbon monoxide on the pregnant woman, fetus, and newborn infant. *Am. J. Obstet. Gynecol.* 129:69–103.

Luria, S. M., and McKay, C. L. 1979. Effects of low levels of carbon monoxide on visions of smokers and nonsmokers. *Arch. Environ. Health* 34:38–44.

McFarland, R. A. 1973. Low level exposure to carbon monoxide and driving performance. *Arch. Environ. Health* 27:355–59.

National Research Council (committee on medical and biological effects of environmental pollutants). 1977. *Carbon monoxide.* Washington, D.C.: National Academy of Sciences.

New Mexico Environmental Improvement Agency. 1977. *Carbon monoxide hazard reduction in recreational vehicles project: Final report.* Atlanta, Ga.: Centers for Disease Control. Contract no. 200-76-0616.

Ott, W., and Flachsbart, P. 1982. Measurement of carbon monoxide concentrations in indoor and outdoor locations using personal monitors. *Environ. Int.* 6:295–304.

Radford, E. P., and Drizd, T. A. 1982. Blood carbon monoxide levels in persons 3–74 years by age, United States, 1976–80. National Center for Health Statistics: *Advance data from vital and health statistics no. 76.* Hyattsville, Md.: Government Printing Office. DHHS Publication no. (PHS) 82-1250.

Roughton, F. J. W., and Darling, R. C. 1944. The effect of carbon monoxide on the oxyhemoglobin dissociation curve. *Am. J. Physiol.* 141:17–31.

Sarma, S. J. M., et al. 1975. The effect of carbon monoxide on lipid metabolism of human coronary arteries. *Atherosclerosis* 22:193–95.

Sheps, D. S. 1985. Lack of effect of 4% carboxyhemoglobin concentration on cardiac function in patients with ischemic heart disease. *J. Am. Coll. Cardiol.* 5:406 (abstr.).

Singh, J., and Scott, L. H. 1984. Threshold for carbon monoxide induced fetotoxicity. *Teratology* 30:253–57.

Sokal, J. A., and Kralkowska, E. 1985. The relationship between exposure duration, carboxyhemoglobin, blood glucose, pyruvate and lactate and the severity of intoxication in 39 cases of acute carbon monoxide poisoning in man. *Arch. Toxicol.* 57:196–99.

Spengler, J. D., and Cohen, M. A. 1985. Emissions from indoor combustion sources. In *Indoor air and human health.* Ed. R. B. Gammage and S. V. Kaye, 261–78. Chelsea, Mich.: Lewis Publishers.

Sterling, T. D.; Dimich, H.; and Kobayashi, D. 1981. Use of gas ranges for cooking and heating in urban dwellings. *J. Air Pollut. Control Assoc.* 32:162–65.

Sterling, T. D.; Dimich, H.; and Kobayashi, D. 1982. Indoor byproduct levels of tobacco smoke: A critical review of the literature. *J. Air Pollut. Control Assoc.* 32:250–57.

Stern, F. B., et al. 1988. Heart disease mortality among bridge and tunnel officers exposed to carbon monoxide. *Am. J. Epidemiol.* 128:1276–88.

Stewart, R. D., et al. 1970. Experimental human exposure to carbon monoxide. *Arch. Environ. Health* 21:154–64.

Stryer, L. 1975. *Biochemistry.* San Francisco: W. H. Freeman.

Theodore, J.; O'Donnell, R. D.; and Back, K. C. 1971. Toxicological evaluation of carbon monoxide in humans and other mammalian species. *J. Occup. Med.* 13:242–55.

U.S. Bureau of the Census. *1980 Census of housing, Vol. 1: Characteristics of housing units, Ch. B: Detailed housing characteristics,* Pt. 1: *United States summary.* Washington, D.C.: Government Printing Office. Publication no. HC80-1-B1.

U.S. Consumer Product Safety Commission. 1980. Commission proposes new CO standard to reduce deaths from unvented gas heaters. Washington, D.C.: News from CPSC, January.

U.S. Department of Health and Human Services. 1987. *Vital statistics of the United States 1984, Vol. 2: Mortality, part A.* National Center for Health Statistics. Hyattsville, Md.: Government Printing Office. DHHS Publication no. (PHS) 87-1122.

U.S. Department of Health, Education, and Welfare. 1979. *Smoking and health: A report of the surgeon general.* Washington, D.C.: Government Printing Office. DHEW Publication no. (PHS) 79-50066.

U.S. Public Health Service. 1982. Carbon monoxide intoxication: A preventable environmental health hazard. *MMWR* 31:529–31.

Verhoeff, A. P., et al. 1983. Detecting indoor CO exposure by measuring CO in exhaled breath. *Int. Arch. Occup. Environ. Health* 53:167–73.

Wallace, L. 1983. Carbon monoxide in air and breath of employees in an underground office. *J. Air Pollut. Control Assoc.* 33:678–82.

Warren, J., et al. 1989. Acute effects of carbon monoxide exposure on individuals with coronary artery disease. Paper 89-54.3, presented at the eighty-second annual meeting of the Air and Waste Management Association, 25–30 June, Anaheim, Calif.

Weiser, P. C., et al. 1978. Effects of low-level carbon monoxide exposure on the adaptation of healthy young men to aerobic work at an altitude of 1,610 meters. In *Environmental stress: Individual human adaptations.* Ed. L. J. Folinsbee et al., 101–10. New York: Academic Press.

Werner, B., et al. 1985. Two cases of acute carbon monoxide with delayed neurological sequelae after a "free" interval. *Clin. Toxicol.* 23:249–65.

Wharton, M., et al. 1989. Fatal carbon monoxide poisoning at a motel. *JAMA* 261:1177–78.

Winter, P. M., and Miller, J. N. 1976. Carbon monoxide poisoning. *JAMA* 236:1502–4.

Wittenberg, J. B. 1970. Myoglobin facilitated oxygen diffusion: Role of myoglobin in oxygen entry into muscle. *Physiol. Rev.* 150:559–636.

Wright, G. R., and Shephard, R. J. 1978. Carbon monoxide exposure and auditory duration discrimination. *Arch. Environ. Health* 33:226–35.

Zimmerman, S. S., and Truxal, B. 1981. Carbon monoxide poisoning. *Pediatrics* 68:215–24.

# 9

# WOOD SMOKE

Marian C. Marbury, Sc.D.

Since the early 1970s, use of wood as a heating fuel has increased substantially. In 1981 approximately 7 percent of homes in the United States used wood as the major or supplementary source of heat, compared with only 1 percent in 1970 (Annandale, Duxbury, and Newman 1983). Increased residential wood use has significantly degraded ambient air quality in several areas of the country, most notably in towns and cities prone to wintertime inversions, such as Vail and Denver, Colorado (Lewis and Einfeld 1985), and Portland, Oregon (Cooper 1980). Research on wood combustion emissions, prompted by the resurgence in wood use, has provided inventories of the pollutants emitted by wood combustion, but data needed for understanding the health consequences of wood burning are still lacking. Few investigations of the effects of wood combustion on indoor air quality have been performed, and data concerning the health effects of domestic exposure to wood smoke remain extremely limited.

Wood is composed primarily of carbon, oxygen, and hydrogen. Under ideal conditions with complete combustion, water and carbon dioxide ($CO_2$) are the primary end products. Nitrogen oxides and sulfur oxides are also formed; nitrogen oxides are primarily from the combination of atmospheric nitrogen with oxygen during high temperature combustion, and sulfur oxides are from oxidation of sulfur in the wood. Incomplete combustion results in emissions of other pollutants such as particulates, organic compounds including polycyclic organic materials, and carbon monoxide (CO) (Quraishi 1985). Emission rates for these pollutants are highly variable and depend on such factors as burn rate, amount of air available for combustion, size of fuel charge, type and size of wood, and the moisture content of the wood (Quraishi 1985).

DeAngelis and colleagues (1980) sampled flue gases from two airtight cast iron stoves (one baffled and one nonbaffled) and a zero-clearance fireplace and per-

Table 9.1 Studies of the Impact of Residential Wood Burning (WB) on Indoor Air Quality

| Study | Findings | Conclusions |
|---|---|---|
| One home with wood stove, 2 with fireplaces (1 WB day in each fireplace), Boston, Mass. (Moschandreas, Zabransky, and Rector 1980) | Indoor TSP[a] and RSP[b] four times higher on WB days; BaP[c] increased fivefold in home with wood stove, and tenfold on 1 WB day in home with fireplace; CO peaks during loading and refiring. | Wood burning a major source of particulate matter emissions in residential environment |
| 19 WB homes, 5 non-WB homes; monitored for 2 weeks, Waterbury, Vt. (Sexton, Spengler, and Treitman 1984) | RSP levels: all NWB homes, 24 $\mu g/m$; NWB homes with unexplainably high levels removed, 18 $\mu g/m$; WB homes without kerosene heater, 24 $\mu g/ml$; WB homes with kerosene heater, 34 $\mu g/m$. | Airtight wood stoves can be installed and operated with negligible release of particles into indoor air; particle concentrations in general vary widely among homes. |
| Experimental house, with 3 airtight and 1 non-airtight wood stove; monitored at least 5 h per test, Truckee, Calif. (Traynor et al. 1987) | Airtight stoves caused short-term CO and particulate peaks during door opening; pollutants emitted by non-airtight stove dependent on operation of stove; submicron particles, 210–1,900 $\mu g/m$; CO, 1.8–14 ppm; BaP, 5.4–150 $\mu g/m$. | Airtight stoves not an important source of pollutants; non-airtight stoves can be a moderately heavy source depending on their mode of operation. |
| 20 homes with wood stoves monitored twice during stove operation and twice when not operating, Madison, Wisc. (Kaaraka, Kanarek, and Lawrence 1987) | CO levels slightly higher during WB (2.2 versus 1.8 ppm); on average, RSP levels were unchanged, but indoor and outdoor RSP increased in rural homes during WB; only 2 BaP measurements above limits of detection (0.32 and 0.12 ng/m). | Use of airtight stoves with adequate drafts not a source of pollution; poor stove quality or loading habits can lead to high short-term levels of contamination. |
| Experimental house with airtight wood stove and fireplace, Norway (Alfheim and Ramdahl 1984) | WB increased PAH[d] level from background of 1–16 ng/m with stove, 206 ng/m with fireplace; stove did not increase mutagenic activity of air; fireplace increased it substantially. | Wood stove had little impact on PAH levels or mutagenic activity; fireplace had considerable impact but still less than tobacco smoke. |
| 12 homes with wood stoves, 12 with fireplaces, sampled during 1 WB and 1 non-WB week, Netherlands (Van Houdt et al. 1986) | WB caused increase in mutagenic activity of indoor air in 8 out of 12 homes with stoves, 12 out of 12 with fireplaces. | Fireplaces consistently cause increased mutagenicity, wood stoves less frequently; reasons for variability are unclear. |

[a]TSP, total suspended particles.
[b]RSP, respirable suspended particles.
[c]BaP, benzo[α]pyrene
[d]PAH, polycyclic aromatic hydrocarbon.

formed a detailed characterization of the emissions. They measured more than one hundred chemical compounds. In addition to the four criteria pollutants (particulate matter, CO, nitrogen oxides, and sulfur oxides) they identified seventeen priority pollutants of the U.S. Environmental Protection Agency, fourteen carcinogenic compounds, six cilia-toxic and mucus-coagulating agents, and four co-carcinogenic agents. Other respiratory irritants, including aldehydes, phenols, and furans, were also detected (Cooper 1980). Emissions of CO and polycyclic organic compounds were higher from the stoves, and emissions of nitrogen oxides were higher from the fireplace. Ramdahl and colleagues (1982) reported that emissions of CO, hydrocarbons, aldehydes, and volatile organic compounds were higher under starved air conditions than under normal conditions.

## EXPOSURE TO WOOD SMOKE

The impact on indoor air quality of residential wood combustion in general, and specific combustion appliances in particular, has not yet been well described (Table 9.1). Indoor air concentrations of wood combustion emissions could be increased directly through leakage of pollutants from appliances or indirectly by entrainment of polluted outdoor air into the indoor environment. The newer airtight stoves operate under negative pressure and would not be expected to leak combustion by-products into the home under normal operating conditions. However, under non-airtight conditions and during starting, stoking, and reloading, pollutants may be emitted indoors.

Moschandreas and co-workers (1980) studied two residences with fireplaces and one with a wood stove over a two-week period. Twenty-four-hour levels of respirable suspended particles were higher inside on wood-burning days than outside on non-wood-burning days. During one wood-burning day, respirable suspended particulate levels ranged from 14.3 to 72.5 $\mu g/m^3$ in the home with the wood stove and averaged 159.9 and 67.6 $\mu g/m^3$ in the two homes with a fireplace. Benzo[a]pyrene levels were five times higher on wood-burning days in the home with the wood stove, averaging 4.7 $ng/m^3$. On the wood-burning day in one of the homes with a fireplace, benzo[a]pyrene levels reached 11.4 $ng/m^3$, compared with an outside concentration of 0.6 $ng/m^3$. CO levels were reported only for the home with the wood stove; although generally below 1 ppm, peaks exceeding 5 ppm were noted during stoking and reloading. The authors concluded that wood burning in a stove or a fireplace could be a significant source of indoor air pollution.

In a more extensive survey, Sexton and co-workers (1984) measured respirable suspended particles inside and outside twenty-four homes, nineteen with wood stoves and five without. When one non-wood-burning home that had exceptionally high levels from an unknown source was removed from the analysis, average concentrations of respirable suspended particles were 18 $\mu g/m^3$ in homes without wood-burning stoves, 24 $\mu g/m^3$ in homes with wood-burning stoves but without kerosene heaters, and 34 $\mu g/m^3$ in homes with both stoves and kerosene heaters. Although the airtightness of the stoves was not discussed explicitly in the text, the authors concluded that their "findings suggest that airtight stoves can be installed, operated, and maintained in such a way that direct release of particles to the indoor environment is negligible."

Investigators in Wisconsin measured nitrogen dioxide ($NO_2$), CO, respirable suspended particles, and benzo[a]pyrene on four separate occasions in twenty homes with wood stoves, twice during the winter when the stove was in use and twice during the summer (Kaaraka, Kanarek, and Lawrence 1987). Most of the stoves were airtight. Indoor $NO_2$ levels were higher during wood burning (13.3 versus 9.8 $\mu g/m^3$), but this increase in levels was attributed to higher outdoor concentrations rather than direct emissions. CO levels were also slightly elevated during wood burning (2.2 versus 1.8 ppm), but again, the increase was not completely attributable to wood burning. One site had a peak of 25.3 ppm which was traced to an incident during which loading the stove had taken an unusually long time. Indoor levels of respirable suspended particles were not significantly different over the whole set of homes during the winter and summer periods although rural homes had increased indoor and outdoor concentrations during wood burning. The investigators could not determine whether the increased indoor concentrations were due to direct emissions or infiltration from outside. Only two sites had detectable benzo[a]pyrene concentrations, 0.32 and 0.12 $ng/m^3$, respectively. Both of these concentrations were detected during non-burn periods.

Traynor and colleagues (1987) measured the effect on indoor air quality of three airtight and one non-airtight wood-burning stoves under experimental conditions. With use of the airtight stoves, the average concentrations of CO varied from 0.4 to 2.8 ppm and of submicron particles from 11 to 36 $\mu g/m^3$. In contrast, average emissions from the non-airtight stove ranged from 1.8 to 14 ppm for CO and 210 to 1,900 $\mu g/m^3$ for submicron particles, with a peak of 10,000 $\mu g/m^3$. Indoor concentrations of five different polycyclic aromatic hydrocarbons were higher when the non-airtight stove was used. Differences in operating conditions caused much greater variability in emissions from the non-airtight wood stove although all the stoves demonstrated higher emissions during starting and reloading.

These studies suggest that airtight wood stoves contribute substantially to ambient air pollution but little to indoor concentrations. Airtight wood stoves are more thermally efficient than other wood-burning appliances. Their slower burn rate results in less complete combustion, causing greater release of CO, particulates, and polycyclic organic materials into the ambient air. However, since airtight stoves operate under negative pressure, pollutant emissions from airtight stoves into indoor air are substantially less than from other wood-burning appliances. Although combustion is more complete in fireplaces, fireplace emissions into indoor air have not been characterized adequately. Non-airtight wood stoves are probably intermediate in completeness of combustion and have the potential to cause significant degradation of indoor air quality although the magnitude of their impact can be significantly affected by the way in which they are operated.

## HEALTH EFFECTS OF WOOD SMOKE

Wood smoke is an extremely complex mixture, both in its physical and chemical properties and in its toxicologic properties. The toxicology of certain individual components of wood smoke, such as benzo[a]pyrene, other polycyclic organic compounds, and nitrogen oxides, has been studied extensively. Little research, however, has been directed toward the toxicology of wood smoke as a complex mixture. *In vitro* experiments demonstrate that emissions from a wood stove induce sister chromatid exchange (Hytonen, Alfheim, and Sorsa 1983) and are mutagenic, as assessed by the Ames *Salmonella* assay (Alfheim and Ramdahl 1984; Van Houdt et al. 1986). Alfheim and Ramdahl (1984) found that mutagenic activity in indoor air increased slightly during heating with an airtight wood stove but increased substantially when wood was burning in an open fireplace. Van Houdt and co-workers (1986) found some increase in the mutagenic activity in indoor air in eight of twelve homes with wood stoves and substantial increases in twelve of twelve homes with fireplaces.

ANIMAL STUDIES

Animal studies have addressed the respiratory effects of wood smoke. Using a rabbit model, Fick and colleagues (1984) studied the effects of wood smoke on pulmonary macrophages. Following acute exposure to Douglas fir wood smoke, respiratory tract cells were recovered by bronchoalveolar lavage, and the functional properties of the alveolar macrophages were studied. Significantly more cells were recovered on lavage of exposed rabbits, compared with controls, and defects in macrophage phagocytic activity, bacterial uptake, and surface adherence were noted. Cell differential counts and macrophage viability and bactericidal processing were not affected. Wong and co-workers (1984) evaluated the response of guinea pigs to Douglas fir smoke with repeated $CO_2$ challenges. Exposure resulted in a decreased ventilatory response to $CO_2$ as measured by changes in tidal volume and respiratory frequency, with complete recovery within three days.

EPIDEMIOLOGIC STUDIES

The epidemiologic evidence on the health effects of wood smoke is also limited (Table 9.2). Most of the available information is derived from investigations in developing countries, where intense smoke exposure results from the use of cooking fires in poorly ventilated dwellings. Smith (1987) has reviewed air pollution and biomass fuels comprehensively from a global perspective. Domestic exposure to smoke from biomass fuels, which include dung and straw in addition to wood, has been implicated as a cause of chronic obstructive lung disease, particularly among women who are responsible for cooking. Master (1974) evaluated a random sample of ninety-four New Guinea natives for the presence of respiratory disease. He reported that the prevalence of chronic lung disease, as measured by the presence of chronic productive cough, dyspnea, and/or abnormal pulmonary findings on physical examination, increased with age and reached 78 percent in

Table 9.2 Studies of the Relationship of Domestic Smoke Exposure to Respiratory Illness

| Study | Findings | Conclusions |
| --- | --- | --- |
| *Adults* | | |
| Prevalence survey of chronic respiratory disease, evaluated by questionnaire and spirometry, 1,284 adults, Papua, New Guinea (Anderson 1979) | Increased chronic respiratory symptoms and decreased pulmonary function with age; 20% of males, 10% of females over 45 years had FEV/FVC < 60%; smoking not associated with pulmonary function. | Exposure to smoke not inquired about; raised as a possible etiologic factor based on its widespread prevalence and exclusion of other factors. |
| Prevalence survey of chronic respiratory disease, evaluated by questionnaire with follow-up spirometry and evaluation on subgroup, 2,826 adults; Nepal (Pandey 1984a, 1984b) | Prevalence of chronic bronchitis was 17.6% among men, 18.9% among women; prevalence increased with increasing hours of exposure to domestic smoke in both sexes regardless of smoking status. | Exposure assessed by questionnaire on average number of hours per day spent near the fireplace; socioeconomic status was homogeneous. |
| Prevalence survey of chronic respiratory disease, evaluated by questionnaire and spirometry, 446 adults, India (Malik 1985) | Overall prevalence of chronic bronchitis 21.7% in men, 19.0% in women; prevalence was 5.8% in nonsmoking men, 5.9% in nonsmoking women. | Exposure to smoke not inquired about; raised as a possible etiologic factor due to large number of hours spent in crowded poorly ventilated dwellings. |
| Prevalence survey of chronic respiratory disease, evaluated by questionnaire and peak flow meters, 2,180 adults, India (Malik 1985) | Prevalence of chronic bronchitis varied with type of cooking fuel: 5% with cow dung and firewood; 2.6% coal and kerosene oil; 1.3% kerosene oil; 1.6% low-pressure gas. | Exposure assessed by type of cooking fuel; smoking and socioeconomic status not addressed. |
| *Children* | | |
| Prevalence survey of respiratory symptoms among 807 children from the Highlands, 843 from a coastal area; supplemented by a 30-week prospective study of 112 children, Papua, New Guinea (Anderson 1978) | Prevalence of most respiratory symptoms similar between the two groups; prospective study showed no differences between 87 children exposed to domestic smoke at night and 25 children who lived in smokefree houses. | Degree of smoke exposure not ascertained in either study; in prospective study, lack of comparability between the two groups not addressed. |

| Description | Results | Comments |
|---|---|---|
| Case-control study of serious lower respiratory illness in infants under 13 months, 132 cases, 18 controls, South Africa (Kossove 1982) | Cases more likely to be exposed to smoke than controls (70 versus 33%); no significant differences in cigarette smoking or other sociodemographic factors; cases 2 months older than controls. | Smoke exposure from open cooking fires averaged 6–7 h/day; some degree of confounding by age likely. |
| Prevalence study comparing respiratory symptoms of 31 children from homes with, and 31 children from homes without, wood stoves, Michigan (Honicky, Osborne, and Akpom 1985) | Prevalence rate ratio, comparing exposed to nonexposed children, was 2.7 for moderate respiratory symptoms and 28.0 for severe symptoms; parental smoking, socioeconomic status similar in both groups. | Measure of exposure a dichotomous variable, reflecting presence or absence of woodstove |
| Prospective follow-up of above study group for three years, by interview at end of each winter period; 10% annual attrition (Osborne and Honicky 1986) | Prevalence of coughing at night, coughing more than 4 days per week, and wheezing ranged from 30–85% in exposed, 0–16% in control. | Analyzed cross-sectionally each year, not longitudinally; measure of exposure as before; data available only in abstract form. |
| Prevalence study comparing respiratory symptoms and acute respiratory illnesses over the past 3 months, 258 schoolage children from homes with wood stoves and 141 from homes without, Massachusetts (Tuthill 1984) | Excess illness (defined as two or more episodes) not associated with wood stove use; also no excess of specific symptoms; no covariates related to either exposure or illness. | Specific questions asked relating to use of wood stove; cigarette smoking not related to respiratory illness, but indices of exposure to formaldehyde were related. |
| Prospective study of about 450 children, aged 0–2 years, exposed to smoke from fireplaces in poorly ventilated huts without chimneys, followed up over two time periods (Pandey, Neupane, and Gautam 1987) | Both studies showed association between increasing hours spent near the fireplace and severe acute respiratory illness; less consistent association seen with milder forms of illness. | Illness and exposure history gathered biweekly by trained lay reporters; measures of effect not calculable from data provided in preliminary report. |
| Prevalence study of respiratory symptoms and medical history, 5,338 children from six U.S. cities (Dockery et al. 1987) | Chest illness in past year associated with presence of wood stove in all six cities (prevalence ratio, 1.32); wheezing and coughing not associated | Exposure variable dichotomous reflecting presence or absence of wood stove; preliminary report. |

adults over forty years of age. In contrast to the usual male preponderance of chronic respiratory disease, the prevalence among women was similar to that of men. Although direct measures of smoke exposure were not obtained, Master concluded from the pathologic changes found on autopsy of one young man that smoke exposure was the most important factor in the early development of respiratory disease.

The work of Anderson in New Guinea (1979), of Pandey in Nepal (1984a, 1984b), and Malik in India (1985) supports these conclusions. Anderson (1979) conducted a prevalence survey of respiratory disease among 1,284 adults in Papua, New Guinea. Chronic respiratory symptoms increased with age, and 20 percent of men and 10 percent of women over the age of forty-five years demonstrated an obstructive defect on spirometry. A measure of exposure to wood smoke was not incorporated into the study design, but the author concluded that smoke exposure was a potential etiologic agent for the excess respiratory symptoms and obstruction.

Pandey (1984a) administered a standardized respiratory symptoms questionnaire in a house-to-house survey of 2,826 permanent residents, who were 20 years of age or older, of two villages in Nepal. Subjects who reported more than an occasional cough were referred for further evaluation. The overall prevalence of chronic bronchitis, which was confirmed in the follow-up examination in 94 percent of these subjects, was 18.3 percent, and chronic bronchitis was equally prevalent in men and women. Data on 1,375 individuals were analyzed further to examine the relationship between prevalence of chronic bronchitis and exposure to domestic smoke, as measured by the average time spent near the fireplace on a daily basis (Pandey 1984b). A dose-response relationship was observed between the prevalence of chronic bronchitis and hours of exposure. This relationship was independent of smoking status. Pandey and colleagues (1985) also evaluated the pulmonary function status of 150 women aged thirty to forty-four from two rural villages in Nepal. Pulmonary function declined as hours of smoke exposure increased in cigarette smokers but not in nonsmokers.

Malik (1985) evaluated the respiratory status of 2,180 adult women with a standardized respiratory questionnaire. Pulmonary function was measured with a peak flow meter. Although the overall prevalence of chronic bronchitis reported in this study was lower than in previous studies, the prevalence of chronic bronchitis among women who cooked on chullas (traditional stoves) with cow dung and firewood was higher (5 percent) than among women who cooked with coal and kerosene (2.6 percent), kerosene oil alone (1.3 percent), or low-pressure petroleum gas (1.6 percent). The peak expiratory flow rate was also lower among the group of asymptomatic women who cooked on chullas. Smoking and socioeconomic status were not reported in this study although most of the women who cook with biomass fuels live in rural areas.

The relationship between domestic smoke exposure and acute respiratory illness has also been examined in children from less developed countries. Anderson (1978) examined 112 children from the highlands of Papua, New Guinea, on a weekly basis for thirty weeks. Children who lived in villages were considered to be exposed to smoke, and children who lived in government housing at the village station were not. The weekly prevalence rates of loose cough and nasal discharge were similar in the two groups, but confounding by socioeconomic status cannot be excluded.

Two studies of children in less developed countries have shown associations between exposure to smoke and lower respiratory illness. Kossove (1982) performed a case-control study of 150 Zulu infants under thirteen months of age, 132 infants with severe lower respiratory disease ("wheezing bronchitis" or pneumonia), and eighteen infants without respiratory disease. More than twice as many cases as controls (70 versus 33 percent) had a history of daily heavy smoke exposure from cooking and/or heating fires. Parental smoking and socioeconomic status were similar in the two groups although the average age of controls was two months younger than cases.

Pandey and colleagues (1987) conducted a prospective study during two observation periods of children aged two years and younger. Acute respiratory illnesses were ascertained biweekly by trained lay reporters and classified by severity (grades I–IV). Although some inconsistency was found between the two periods in the relationship between mild illnesses and hours of smoke exposure, both studies showed a strong positive association between the incidence of more severe respiratory illness and hours of exposure to wood smoke.

Cancer of the respiratory tract might plausibly be associated with domestic smoke exposure, but the relevant evidence is quite limited. Ecologic studies have suggested that rates of nasopharyngeal cancer are higher in the Kenyan highlands, where cooking is performed indoors, than in hotter parts of Kenya, where cooking is performed outdoors. Other studies of nasopharyngeal cancer, however, have not demonstrated this relationship (DeKoning, Smith, and Last 1985). High lung cancer mortality rates among women living in Xuan Wei County in China prompted investigators to examine the relationship between lung cancer occurrence and fuel type (Mumford et al. 1987). Comparing lung cancer rates among communes that used different types of fuel, the investigators concluded that lung cancer was related to the burning of "smokey coal" that emits high concentrations of polycyclic aromatic hydrocarbons. Lung disease mortality was substantially lower in communes burning wood and smokeless coal. Although a relationship between cancer and wood smoke remains highly speculative, it is plausible in light of the known toxicology of the constituents of wood smoke and needs further investigation.

Although these studies implicate exposure to smoke as an important etiologic factor in the development of both acute and chronic respiratory illness in developing countries, their relevance to the U.S. experience with residential use of wood stoves and fireplaces is questionable. In addition to differences in type of fuel used, emissions from an unvented open fire are several orders of magnitude higher than emissions from modern wood combustion appliances. In a small pilot study, Smith and colleagues (1983) measured the personal exposures to particulates and benzo[a]pyrene among women cooking food on simple stoves using biomass fuels. During cooking periods, total suspended particulate exposures averaged nearly 7 mg/m$^3$ and benzo[a]pyrene exposures about 4,000 ng/m$^3$, the equivalent of smoking about twenty packs of cigarettes per day. These concentrations markedly exceed the fireplace benzo[a]pyrene concentrations of 11 and 19 ng/m$^3$ as measured by Moschandreas and colleagues (1980).

Unfortunately, the epidemiologic data relevant to the United States are sparse and inconsistent. One case report described a seven-month old infant who had recurrent serious episodes of wheezing and pneumonia, temporally related to being in his parents' or grandparents' homes, both having wood stoves (Honicky, Akpom, and Osborne 1983) The episodes resolved when use of the wood stoves was discontinued. This case prompted the same investigators to conduct a prevalence study of respiratory symptoms among thirty-one children, aged one to seven years, living in homes with wood stoves and thirty-one children, matched for age and sex, from homes with other types of heating (Honicky, Osborne, and Apkom 1985). Using a standardized respiratory symptoms questionnaire, information on demographic factors, sources of home heat, other potential sources of indoor pollutants such as tobacco smoking, past medical history, and occurrence of respiratory symptoms over the past winter was obtained from subjects' parents. Symptoms were scored dichotomously (ever or never present) and graded according to severity. The exposed group experienced significantly more moderate and severe respiratory symptoms: 84 percent of children in the exposed group reported at least one severe symptom as compared with 3 percent of the nonexposed group. These findings were not altered by consideration of potentially confounding factors. Follow-up examination of these children after two and three years showed that the respiratory symptoms persisted among the exposed group (Osborne and Honicky 1986). Over this time span, five families stopped using a wood stove; in all five cases the children's respiratory symptoms disappeared.

Although these findings are provocative, they have not yet been confirmed. Tuthill (1984), using a similar design, asked four hundred parents in western Massachusetts about their youngest elementary schoolchild's respiratory symptoms and illnesses over the previous winter months. Twenty-three percent of children from homes with wood stoves had had two or more acute respiratory illnesses, compared with 20 percent of children from homes without wood stoves. Wood stove use was also unrelated to fever, sore throat, runny nose, cough, or wheeze.

Wood stove use was also investigated in a cohort of six thousand schoolchildren participating in a nationwide study of air pollution in six cities (Dockery et al. 1987). Use of a wood stove was associated with a 32 percent increase in respiratory illness of sufficient severity to keep the child from normal activities for three or more days. This association was found in all six cities, although it was weakest in Portage, Wisconsin, the city with the highest prevalence of wood stoves. Physician-diagnosed respiratory illness before the age of two years, bronchitis in the previous year, chronic cough for three months of the year or more, and persistent wheeze were not associated with use of a wood stove.

Differences in the study populations, type of wood burned, or wood stove used or ascertainment of illness may explain the disparate findings of these studies. Honicky and co-workers (1985) studied preschool children, who usually spend more time at home than do children who are in school, and thus have higher exposures to pollutants in the home. Although questionnaires were used in each study to obtain data on recent respiratory symptoms, differences in questionnaire design might have produced different results. The lack of information on the effect of wood stoves on indoor air quality adds to the difficulty of interpreting these studies. Emission studies that have monitored particulates, CO, and $NO_2$ have not found a significant impact of airtight wood stoves on indoor air concentrations of these pollutants. Thus, the biologic basis for the positive findings of Honicky and colleagues (1985) and of Dockery and colleagues (1987) is uncertain. However, some unmeasured component of wood smoke, such as acrolein or another toxic aldehyde, may be emitted at sufficiently high concentrations to cause respiratory disease.

Although no epidemiologic studies have examined the effect of domestic exposure to wood smoke on adults in the United States, a case of interstitial lung disease attributed to wood smoke has been reported (Ramage et al. 1988). The subject was a sixty-one-year-old woman who developed increasingly severe shortness of breath over the period of a year. The patient's lungs contained a large number of carbonaceous particulates and fibers, with inflammation and fibrosis surrounding them. An evaluation of the patient's home implicated a malfunctioning wood-burning radiant heater as the source of the particles.

Another potential hazard of wood-burning stoves is illustrated by a case report of a Wisconsin family that experienced arsenic poisoning (Peters et al. 1984). All eight family members experienced recurring health problems involving the eyes, respiratory system, central nervous system, blood, reproductive system, skin, and hair loss. Symptoms improved during the summer but then became progressively worse each winter over a three-year period. When hair analysis revealed elevated arsenic levels, a thorough environmental evaluation of the house implicated the burning of chromium-copper-arsenate-treated wood as the major arsenic source.

Wood smoke exposure may also occur in the workplace. In a small preliminary survey of restaurant broiler cooks in Utah, the prevalence of respiratory symptoms in thirteen mesquite broiler cooks was compared with the prevalence in seventeen gas flame broiler cooks (Johns et al. 1986). Symptoms suggestive of any respiratory irritation were significantly higher in the mesquite broiler cooks. The prevalence of symptoms suggestive of either upper or lower respiratory tract irritation was also higher in the mesquite broiler group although the differences did not meet statistical significance. Although the small sample size prevented the authors from considering the effect of cigarette smoking, the differences are unlikely to be due solely to this factor.

## SUMMARY

The current data base regarding the impact of wood combustion appliances on indoor air quality and the effect of these emissions on health is inadequate. Use of wood stoves may increase in the future if prices of oil and natural gas rise. Although the need to control ambient emissions became obvious in the 1970s, we do not yet have sufficient information to determine whether more effort to control indoor emissions is also warranted. A trial of discontinuance of wood stove use is certainly warranted in cases of children with recurrent respiratory symptoms. However, we do not yet have sufficient data on the relationship between respiratory symptoms and the use of a wood stove to recommend that all parents with wood stoves discontinue their use.

## REFERENCES

Alfheim, I., and Ramdahl, T. 1984. Contribution of wood combustion to indoor air pollution as measured by mutagenicity in *Salmonella* and polycyclic aromatic hydrocarbon concentration. *Environ. Mutagen.* 6:121–30.

Anderson, H. R. 1978. Respiratory abnormalities in Papua, New Guinea children: The effects of locality and domestic wood smoke pollution. *Int. J. Epidemiol.* 7:63–72.

Anderson, H. R. 1979. Respiratory abnormalities, smoking habits and ventilatory capacity in a highland community in Papua, New Guinea: Prevalence and effect on mortality. *Int. J. Epidemiol.* 8:127–35.

Annandale, D. D.; Duxbury, M. L.; and Newman, P. G. 1983. Wood: The growing fuel of the future. *Search* 14:263–68.

Cooper, J. A. 1980. Environmental impact of residential wood combustion emissions and its implications. *JAPCA* 30:855–61.

DeAngelis, D. G.; Ruffin, D. S.; and Reznik, R. B. 1980. Preliminary characterization of emissions from wood-fired residential combustion equipment. Washington, D.C.: Government Printing Office. Publication no. EPA/600/7-80/040.

DeKoning, H. W.; Smith, K. R.; and Last, J. M. 1985. Biomass fuel combustion and health. *Bull. WHO* 63:11–26.

Dockery, D. W., et al. 1987. Associations of health status with indicators of indoor air pollution from an epidemiologic study in six U.S. cities. In *Indoor air 1987, Vol. 2: Environmental tobacco smoke, multicomponent studies, radon, sick buildings, odours and irritants, hyperactivities and allergies.* Ed. B. Seifert et al., 203–7. Berlin: Institute for Water, Soil, and Air Hygiene.

Fick, R. B., et al. 1984. Alterations in the antibacterial properties of rabbit pulmonary macrophages exposed to wood smoke. *Am. Rev. Respir. Dis.* 129:76–81.

Honicky, R. E.; Akpom, C. A.; and Osborne, J. S. 1983. Infant respiratory illness and indoor air pollution from a wood-burning stove. *Pediatrics* 71:126–28.

Honicky, R. E.; Osborne, J. S., III; and Apkom, C. A. 1985. Symptoms of respiratory illness in young children and the use of wood-burning stoves for indoor heating. *Pediatrics* 75:587–93.

Hytonen, S.; Alfheim, I.; and Sorsa, M. 1983. Effect of emissions from residential wood stoves in SCE induction in CHO cells. *Mutat. Res.* 118:69–75.

Johns, R. E., Jr., et al. 1986. Respiratory effects of mesquite broiling. *J. Occup. Med.* 28:1181–84.

Kaaraka, P.; Kanarek, M. S.; and Lawrence, J. R. 1987. Assessment and control of indoor air pollution resulting from wood-burning appliance use. In *Indoor air 1987, Vol. 1: Volatile organic compounds, combustion gases, particles and fibers, microbiological agents.* Ed. B. Seifert et al., 425–29. Berlin: Institute for Water, Soil, and Air Hygiene.

Kossove, D. 1982. Smoke-filled rooms and lower respiratory disease in infants. *S. Afr. Med. J.* 61:622–24.

Lewis, C. W., and Einfeld, W. 1985. Origins of carbonaceous aerosol in Denver and Albuquerque during winter. *Environ. Int.* 11:243–47.

Malik, S. K. 1985. Exposure to domestic cooking fuels and chronic bronchitis. *Indian J. Chest Dis. Allied Sci.* 27:171–74.

Master, K. M. 1974. Air pollution in New Guinea: Cause of chronic pulmonary disease among stone-age natives in the highlands. *JAMA* 228:1653–55.

Moschandreas, D. J.; Zabransky, J.; and Rector, H. E. 1980. The effects of wood burning on the indoor residential environment. *Environ. Int.* 4:463–68.

Mumford, J. L., et al. 1987. Lung cancer and indoor exposure of unvented coal and wood combustion emissions in Xuan Wei, China. In *Indoor air 1987, Vol. 3: Developing countries, guaranteeing adequate indoor air quality, control measures, ventilation effectiveness, thermal climate and comfort, policy and strategies.* Ed. B. Seifert et al., 8–14. Berlin: Institute for Water, Soil, and Air Hygiene.

Osborne, J. S., and Honicky, R. E. 1986. Chronic respiratory symptoms in young children and indoor heating with a woodburning stove. *Am. Rev. Respir. Dis.* 133:300 (abstr.).

Pandey, M. R. 1984a. Prevalence of chronic bronchitis in a rural community of the hill region of Nepal. *Thorax* 39:331–36.

Pandey, M. R. 1984b. Domestic smoke pollution and chronic bronchitis in a rural community of the hill region of Nepal. *Thorax* 39:337–39.

Pandey, M. R., et al. 1985. Domestic smoke pollution and respiratory function in rural Nepal. *Tokai J. Exp. Clin. Med.* 10:471–81.

Pandey, M. R.; Neupane, R. P.; and Gautam, A. 1987. Domestic smoke pollution and acute respiratory infection in Nepal. In *Indoor air 1987, Vol. 3: Developing countries, guaranteeing adequate indoor air quality, control measures, ventilation effectiveness, thermal climate and comfort, policy and strategies.* Ed. B. Seifert et al., 25–29. Berlin: Institute for Water, Soil, and Air Hygiene.

Peters, H. A., et al. 1984. Seasonal arsenic exposure from burning chromium-copper-arsenate-treated wood. *JAMA* 251:2392–96.

Quraishi, T. A. 1985. Residential wood burning and air pollution. *Int. J. Environ. Studies* 24:19–33.

Ramage, J. E., Jr., et al. 1988. Interstitial lung disease and domestic wood burning. *Am. Rev. Respir. Dis.* 137:1229–32.

Ramdahl, T., et al. 1982. Chemical and biological characterization of emissions from residential stoves burning wood and charcoal. *Chemosphere* 116:601–11.

Sexton, K.; Spengler, J. D.; and Treitman, R. D. 1984. Effects of residential wood combustion on indoor air quality: A case study in Waterbury, Vermont. *Atmos. Environ.* 18:1371–83.

Smith, K. R. 1987. *Biofuels, air pollution and health: A global review.* New York: Plenum.

Smith, K. R.; Aggarwal, A. L.; and Dave, R. M. 1983. Air pollution and rural biomass fuels in developing countries: A pilot village study in India and implications for research and policy. *Atmos. Environ.* 17:2343–62.

Traynor, G. W., et al. 1987. Indoor air pollution due to emissions from wood-burning stoves. *Environ. Sci. Technol.* 21:691–97.

Tuthill, R. W. 1984. Woodstoves, formaldehyde and respiratory disease. *Am. J. Epidemiol.* 120:952–55.

Van Houdt, J. J., et al. 1986. Contribution of wood stoves and fire places to mutagenic activity of airborne particulate matter inside homes. *Mutat. Res.* 171:91–98.

Wong, K. L., et al. 1984. Evaluation of the pulmonary effects of wood smoke in guinea pigs by repeated $CO_2$ challenges. *Toxicol. Appl. Pharmacol.* 75:69–80.

# 10

# FORMALDEHYDE

Marian C. Marbury, Sc.D.
Robert A. Krieger, Ph.D.

Few indoor air pollutants have provoked more public, regulatory, or scientific controversy in the past ten years than formaldehyde (Graham, Green, and Roberts 1988). In the late 1970s, numerous reports described the adverse health effects in residents of homes insulated with urea-formaldehyde foam insulation (UFFI). By 1979, two state agencies in Massachusetts had received more than 350 complaints of adverse health effects (Walker et al. 1987). These reports generated intense public concern and spurred awareness of the ubiquity of formaldehyde in consumer products and residences. This concern was fueled by a report in 1979 from the Chemical Industry Institute of Toxicology (CIIT) that formaldehyde exposure caused nasal cancer in rats (Kerns, Donofrio, and Pavkov 1983).

The regulatory response to the evidence of adverse effects of formaldehyde has varied in speed and intensity. Massachusetts banned further installation of UFFI as early as 1979 (Walker et al. 1987). The Consumer Products Safety Commission followed suit, issuing a ban on UFFI in 1982 (Ashford, Ryan, and Caldant 1983). Other federal agencies were slower to act. The U.S. Environmental Protection Agency (EPA) did not take definitive action until April 1987, when it officially classified formaldehyde as a probable human carcinogen and performed an assessment of the health risks of formaldehyde to garment workers and home residents (U.S. EPA 1987). In a similarly slow response, the Occupational Safety and Health Administration (OSHA) initially declined to change the workplace standard of 3 parts per million (ppm) in effect in 1980. This standard was not revised until 1988, when, under threat of a contempt of court citation from the U.S. Court of Appeals, OSHA issued a new standard of 1 ppm with a short-term exposure limit of 2 ppm.

The public controversy over formaldehyde has been mirrored by scientific controversy. Numerous toxicologic, clinical, and epidemiologic investigations have been conducted over the past ten years and their results extensively reviewed and debated (National Research Council [NRC] 1981; Hart, Terturro, and Neimeth 1984; Nelson et al. 1986; U.S. EPA 1987; Council on Scientific Affairs 1989). Scientific consensus has not been reached on the human carcinogenicity of low-level exposure to formaldehyde or on the ability of formaldehyde to induce respiratory sensitization (Hart, Terturro, and Neimeth 1984). Nonetheless, with the virtual freeze in installation of UFFI and the development of product standards regulating the amount of formaldehyde that can be emitted by consumer products, much of the public concern about formaldehyde seems to have abated (Mage and Gammage 1985).

This chapter provides an overview of what is known about formaldehyde, indicates where the controversies lie, and discusses some of the important studies in more detail. Of necessity, literature citation has been selective rather than comprehensive. Every effort has been made, however, to provide a balanced view of the issues.

## EXPOSURE TO FORMALDEHYDE

Formaldehyde, the simplest chemical in the aldehyde family, is a one-carbon compound with the formula HCHO. Existing in both gaseous and liquid states, it readily polymerizes at normal room temperatures. Gaseous formaldehyde is colorless with a characteristic pungent odor. Formalin, which contains about 37 percent (by weight) dissolved formaldehyde in water, is a clear colorless liquid. It usually contains 6–15 percent methanol to prevent polymerization (U.S. EPA 1987).

Formaldehyde has been in widespread industrial use since World War II, with annual production increasing from one billion to more than five billion pounds during this period (Mage and Gammage 1985). Numerous sources of formaldehyde are present in the indoor environment. Formaldehyde is most commonly found in the form of urea- and phenol-formaldehyde resins. Urea-formaldehyde (UF) resins are used to treat many consumer products; facial tissues, paper towels, grocery bags, and other paper products are treated with these resins to increase their wet strength. UF resins are also used as stiffeners, water repellants, and wrinkle resisters, and thus formaldehyde may be emitted from permanent-press clothing, carpet backings, floor coverings, and adhesive binders. Formaldehyde is also emitted by gas stoves, is present in tobacco smoke, and is a constituent of numerous other consumer products, such as cosmetics and detergents (Mage and Gammage 1985).

Formaldehyde is also used in building materials and as a component of UFFI. Formaldehyde resins exhibit good bonding properties, and thus UF resins, in particular, have been used as a glue for plywood, which is made by gluing thin sheets of wood together; they are also used as a component of particleboard, which is manufactured by cooking small particles of wood with the resin and then pressing the particles into sheets. Both plywood and particleboard are used extensively in the manufacture of new furniture and cabinets and are also important building materials in mobile homes.

UFFI, a major source of residential formaldehyde exposure in the past, was used widely in the 1970s because it provided one of the few methods for insulating existing homes effectively. To make UFFI, partially polymerized UF resin was mixed with a foaming agent and an acid catalyst under pressure. The foam was then injected into wall cavities through small holes. After installation, formaldehyde was normally emitted for a few days as the foam hardened (or cured). However, if UFFI was not properly formulated or mixed—for example, if too much formaldehyde was used in the resin-concentrate solution—then the release of formaldehyde could be sustained over a longer period of time. The adverse publicity about UFFI and a large number of lawsuits against insulators have virtually ended the use of UFFI as an insulation material.

As would be anticipated from the sources of formaldehyde described previously, the highest indoor concentrations of formaldehyde have been found in homes insulated with UFFI; in new homes with new furnishings, particularly homes that are tightly sealed; and in manufactured and mobile homes, which combine extensive use of plywood, a high surface area to air ratio, and a low ventilation rate. Within these and other types of structures, however, formaldehyde concentrations vary extensively. In a particular dwelling, determinants of the formaldehyde concentration are the age of the residence, the specific formaldehyde sources, and the ambient temperature and humidity. Formaldehyde emissions result from the release of unreacted formaldehyde in formaldehyde-containing resins and the decomposition of the resins. The first half-life of formaldehyde in mobile homes and new homes with particleboard and plywood is generally four to five years; the half-life in homes with UFFI is one year (Hart, Terturro, and Neimeth 1984). High heat and humidity also contribute to formaldehyde release, and as a consequence, the highest indoor formaldehyde concentrations occur in the summer.

Numerous potential sources of formaldehyde also exist in office buildings and include insulation, new furniture and furnishings, carpets, carbonless copy paper, and tobacco smoke. Measurements of formaldehyde concentrations have not been performed systematically in office buildings but have been taken to evaluate building-related illness. Breysse (1985) reported that concentrations ranged from 0.01 to 0.30 ppm in twenty health hazard evaluations conducted in problem buildings. Although formaldehyde has been implicated as the causative agent in 4 percent of episodes of building-related illness investigated by the National Institute of Occupational Safety and Health (Melius et al. 1984), the true contribution of formaldehyde to the problem of building-related illness is not known.

Surveys of residential formaldehyde concentrations have been conducted in the past ten years by federal, state, and university investigators (Table 10.1). The results of these surveys cannot be readily compared because of differences in methods of selecting the study population (random sample versus volunteers) and

Table 10.1  Surveys of Formaldehyde in Residential Settings

| Study Design | Number and Type of Dwellings | HCHO Results (ppm) Mean (Median) | Range |
|---|---|---|---|
| Investigated by Minnesota Department of Health at resident physician's request (Ritchie and Lehnen 1985) | 397 mobile homes | 0.4 | 0.02–3.69 |
|  | 489 conventional homes (34% w/UFFI; no difference) | 0.14 | 0.01–5.62 |
| Convenience sample of Houston, Tex. homes (Stock and Mendez 1985) | 78 residences: conventional and energy-efficient homes, apartments, condos | 0.07 | 0.008–0.29 |
| 65 volunteers from random sample of 208 Wisconsin homes (Hanrahan 1984) | 65 mobile homes | 0.16 | <0.10–0.80 |
| Investigated by Wisconsin Division of Health at resident request (Dally et al. 1981) | 65 mobile homes | 0.35 | <0.10–3.68 |
|  | 14 UFFI homes | 0.10 | 0.10–0.28 |
|  | 13 UF wood products | 0.10 | 0.10–0.92 |
| Random sample of California homes (Sexton, Liu, and Petreas 1986) | 663 mobile homes, summer | 0.072 | <0.10–0.46 |
|  | 523 mobile homes, winter | 0.078 | 0.17–0.31 |

in the measurement techniques. (Proper sampling technique is another entire issue; see, for example, Godish [1985].) The EPA has recently summarized the results of studies conducted since 1982 on random population samples. This review showed that the average concentrations of formaldehyde in mobile homes range between 0.2 and 0.5 ppm, and in conventional homes between 0.03 and 0.09. Higher levels may be found in conventional homes with plywood paneling or with new furnishings (U.S. EPA 1987).

## TOXICOLOGY

Formaldehyde can enter the body through inhalation, ingestion, and dermal absorption. Data from animal studies suggest that the absorption rate from inhalation exposures is high. Because of formaldehyde's water solubility, more than 95 percent is retained in the upper respiratory tract of dogs (Egle 1972) and 98 percent in the nasal passages of rats (Dallas et al. 1985). Oral absorption in animals also occurs rapidly and efficiently (Malorny, Rietbrock, and Scheider 1965). In contrast, dermal absorption appears to be an inefficient exposure pathway. Depending on the animal species and the test conditions, dermal absorption ranges from 6 to 10 percent in experiments (Robbins et al. 1984).

Once absorbed, formaldehyde either oxidizes rapidly to formate and carbon dioxide ($CO_2$) or combines with tissue constituents. The major oxidative process is dependent upon the enzyme formaldehyde dehydrogenase, which oxidizes formaldehyde-glutathione adduct with $NAD^+$ to form NADH and $S$-formylgluta-thione. Hydrolase then reacts further with $S$-formylglutathione to produce formate and glutathione (Strittmatter and Ball 1955; Ulsamer et al. 1984). Formaldehyde is also oxidized by either a nonspecific dehydrogenase, a catalase, or other less important pathways (Palese and Tephley 1975). Formaldehyde is metabolized quite rapidly. Studies in primates demonstrate a half-life of formaldehyde in plasma of 1.5 minutes following infusion. Experimental studies of humans have also indicated that formaldehyde blood concentrations do not increase following inhalation of 2 ppm for forty minutes (Heck et al. 1985). Because formaldehyde is principally absorbed in the respiratory tract and metabolism of absorbed formaldehyde is rapid, several expert panels have concluded that the respiratory tract is the primary target following inhalation of formaldehyde and that formaldehyde itself is unlikely to cause adverse effects at sites that are distant from exposure (Hart, Terturro, and Neimeth 1984; U.S. EPA 1987).

In addition to being oxidized, absorbed formaldehyde can also bind electrophilically with macromolecules, including proteins, DNA, and RNA. This binding may result in formation of reversible adducts or irreversible cross-links with the macromolecules. *In vitro* studies of the effect of formaldehyde on human bronchial cells have demonstrated that formaldehyde can also induce single-strand breaks in DNA and inhibit the repair of breaks induced by ionizing radiation (Grafstrom et al. 1983).

The specific mechanisms by which formaldehyde exerts its toxic effects have not yet been identified. At the cellular level, the toxic effects of formaldehyde may be due to the action of monomethylol-amino acid intermediates formed by reactions with amino acids. These intermediates are known to have toxic effects and can cause DNA strand breaks (Poverenny et al. 1975). The sensory irritation caused by formaldehyde is thought to result from stimulation of the afferent trigeminal nerve, which induces a burning sensation and other reflexive responses (Barrow, Steinhagen, and Chang 1983). Formaldehyde also damages the mucociliary clearance system and the epithelial cell layer of the respiratory tract (Starr et al. 1984). The cytotoxic effect of formaldehyde exposure produces abnormal cell replication (metaplasia and hyperplasia) in the upper respiratory tract of some test animals. In *in vitro* experiments, formaldehyde causes genetic damage in a wide variety of test systems, including gene mutations, sister chromatid exchanges (SCE), and chromosome aberrations, as well as the single-strand breaks in DNA and DNA-protein cross-links mentioned previously (Hart, Terturro, and Neimeth 1984).

In 1979, the CIIT reported that rats exposed to formaldehyde developed nasal cancer, a tumor rarely found in control animals. In this bioassay, Kerns and co-workers (1983) exposed groups of 240 mice and 240 rats to four different concentrations of formaldehyde gas for six hours a day, five days a week, for two years. Squamous cell carcinomas developed in the nasal cavities of two mice and 103 rats exposed to 14.3 ppm and of two rats exposed to 5.6 ppm. Small numbers of polypoid adenomas, which are benign tumors, were also observed at each dose level. These results have been confirmed in subsequent studies (Albert et al. 1982; Tobe et al. 1985).

Data regarding the effect of formaldehyde on the reproductive system have been much less consistent. The consensus panel, an expert panel gathered by the federal government to review all the available data on formaldehyde, noted that animal studies had not shown a teratogenic response to formaldehyde (Hart, Terturro, and Neimeth 1984). One study in which mice were intubated demonstrated no treatment-related difference in malformations, even at doses sufficiently high to kill 50 percent of the dams. In another study, pregnant beagles were fed hexamethylenetetramine, a substance that is metabolized to formaldehyde; again, no malformations were found. Studies of germ cell effects in animals have not provided consistent data. Other studies have demonstrated effects, such as embryo resorption, that are difficult to relate to humans (Overman 1985).

## HUMAN HEALTH EFFECTS OF FORMALDEHYDE

Numerous adverse health consequences have been ascribed to formaldehyde, ranging from well-documented effects such as eye and nose irritation, to more controversial claims including menstrual irregularity, chronic respiratory disease, and neuropsychological deficit. The evidence for these effects is variable in quality and consistency. Although no biologic mechanism is currently known by which formaldehyde might exert an effect at sites distant to the point of absorption (Hart, Terturro, and Neimeth 1984), a toxic metabolite of formaldehyde could be responsible. Data on human health effects derive largely from surveys of residents of mobile homes or homes insulated with UFFI (Table 10.2) and from epidemiologic and clinical investigations of occupationally exposed workers.

### CARCINOGENICITY

Although the evidence regarding the carcinogenicity of formaldehyde in rodents is unequivocal, the extrapolation of these results to humans has been controversial (Starr and Gibson 1985; Nelson et al. 1986; Bolt 1987). Unfortunately, human epidemiologic studies do not fully resolve this controversy.

Numerous studies of formaldehyde-exposed populations to assess carcinogenicity have now been performed. With the exception of a single study of mobile home residents, these investigations have focused on formaldehyde-exposed professional and occupational groups, and cancer of the respiratory tract has been the health outcome of primary concern.

Cohort studies, in which the mortality pattern of a group of formaldehyde-exposed workers is monitored over time, have not shown an excess of nasal cancer (Table 10.3). Since the baseline incidence of this cancer is quite low in human populations, however, these studies have been too small to detect anything less than a tenfold increase. Even the largest of the studies had only an 80 percent chance, as calculated by the authors, of detecting a fourfold increase (Blair et al.

Table 10.2  Surveys of Occupants Living or Working in Mobile Homes
or Homes with UFFI

| Study Population | Findings[a] Symptom | % | Comments |
|---|---|---|---|
| 424 adults and 99 children living in 334 mobile homes; complaint investigations, Washington State (Breysse 1980) | Eye irritation<br>Throat irritation<br>Chronic headache<br>Chronic cough<br>Memory lapse/drowsiness | 58A, 41C<br>66A, 62C<br>40A, 16C<br>9A, 33C<br>24A, 7C | Formaldehyde levels, 0.03–1.77 ppm; no control group; exposure response not examined |
| 256 adults and children living in 65 mobile homes or 35 other structures; complaint investigations, Wisconsin (Dally et al. 1981) | Eye irritation<br>Throat irritation<br>Headache<br>Cough<br>Difficulty sleeping<br>Wheezing | 68<br>57<br>53<br>51<br>38<br>20 | Formaldehyde levels, 0.0–3.68 ppm; no control group; exposure response not examined |
| 162 residents of 68 homes with UFFI; complaint investigations, Connecticut (Sardinas et al. 1979) | Eye irritation<br>Nose/throat/lung irritation<br>Headache<br>No apparent relationship between symptoms and crude formaldehyde level | 39<br>48<br>17 | Formaldehyde levels, 0.0–10 μg/liter with detectable and nondetectable levels |
| Unknown number of residents in 443 families living in mobile homes; complaint investigations, Texas (Norsted, Kozinetz, and Annegers 1985) | No difference in symptom prevalence in families living in homes with and without detectable levels | | Formaldehyde levels, 0.0–8 ppm; comparison of homes with detectable and nondetectable levels |
| 1,396 residents of UFFI homes and 1,395 residents of non-UFFI homes; retrospective cohort, New Jersey (Thun, Lakat, and Altman 1982) | Exposed more likely to report wheezing than nonexposed<br>Wheezing<br>  Exposed<br>  Nonexposed<br>Burning skin<br>  Exposed<br>  Nonexposed<br>Subgroup, in whose homes odor persisted >7 days after foam installed, had higher symptom incidence | <br><br>0.6<br>0.1<br><br>0.7<br>0.1 | Population-based study; formaldehyde concentrations not measured |
| 70 exposed employees of 7 mobile home care centers and 34 nonexposed employees of 3 permanent structures, Denmark (Olsen and Dossing 1982) | Exposed reported significantly more symptoms than nonexposed<br>Menstrual irregularities<br>  Exposed<br>  Nonexposed<br>Excessive thirst<br>  Exposed<br>  Nonexposed<br>Eye irritation<br>  Exposed<br>  Nonexposed<br>Headache<br>  Exposed<br>  Nonexposed | <br><br>35<br>0<br><br>60<br>5<br><br>55<br>15<br><br>80<br>50 | Formaldehyde levels in mobile day care centers, 0.24–0.55 ppm; permanent structures, 0.05–0.11 ppm |

(*continued*)

Table 10.3  (*continued*)

| Study Population | Findings[a] | | Comments |
|---|---|---|---|
| | Symptom | % | |
| 21 exposed workers in mobile home office and 18 nonexposed workers in another office, Illinois (Main and Hogan 1983) | Exposed reported significantly more symptoms | | Formaldehyde levels in offices, 0.12–1.6 ppm |
| | Eye irritation | | |
| | Exposed | 81 | |
| | Nonexposed | 17 | |
| | Throat irritation | | |
| | Exposed | 57 | |
| | Nonexposed | 22 | |
| | Fatigue | | |
| | Exposed | 81 | |
| | Nonexposed | 22 | |
| | Headache | | |
| | Exposed | 76 | |
| | Nonexposed | 11 | |
| | No difference in pulmonary function | | |

[a]A, adults; C, children.

1986). In addition, any elevated risk would not have been detected if the period between exposure and development of nasal cancer, the latent period, exceeded the follow-up interval in these studies.

Case-control studies, in which the exposure histories of people with a particular disease are compared with the exposure histories of people without the disease, provide a more sensitive method for investigating the etiology of a rare cancer. Several case-control studies have been conducted to examine the association between formaldehyde exposure and sinonasal cancer, nasopharyngeal cancer, or both. In five of these studies, formaldehyde exposure was not assessed directly; instead, the likelihood of exposure was based on an industrial hygienist's evaluation of the subjects' occupational history. Both Hayes and colleagues (1986) and Olsen et al. (1984) reported a statistically significant association between imputed formaldehyde exposure and sinonasal cancer. Nasopharyngeal cancer was not considered in the former study and was not found to be associated with formaldehyde exposure in the latter. The findings of an association between formaldehyde exposure and sinonasal cancer were not confirmed in studies by Hernberg et al. (1983), Vaughan and colleagues (1986a), or Roush and co-workers (1987), although the latter two studies did find nonsignificant associations between formaldehyde exposure and nasopharyngeal cancer after a latency period of at least twenty years. In another case-control study of sinonasal cancer, Brinton and colleagues (1985) reported an association between nasal cancer and previous employment in textile manufacturing, an industry in which the use of formaldehyde is widespread. In the study by Brinton and co-workers, formaldehyde exposure was directly asked about, however, and cases reported a history of exposure less frequently than controls.

Table 10.3   Studies of Formaldehyde-Exposed Cohorts and Cancer

| Study | Findings | Comments |
|---|---|---|
| Cohort study of pathologists, Great Britain (Harrington and Shannon 1975) | SMR elevated for lymphoma and hematopoietic neoplasms (211) but not for leukemia | Less than 10% of cohort deceased; less than 20 years of follow-up |
| Proportional mortality study of embalmers, New York (Walrath and Fraumeni 1983) | PMR[a] significantly elevated for cancers of skin (221) and colon (143); nonsignificantly for cancers of brain (156) and kidney (150), and leukemia (140) | Limitations of PMR methodology |
| Proportional mortality study of embalmers, California (Walrath and Fraumeni 1983) | PMR significantly elevated for cancers of colon (188), brain (191), and prostate (176), and leukemia (174); nonsignificantly for bladder cancer (138) | Limitations of PMR methodology |
| Cohort study of pathologists, Great Britain (Harrington and Oakes 1984) | SMR significantly elevated for brain cancer (300) but not lymphoma | Less than 5% of cohort deceased; 6 years of follow-up |
| Cohort study of anatomists, U.S. (Stroup, Blair, and Erickson 1986) | SMR elevated for brain cancer (271, 95% CI[b] = 130–499) and leukemia (148, 95% CI = 71–272) | Excess brain cancer persisted when psychiatrists used as a reference group |
| Cohort study of undertakers, Canada (Levine, Andjelkovich, and Shaw 1984; Levine et al. 1984) | SMR nonsignificantly elevated for brain cancer (115) and leukemia (160) | 20 years of follow-up |
| Proportional mortality study of chemical plant employees, Massachusetts (Marsh 1982) | PMR nonsignificantly elevated for cancers of digestive organs (152) among formaldehyde-exposed workers; no data reported on brain cancer and leukemia | No evidence of trend of mortality in relation to exposure |
| Cohort study of chemical plant employees, United States (Marsh 1983) | SMR significantly elevated for cancers of genitourinary tract (169); SMR for leukemia not elevated; no data for brain cancer | Case-control study within cohort showed no association between genitourinary cancer and a general plant exposure |
| Cohort study of chemical plant employees, Great Britain (Acheson et al. 1984) | SMR for lung cancer significantly elevated (124) in one of six plants with highest levels | Retrospective assessment made of level of exposure |
| Cohort study of industrial workers with formaldehyde exposure, U.S. (Blair et al. 1986) | SMR significantly elevated for nasopharyngeal cancer (318); SMR nonsignificantly elevated for lung cancer (111) and Hodgkin's disease (142); lung cancer significantly elevated in men with 20+ years latency (132) | Largest study reported to date; retrospective assessment of exposure level |

(*continued*)

Table 10.3  (*continued*)

| Study | Findings | Comments |
|-------|----------|----------|
| Cohort study of garment workers, U.S. (Brinton, Blot, and Fraumeni 1985) | SMR significantly elevated for buccal cavity (343) and connective tissue cancer (364) | Retrospective assessment of exposure level |
| Cohort study of workers in a resin manufacturing plant (Bertazzi et al. 1986) | SMR for lung cancer significantly elevated (236) | Incomplete ascertainment of exposure history makes interpretation difficult |

[a]PMR, proportional mortality ratio.
[b]Confidence interval.

Although the studies described above considered only occupational sources of formaldehyde exposure, Vaughn and co-workers (1986b) also inquired about residential exposure to formaldehyde, including whether subjects had ever lived in a mobile home. Associations were not found between residence in a mobile home and cancer of the oropharynx or hypopharynx, or cancer of the sinus and nasal cavity. However, an increased risk of nasopharyngeal cancer was associated with living in a mobile home. Residence in a mobile home for one to nine years was associated with a relative risk of 2.1 (95 percent confidence interval = 0.7, 6.6), increasing to 5.5 (95 percent confidence interval = 1.6, 19.4) for residence exceeding nine years. Although these results were based on only eight exposed cases of nasopharyngeal cancer, the association persisted after control for effects of other factors, including cigarette smoking, alcohol consumption, and race.

Although an increase of nasal cancer has not been demonstrated in cohort studies of formaldehyde-exposed populations, two recent studies provide evidence of a possible relationship between formaldehyde and buccal-pharyngeal cancer. Unlike rats, humans are not obligate nose breathers, and consequently the buccal cavity is a biologically plausible site for formaldehyde-induced cancer. Blair and co-workers (1986, 1987) studied more than 26,000 workers employed in ten different plants in which formaldehyde was either used or produced. Initially, they reported a statistically significant excess of nasopharyngeal cancers with a standardized mortality ratio (SMR) of 318 (an SMR of 318 indicates that the mortality rate of nasopharyngeal cancer was 3.18 times higher in the formaldehyde-exposed group than in a nonexposed comparison group) and a nonsignificant excess of oropharyngeal cancer (SMR = 192). Further analysis (Blair et al. 1987) demonstrated that among workers who were simultaneously exposed to particulates, the SMR increased from 192 in the low-exposure category to 403 in the middle- and 746 in the high-exposure category. A similar trend was not present in workers who were not exposed to particulates or in cases of oropharyngeal cancer. However, four of the seven cases of nasopharyngeal cancer were among workers from one plant, a pattern suggesting that the exposure environment may have been unique in that plant.

Stayner and co-workers (1988) reported an increased risk of buccal cavity cancer (SMR = 343) but not pharyngeal cancer among a cohort of formaldehyde-exposed garment workers. The risk was highest among workers with a long duration of employment and follow-up. Although a significant excess of cancer of the tonsils was also reported, the small number of deaths restricted the ability to examine exposure trends.

The occurrence of lung cancer has also been examined in the formaldehyde-exposed cohorts, and an excess of lung cancer has been found in three. Acheson and co-workers (1984) studied seven thousand men employed in six different chemical and plastics factories. They found a 24 percent increase in lung cancer in one of the factories when national mortality rates were used as the standard of comparison. The investigators discounted the significance of these results because the elevation was confined to one of the factories and was not significant when local rates were used for comparison. However, the local rates were for the period 1968–78 whereas the study period included earlier years, when rates were lower. Consequently, use of these local rates might have overestimated the number of expected deaths. In addition, the lung cancer risk was greatest among men who started employment between 1935 and 1946, when exposures were highest, and the risk was elevated only among men in the high-exposure category.

Blair and colleagues (1986), in their study of formaldehyde-exposed workers, reported a small and not statistically significant excess of lung cancer. There was a statistically significant 32 percent increase among workers with more than twenty years since their first exposure. The investigators minimized the significance of this finding, noting that the excess did not increase either with estimates of intensity or duration of exposure or with cumulative exposure. Bertazzi and co-workers (1986), in a study of 1,332 men employed in a resins manufacturing plant, reported a statistically significant increase in lung cancer (SMR = 236) which persisted with comparison with local rates (SMR = 186). The excess could not definitely be attributed to formaldehyde as the risk was highest in the group whose exposure to formaldehyde was unknown, and the excess risk was not clearly related to either length of employment or latency.

These three studies show an excess risk of lung cancer in formaldehyde-exposed workers, but the evidence is not sufficient to establish a causal relationship between formaldehyde and lung cancer. The lack of a trend in the relationships between increasing exposure and excess risk may be due to misclassification of exposure or to the instability of comparisons based on the stratification of a small number of deaths. Alternatively, other exposures, either at the workplace or from personal habits such as smoking, may be responsible for the excess risk of lung cancer. Studies of formaldehyde-exposed professional groups, such as embalmers (Walrath 1983; Walrath and Fraumeni 1983; Levine, Andjelkovich, and Shaw 1984; Levine et al. 1984), anatomists (Stroup, Blair, and Erickson 1986), and pathologists (Harrington and Shannon 1975; Harrington and Oakes 1984) have not shown an excess of lung cancer.

Cancers of other sites have also been examined. Studies of the aforementioned professional groups, but not of formaldehyde-exposed industrial workers (Marsh

1982; Fayerweather, Pell, and Bender 1983; Acheson et al. 1984; Blair et al. 1986), have demonstrated significant excesses of brain cancer (Walrath 1983; Walrath and Fraumeni 1983; Harrington and Oakes 1984; Stroup, Blair, and Erickson 1986); excess leukemia has also been found in embalmers (Walrath 1983; Walrath and Fraumeni 1983; Levine, Andjelkovich, and Shaw 1984), anatomists (Stroup, Blair, and Erickson 1986), garment workers (Stayner et al. 1988), and one cohort of chemical workers (Bertazzi et al. 1986). Small excesses of Hodgkin's disease (Blair et al. 1986) and prostate (Walrath 1983), skin (Walrath and Fraumeni 1983), kidney (Walrath and Fraumeni 1983), connective tissue (Stayner et al. 1988), and digestive system cancers have been reported from individual studies (Marsh 1982; Walrath 1983; Walrath and Fraumeni 1983; Bertazzi et al. 1986) but have not been confirmed by other studies. As formaldehyde is rapidly metabolized and cleared from the plasma, the hypothesis that it causes cancer at sites distant from the point of absorption would not seem to have strong biologic plausibility (Hart, Terturro, and Neimeth 1984).

CARCINOGENIC RISK ASSESSMENT

Several scientific groups have described the evidence linking formaldehyde exposure to cancer in humans as "limited" (Hart, Terturro, and Neimeth 1984; Nelson et al. 1986; U.S. EPA 1987) and have concluded that the original study of nasal cancer in rats provides the most suitable data for quantitative risk estimation (Hart, Terturro, and Neimeth 1984; U.S. EPA 1987). Risk estimation requires both the selection of a model to extrapolate from observed effects at high doses to the lower doses anticipated from human exposures, and an understanding of the toxic mechanisms by which formaldehyde causes cancer.

The CIIT has argued that use of a simple linear extrapolation model overestimates the carcinogenic risk posed by formaldehyde (Starr and Gibson 1985; Swenberg et al. 1985). Based on an understanding of the toxic mechanisms of formaldehyde and the relationship between the administered dose (exposure) and dose to the target tissue, the CIIT proposes that the carcinogenic effect of formaldehyde demonstrable at high concentrations is unlikely to occur at low concentrations.

Based on experiments conducted at the CIIT, the CIIT asserts that the cell proliferation and hyperplasia following formaldehyde cytotoxicity are essential steps in the carcinogenic process, as formaldehyde binds only to single-stranded DNA. Since DNA in this form is more common during DNA replication with cellular proliferation, formaldehyde has a greater chance of binding to DNA during cell proliferation. It follows that errant DNA synthesis and expansion of initiated cell populations to neoplasia are also related to cell proliferation (Starr and Gibson 1985). Further, cytotoxicity and the resultant cell proliferation are related more closely to intensity of exposure than to duration, which implies that exposure to a high concentration for a short period is more carcinogenic than the same total dose delivered over a longer period of time.

The CIIT has also argued that the relationship between the administered dose and the dose to the target tissue is not linear over a range of concentrations. They contend that several respiratory defense mechanisms, which are overwhelmed by high concentrations, effectively minimize the amount of formaldehyde reaching target tissue at low concentrations. The defense of primary importance is the mucociliary apparatus, specifically the layer of mucus which flows continuously over the nasal epithelium. Formaldehyde readily reacts with the albumin component of mucus. At low concentrations, the binding reaction coupled with mucus clearance effectively prevents formaldehyde from reaching the epithelium. At higher concentrations, mucociliary function is inhibited, and large areas of the mucous blanket are immobilized, effectively removing this defense mechanism (Swenberg et al. 1985).

The CIIT concludes that these findings collectively suggest that the administered dose is a poor measure of delivered dose, which is of greater biologic relevance. The CIIT argues that a better measure of delivered dose is the amount of formaldehyde covalently bound to respiratory mucosal DNA, which also exhibits a nonlinear relationship with the administered dose. The use of bound formaldehyde as the measure of exposure lowers the estimates of risk from formaldehyde exposure by a factor of fifty-three at concentrations of 1 ppm or less, regardless of the specific mathematical dose-response model employed (Swenberg et al. 1985).

The appropriateness of this approach for quantitative risk assessment has been disputed, however, and the EPA chose not to consider it in assessing risks of formaldehyde to garment workers and to the general population (U.S. EPA 1987). The EPA stated that some evidence from mutagenicity studies suggests a linear relationship between formaldehyde exposure and point mutations, chromosome aberrations, and DNA damage. The EPA also asserted that the relationship between cellular proliferation and carcinogenesis had not been demonstrated unequivocally. Furthermore, the agency regarded the data on DNA adducts as an inappropriate basis for use in risk assessment.

As a result, the EPA concluded that the data provided by the CIIT were not sufficiently compelling to warrant deviation from the standard risk assessment procedure, which includes use of the linearized multistage model. Using this model, the EPA estimated that the upper bound estimate for the lifetime excess risk of developing cancer is three per ten thousand for garment workers exposed to formaldehyde concentrations of 0.17 ppm, two per ten thousand for mobile home residents exposed to 0.10 ppm for ten years, and one per ten thousand for residents of conventional homes exposed to 0.07 ppm for ten years. These estimates are upper bounds; the maximum likelihood, or point, estimate is substantially lower, particularly at low concentrations. The EPA stated that the lower bound estimate, as always, could be zero, but they noted the excess cancer incidences reported in various epidemiologic studies were consistent with these upper bound estimates (U.S. EPA 1987).

GENOTOXICITY

As a phenomenon closely related to carcinogenicity, the genotoxicity of formaldehyde has also received attention. Data concerning the *in vivo* genotoxicity of formaldehyde in human studies are not consistent (Table 10.4) (Hart, Terturro, and Neimeth 1984). Yager and colleagues (1986) measured sister chromatid exchange (SCE) in the peripheral lymphocytes of eight anatomy students, before and after a ten-week anatomy class, during which they were exposed to formaldehyde embalming solution. The investigators reported a statistically significant overall increase in SCE which exceeded 20 percent in three students. Breathing zone samples of formaldehyde taken during the class were 1.2 ppm. Mierauskiene and Lekevicius (1985) found a statistically significant increase in chromosome aberrations (2.8 versus 1.3 percent) in fifty workers exposed to phenol, styrene, and formaldehyde, compared with twenty-five workers without such exposure. Bauchinger and Schmid (1985) studied the lymphocytes of twenty exposed and unexposed male paperworkers. The exposed paperworkers had a significantly elevated prevalence of dicentrics or of dicentrics and ring chromosomes. This excess was concentrated among the eleven most highly exposed workers. Other chromosomal aberrations and SCE values did not differ between the exposed and control groups.

Other studies of genetic effects have not been confirmatory. Fleig and coworkers (1982) found no statistically significant differences in chromosomal aberrations between fifteen workers with twenty-three to thirty-five years of exposure

Table 10.4  Studies of Genotoxicity in Formaldehyde-Exposed Populations

| Study Population | End Point(s) | Findings |
|---|---|---|
| 15 workers engaged in HCHO manufacture and 15 matched controls (Fleig et al. 1982) | Chromosomal aberrations | No difference in number of aberrations between groups |
| 6 pathology workers and 5 nonexposed controls (Thomson, Shackleton, and Harrington 1984) | Chromosomal aberrations, SCE | Exposed group had nonsignificant increase in aberrations, no differences in SCE frequency |
| 11 hospital autopsy service workers and 11 matched controls (Ward et al. 1984) | Sperm count and morphology, fluorescent body frequency | Exposed group had decreased sperm count, more abnormal morphology; differences not significant |
| 50 workers exposed to HCHO, phenol, styrene and 25 nonexposed controls (Mierauskiene and Lekevicius 1985) | Chromosomal aberrations | Exposed had twice the frequency of aberrations, independent of age and smoking |
| 20 papermakers exposed to HCHO and 20 nonexposed workers as controls (Bauchinger and Schmid 1985) | Chromosomal aberrations, SCE | Frequency of dicentrics or dicentrics and ring chromosomes significantly increased for most heavily exposed group |
| 19 HCHO-exposed hospital autopsy service workers and 20 matched controls (Connor, Ward, and Legator 1985) | Urine mutagenicity | No difference in mutagenicity between the two groups |
| 8 students, studied before and after a 10-week anatomy class (Yager et al. 1986) | SCE | Small but significant increase in SCEs after exposure |

to formaldehyde manufacture and processing and a matched unexposed control group from the same workplace. Exposures had not exceeded 1 ppm in this workplace for eleven years prior to this study. Thomson and colleagues (1984) studied members of a pathology staff, six recently exposed to formaldehyde at peak concentrations exceeding 6 ppm. In these six, the frequency of chromosomal aberrations was increased, but not significantly in comparison with five nonexposed workers. SCE values did not differ between the two groups. Ward and co-workers (1984) evaluated sperm count, sperm morphology, and fluorescent body frequency in eleven autopsy service workers and eleven nonexposed controls. Formaldehyde concentrations were between 0.61 and 1.32 ppm as a time-weighted average, with peaks up to 5.8 ppm. The mean sperm count of exposed workers was lower (62.9 versus $87.4 \times 10^6/$ml), and the percentage of abnormal sperm morphology was higher among nonexposed workers (53.3 versus 44.5 percent), but these differences were not statistically significant. Finally, Connor and colleagues (1985) did not find an increase in the urine mutagenicity of nineteen workers exposed to formaldehyde on an autopsy service when compared with twenty nonexposed workers.

Inconsistency among these results may be due to differences in the outcomes measured, in study techniques, or in study populations. More importantly, because formaldehyde is oxidized so rapidly, neither peripheral lymphocytes nor germ cells should be targets for formaldehyde. The positive studies, therefore, must be confirmed before much weight can be given to them.

IRRITATION OF THE EYES AND UPPER RESPIRATORY TRACT

Formaldehyde is indisputably a mucous membrane irritant that causes discomfort of the eyes, nose, and throat. Symptoms of irritation have been reported by residents of mobile homes and homes insulated with UFFI (Table 10.2), by subjects exposed to formaldehyde in environmental chambers (Sauder et al. 1986; Schachter et al. 1986; Kulle et al. 1987), and by employees exposed in the workplace (Schoenberg and Mitchell 1975; Alexandersson, Hedenstierna, and Kolmodin-Hedman 1982; Alexandersson and Hedenstierna 1989; Horvath et al. 1988). Formaldehyde induces sensory irritation through stimulation of the afferent trigeminal nerve as well as other reflexive responses. Questions remain, however, about the concentrations of formaldehyde necessary to elicit these responses.

Questionnaire surveys of symptoms have been performed on residential populations, usually selected because of health complaints attributed to formaldehyde exposure from UFFI or to offgasing from building materials. These surveys show seemingly high prevalences of both respiratory and nonrespiratory symptoms. However, the investigations of complaints in Washington (Breysse 1980), Wisconsin (Dally et al. 1981), Connecticut (Sardinas et al. 1979), and Texas (Norsted, Kozinetz, and Anneggers 1985) cannot be readily interpreted because of methodologic problems. Comparison populations were not evaluated in two studies (Breysse 1980; Dally et al. 1981), bias may have resulted from the selection of complaining subjects, and formaldehyde measurements were obtained only once, although formaldehyde concentrations vary with ambient heat and humidity. A Canadian study involving comparison of symptoms in two formaldehyde-exposed groups illustrates the potential for reporting bias (Morgan 1984). In this study, subjects from homes insulated with UFFI were compared with pathology laboratory employees, who are presumably exposed to higher concentrations of formaldehyde than were the persons from the UFFI-insulated homes. The prevalences of symptoms related to upper respiratory irritation were similar in the two groups, but vague symptoms characteristic of anxiety, such as headache, loss of libido, anorexia, and malaise, were substantially higher in the subjects from homes with UFFI. The questionnaire surveys of symptom prevalence provide documentation, however, that formaldehyde exposure occurs in the domestic environment and that individual response to exposure is variable.

Thun and colleagues (1982) used a more informative and less biased design in a study of 1,396 residents of homes insulated with UFFI and 1,395 residents of homes without UFFI. Subjects were selected from a roster of homes that had been insulated with UFFI rather than on the basis of symptom status. By telephone interview, the investigators ascertained symptom prevalence over the previous year and the timing of symptom onset in relation to installation of UFFI. The reported incidence of all symptoms was low, and only wheezing and burning skin were significantly more frequent in residents of homes with UFFI. Subjects who reported that odor had persisted for more than seven days after UFFI installation had the highest incidence of symptoms.

To assess the persistence of symptoms among residents of older homes with particleboard, Daugbjerg (1989) sent questionnaires to the parents of three groups of children living in homes that had varying amounts of particleboard: 254 children from homes with large amounts, 144 from homes with small amounts, and 574 from homes free of particleboard. Living in a home with a large amount of particleboard was found to be a risk factor for coughing, eye and nose irritation, and wheezy bronchitis among children zero to five years of age but not among older children. A large amount of particleboard was also a risk factor for headache, throat irritation, and a need for daily asthma medication for all children. Living in a home with a small amount of particleboard was not a risk factor for any respiratory symptoms. Environmental measurements were not obtained.

In the most comprehensive study performed to date of the health effects of UFFI Broder and colleagues (1988a, 1988b, 1988c) studied 1,726 subjects from 571 homes insulated with UFFI and 720 controls from 231 homes not insulated with UFFI at two intervals a year apart. In addition to the administration of health questionnaires, study methods included the measurement of nasal airway resistance, pulmonary function, and sense of smell; patch tests for sensitivity to formaldehyde and to UFFI; and nasal surface cytology. Most of the subjects were reevaluated one year later. At the one-year follow-up, two-thirds of the subjects originally living in homes insulated with UFFI had either removed the UFFI or had taken some other remedial action (Broder et al. 1988c). The average formaldehyde concentration was 0.043 ppm in UFFI houses and 0.035 ppm in control houses; the average age of the UFFI was 4.6 years (Broder et al. 1988b). At the initial survey, subjects from the UFFI homes had more nasal symptoms than controls, but nasal resistance and the distribution of smell threshold were similar in the two groups (Broder et al. 1988b). Throat and eye complaints were also more frequent in the UFFI-exposed subjects, and the subjects from UFFI homes also reported an increased prevalence of skin irritation, cough, sputum, wheeze, headache, dizziness, tiring easily, troubled hearing, increased thirst, nausea, diarrhea, constipation, menstrual trouble, and arthritis. The excess symptom prevalence occurred primarily among those who intended to have the UFFI removed from their homes.

Positive dose-response relationships between formaldehyde concentration and many of these symptoms were found among the subjects from UFFI homes but not among the control subjects. When 135 subjects whose mean formaldehyde concentration exceeded 0.08 ppm were eliminated, the exposure-response relationship persisted only for cough and sputum. The authors interpreted the presence of a dose response only among subjects from UFFI homes as evidence that the excess symptom prevalence was due to a combination of formaldehyde and some unidentified UFFI-associated factor rather than formaldehyde alone.

At follow-up one year later, the prevalence of nasal symptoms dropped in the groups removing the UFFI or taking some other action (Broder et al. 1988c). The prevalence of nasal and other symptoms declined to the level in the UFFI-exposed group who took no action, but a small excess persisted relative to the controls. The reduction of symptom rates was not associated with changes in formaldehyde levels. Overall, the investigators concluded that their study supported a causal relationship between impaired health and living in a house with UFFI, but they considered the demonstrated health effects to be relatively minor and reversible.

These studies demonstrate the difficulty of quantitating the irritative potential of formaldehyde. The EPA concluded that existing population studies did not provide an adequate basis for risk assessment because of their limitations; evidence from clinical studies was also judged insufficient because study subjects were volunteers, and study sizes were small (U.S. EPA 1987). Instead, the EPA affirmed the more qualitative conclusion that 95 percent of people respond to concentrations of 0.1–3.0 ppm and that fewer responses are expected to be associated with lower concentrations.

LOWER RESPIRATORY TRACT EFFECTS

Based on studies of occupationally and domestically exposed populations, formaldehyde has been reported to cause respiratory symptoms, acute and chronic reduction of lung function, and asthma. Questionnaire symptom surveys performed on populations selected because of their complaints about formaldehyde exposure have shown seemingly high prevalences of respiratory and nonrespiratory symptoms. These findings have been interpreted as evidence that formaldehyde might be a lower respiratory tract irritant and also be capable of inducing a specific sensitization reaction. These potential effects of formaldehyde have been more adequately investigated in clinical and epidemiologic studies of both acute and chronic effects.

Effects of acute formaldehyde exposure on the lung function level of asthmatics and healthy nonsmoking volunteers have been evaluated in chamber studies (Table 10.5). Three studies of asthmatics showed no changes in pulmonary function following exposures of up to 3 ppm formaldehyde, either at rest (Harving et al. 1986) or during moderate exercise (Sheppard, Eschenbacker, and Epstein 1984; Green et al. 1987). Studies of healthy nonsmokers exposed to up to 3 ppm formaldehyde either at rest or during moderate exercise have similarly found no effect of exposure (Schachter et al. 1986; Kulle et al. 1987). Some evidence suggests, however, that exposure during more intense exercise may produce a small and transient bronchoconstriction. Sauder and colleagues (1986) exposed nine volunteers to 3 ppm formaldehyde for three hours during intermittent exercise and found a 2 percent decrease in $FEV_1$ and a seven percent decrease in $FEF_{25-75}$. The reductions were no longer apparent at 60 and 180 minutes. These findings were replicated by Green and co-workers (1987), who exposed twenty-two healthy volunteers to 3 ppm formaldehyde for one hour during intermittent heavy exercise. By increasing respiratory rate and depth, heavy exercise may plausibly increase the dose and the deposition of formaldehyde in the lower respiratory tract. Increases in upper respiratory symptoms of irritation were also reported uniformly in these studies.

The acute effects of UFFI offgas on pulmonary function in nonasthmatics has been examined in a clinical study by Day and colleagues (1984). They studied nine residents of UFFI-insulated homes, who attributed their nonrespiratory symptoms to UFFI, and nine subjects who were either asymptomatic or living in homes without UFFI. Lung function, as assessed by spirometry, did not change after exposure either to 1 ppm formaldehyde or to UFFI offgas that contained 1.2 ppm formaldehyde. Although these clinical investigations have evaluated only small numbers of subjects, the findings suggest that in most cases, symptoms of lower respiratory irritation experienced by residents of mobile homes or houses insulated with UFFI are unlikely to result solely from formaldehyde.

Epidemiologic approaches have also been used to examine the relationship between pulmonary function and residential formaldehyde exposure. Norman and co-workers (1986), using data gathered during a previous study in Canada, identified children who had been living in homes insulated with UFFI. Two children from homes with conventional insulation were matched to each exposed child (n = 29) on the basis of nine variables that had been shown to predict pulmonary function. No association was found between residence in a home insulated with UFFI and respiratory function or symptoms. Measurements of formaldehyde were not made.

In the study of UFFI exposure reported by Broder et al. (1988a, 1988b, 1988c) differences in ventilatory function between the UFFI-exposed and nonexposed subjects were not present at either the initial or follow-up surveys. Cross-sectional

| Study Design and Population | Findings |
| --- | --- |
| 7 mild asthmatics, exposed to 1 and 3 ppm HCHO at rest and during moderate exercise for 10 min (Sheppard, Eschenbacker, and Epstein 1984) | No increase in specific airways resistance before and after exposure |
| 15 healthy volunteers, exposed to 9 and 2 ppm HCHO at rest and during moderate exercise for 40 min (Schachter et al. 1986) | No changes in $FEV_{1.0}$, FVC, $MEF_{50}$, $MEF_{40}$, airway resistance; follow-up of 3 subjects showed no late responses; irritative symptoms increased |
| 9 healthy volunteers, exposed to 3 ppm HCHO for 3 h during intermittent heavy exercise (Sauder et al. 1986) | 2% decrease in $FEV_{1.0}$ and 7% decrease in $MEF_{25-75}$ at 30 min, no longer present at 60 and 180 min |
| 15 subjects with bronchial hyperreactivity exposed to 0.85, 0.12, and 0 mg/m³ for 90 min at three different times (Harving et al. 1986) | No changes in $FEV_{1.0}$, airways resistance, or functional residual capacity or symptoms of asthma |
| 22 healthy volunteers, exposed to 0 and 3 ppm HCHO during intermittent heavy exercise; 16 asthmatics exposed at rest and moderate exercise for 1 h (Green et al. 1987) | Healthy volunteers had small but statistically significant decreases in $FEV_{1.0}$, FVC, and $FEV_{3.0}$; asthmatics showed no changes; 13% of study group showed changes >10% |
| 19 healthy volunteers exposed to 0–3 ppm HCHO at rest, 2.0 ppm during exercise (Kulle et al. 1987) | Dose response for irritation symptoms; nasal flow resistance increased at 3.0 ppm; no changes in pulmonary function or bronchial hyperreactivity |
| 9 subjects with previous complaints from UFFI and 9 controls, exposed to 1 ppm HCHO and UFFI offgas for 90 and 30 min, respectively (Day et al. 1984) | No changes in $FEV_{1.0}$, FVC, or MMEF either immediately or 8 h after exposure |

studies conducted in occupational settings, where exposures are usually higher and more readily quantified than in the residential setting, also supply information on formaldehyde and lung function. Levine and co-workers (Levine et al. 1984) surveyed ninety embalmers attending a continuing education course and found that levels of spirometric parameters were not reduced in comparison with standard reference populations. The pulmonary function of subjects with higher exposures, as estimated by the number of embalmings performed, was similar to that of subjects with lower exposures. The pulmonary function of fourteen policemen, who worked in mobile trailers with formaldehyde concentrations ranging from 0.12 to 1.6 ppm, was evaluated by Main and Hogan (1983). Decrements in function were not found when the values were compared either with a standard reference population or with a nonexposed control population. Pre- and postexposure pulmonary function were not evaluated in either study.

At least four studies have surveyed the pulmonary function of workers in industrial environments in which formaldehyde exposure was accompanied by exposure to particulates. Each demonstrated transient decreases in pulmonary function as measured by pre- and postshift spirometric evaluation (Schoenberg and Mitchell

1975; Gamble et al. 1976; Alexandersson, Hedenstierna, and Kolmodin-Hedman 1982; Horvath et al. 1988). Only one of these four studies reported lower baseline spirometric values for exposed workers, which the investigators interpreted as providing evidence of a persistent effect of exposure (Schoenberg and Mitchell 1975). Another study did not find changes in pulmonary function across shift among exposed workers but did report that the baseline spirometric values were lower (Alexandersson and Hedenstierna 1988).

The most informative of these investigations was conducted in Wisconsin by Horvath and colleagues (Horvath et al. 1988). These investigators evaluated pre- and postshift pulmonary function of 109 workers employed in a particleboard or molded products operation and of 254 workers employed in two other plants not using formaldehyde. Formaldehyde exposures were estimated for each participant from active and passive monitoring. Formaldehyde concentrations ranged from 0.17 to 2.93 ppm, with a median of 0.62 ppm. Across the work shift, both the $FEV_1$ and the $FEV_1/FVC$ ratio dropped significantly in the exposed group. A reduction in $FEV_1$ and FVC of similar magnitude was also found in the control group. The investigators attributed this unexpected finding in both groups to diurnal variation in lung function. The exposed workers also demonstrated statistically significant decreases in $FEF_{25-75}$, $FEF_{50}$, and $FEF_{75}$. These parameters, as well as the FEV/FVC ratio, were positively correlated with measured formaldehyde concentrations. In addition, the investigators reported a significant association between formaldehyde exposure and symptoms of cough, chest complaints, phlegm, burning nose, stuffy nose, itchy nose, sore throat, burning eyes, and itchy eyes.

The investigators attempted to assess the bias that may have resulted from selective withdrawal from the work force of formaldehyde-sensitive individuals. To evaluate this bias, Horvath and co-workers determined the reasons for the departure of fifty-four former employees from the company; only two employees had left for reasons related to respiratory health, both because of exacerbations of preexisting respiratory conditions.

In summary, the available evidence suggests that exposure to formaldehyde at levels up to 3 ppm does not result in permanent pulmonary impairment. In certain working conditions, transient reductions in lung function of uncertain clinical significance have been demonstrated. These deficits have been detected in industrial settings in which formaldehyde exposure occurred along with exposure to particulates. Adsorption of formaldehyde onto particulates may result in deposition of the formaldehyde in the lower respiratory tract rather than absorption onto the mucosa of the upper respiratory tract. Alternatively, physical exertion in an industrial setting may increase minute ventilation and thereby increase both the dose and deposition of formaldehyde in the lower respiratory tract.

Formaldehyde has been shown to cause occupational asthma (Popa et al. 1969; Hendrick and Lane 1977; Hendrick et al. 1982) although the mechanism of effect is uncertain. Formaldehyde might induce asthma through specific immunologic sensitization or exacerbate preexisting asthma by causing bronchoconstriction through nonspecific irritation (Imbus 1985). Medical and nonmedical publications (anonymous *Lancet* editorial 1981; Breysse 1981) have raised concern that residential formaldehyde exposure could also be associated with asthma. These concerns are supported by surveys of formaldehyde-exposed populations that have reported high prevalences of wheezing, chest tightness, and other symptoms compatible with asthma. However, cases of asthma resulting from domestic exposure to formaldehyde have not been published. In a unique documented case of a woman who developed asthma after installation of UFFI, the offending agent was found to be UFFI dust rather than formaldehyde (Frigas, Filley, and Reed 1981).

Several case series provide evidence on the role of formaldehyde as a cause of asthma. In each series, subjects referred to a clinical facility for investigation of suspected formaldehyde-induced asthma were evaluated with bronchial provocation tests. Nordman and colleagues (1985) reported that 12 of 230 workers referred to the Finnish Institute of Occupational Health had a positive bronchial provocation test when exposed to formaldehyde at 2 ppm. In England, Burge and coworkers (Burge et al. 1985) described fifteen workers evaluated for occupational asthma. The authors concluded that three subjects showed specific hypersensitivity to formaldehyde, two were affected through irritant mechanisms, and the remaining ten subjects were probably affected by other agents.

Frigas and co-workers (1984) evaluated thirteen subjects who believed they had developed asthma secondary to formaldehyde exposure in their work or home environments. As none of the subjects responded to formaldehyde challenge, the investigators questioned the importance of formaldehyde as a cause of asthma at levels below 3 ppm, the range generally encountered in the domestic environment. However, because this series comprised only thirteen subjects, firm conclusions on the role of formaldehyde cannot be drawn from its results.

Studies of immunologic function have not helped to resolve whether formaldehyde causes disease through immunologic mechanisms. Although IgE antibody has been produced against other chemicals known to be allergens, specific IgE antibodies to gaseous formaldehyde have not been demonstrated (Hart, Terturro, and Neimeth 1984; Imbus 1985). Two investigative groups have demonstrated the presence of antibodies against formaldehyde-human serum albumin conjugates in some formaldehyde-exposed persons (Patterson et al. 1986; Thrasher et al. 1987). The clinical significance of these antibodies has not been established.

Pross and colleagues (1987) conducted a comprehensive immunologic investigation of twenty-three subjects with asthmalike symptoms attributed to the subjects' living in UFFI-insulated homes and four asthmatics who served as controls, who lived in conventionally insulated homes. The subjects were exposed in an environmental chamber to placebo, dust, formaldehyde, and UFFI offgas at levels usually found in UFFI-insulated homes. A broad range of immunologic parameters was evaluated. At the base line, the data for the UFFI-exposed subjects and the controls were similar. Minor changes were noted in some tests after UFFI exposure; only transient increases in eosinophil and basophil count, a slight increase in the T8 (suppressor) cell population, and a decrease in the NK (natural killer) cell response to low concentrations of interferon were detected. Although this study provides some evidence that formaldehyde is not a potent immunotoxin, interpretation of the data is limited by the small size of the study and the investigators' failure to characterize the study subjects adequately. It is unclear whether the subjects had documented asthma, and if so, whether their symptoms had any objective relationship to UFFI exposure.

Collectively, these studies suggest that asthma may be attributed mistakenly to formaldehyde exposure and that the incidence of true formaldehyde-induced asthma may be low. Although not widely available, specific bronchial provocation testing with formaldehyde is essential for diagnosis. A careful clinical history is important for raising initial concern about formaldehyde-related asthma but by itself may be misleading.

OTHER EFFECTS

Questionnaire surveys of symptoms in subjects concerned about formaldehyde exposure have suggested that formaldehyde may have an adverse effect on both the central nervous system and the female reproductive system (Table 10.2). More formal studies of these effects have been preliminary in nature, and current understanding of the metabolism of formaldehyde suggests that formaldehyde per se is unlikely to have a significant impact on either system. Consequently, studies of the relationship between formaldehyde exposure and these two organ systems will be discussed only briefly.

Olsen and Dossing (1982) reported that day-care workers in mobile homes, compared with day-care workers in permanent structures, experienced significantly more symptoms of headache and unnatural fatigue, but memory and concentration did not differ in the two groups. Kilburn and co-workers (1985) compared the frequency of neurobehavioral, mucous membrane, and respiratory symptoms among seventy-six histology technicians exposed to formaldehyde and fifty-six secretaries and clerks. The histology technicians were more likely to have experienced disturbances of memory, sleep, balance, mood, concentration, and appetite. Each technician estimated the average number of hours per day of exposure to formaldehyde. The prevalence of most symptoms increased with lengthening exposure. Of forty-four technicians who completed a twenty-item depression scale, four had scores suggesting depression. Limitations in the study design preclude attaching much significance to these results until they have been replicated independently.

In order to measure neuropsychological symptoms objectively, Schencker and co-workers (1982) used standardized neuropsychological tests in a study of twenty-four residents of six homes insulated with UFFI. Nine of twenty-three subjects reported neuropsychological symptoms, including memory difficulty, headaches, difficulty concentrating, and emotional lability. Complaints of memory loss were not validated by formal tests. However, eleven of the fourteen tested subjects demonstrated a deficit in their attention, and nine of those eleven also had elevated depression scores. Although the use of objective tests of neuropsychological function represents an improvement over questionnaire assessment of symptoms alone, the results of this study are nonetheless limited by the lack of a comparison population and the small number of study subjects.

These cross-sectional epidemiologic studies involved small numbers of subjects, and their results are not definitive. Further laboratory investigation is needed to establish biologic mechanisms that may underlie the neuropsychological effects of formaldehyde. Formaldehyde might exert a direct toxic effect on the central nervous system. Alternatively, its odor could make individuals more aware of symptoms and more likely to attribute significance to them (Hart, Terturro, and Neimeth 1984).

Although the data base concerning relationships between formaldehyde exposure and adverse reproductive outcomes is not complete, available evidence suggests that formaldehyde does not pose a teratogenic risk to humans (Hart, Terturro, and Neimeth 1984; U.S. EPA 1987). Only a few studies of the relationship between formaldehyde exposure and reproductive outcomes in humans have been published. As described in the report of the consensus panel (Hart, Terturro, and Neimeth 1984), Shumilina studied female workers who were and were not exposed to UF resins. The author concluded that exposed women had three times the prevalence of menstrual disorders and a higher proportion of babies weighing between 2,500 and 3,000 grams, but the translation of the article did not provide sufficient information for the consensus panel to assess the methodologic adequacy of the study.

An increase in menstrual disorders among women exposed to formaldehyde was noted by Olsen and Dossing (1982) in a prevalence survey of women working in mobile homes. In this study, 35 percent of exposed women reported menstrual irregularities as compared with 0 percent of the control group. Finally, Hemminki and co-workers (1982) did not find an increased rate of spontaneous abortions among hospital staff who sterilized hospital instruments with formaldehyde.

The biologic significance of the reported association between formaldehyde exposure and menstrual irregularity remains to be elucidated. Menstrual irregularity cannot be investigated readily, and little is known about its etiology. At present, biologic mechanisms by which formaldehyde could affect menstrual regularity have not been identified.

## SUMMARY

Since formaldehyde was first identified as an animal carcinogen, substantial research effort and money have been expended to investigate the human health consequences of exposure to this pollutant. Much has been learned about sources of formaldehyde in the domestic environment, and control technology has been developed to reduce concentrations from these sources. Significant progress has also been made in understanding acute human responses to formaldehyde exposure.

As for many environmental pollutants, the chronic effects of formaldehyde exposure have not been readily identified. Epidemiologic studies are unlikely to resolve fully the issue of formaldehyde's human carcinogenicity, and establishing a "safe" dose will depend on further refining our risk assessment models. Progress has been made, however, in elucidating the underlying mechanisms of formaldehyde carcinogenicity and in understanding the relationship between the administered and delivered doses. This progress represents a major step in understanding the toxicology of inhaled pollutants in general.

The most important lesson of formaldehyde is that prudent public health measures need not wait for the full resolution of scientific issues. Complete understanding of the human health effects of this pollutant will probably never be achieved. Nonetheless, exposure to formaldehyde in the residential setting has been mitigated to the extent that the urgency of further research has also diminished.

## REFERENCES

Acheson, E. D., et al. 1984. Formaldehyde in the British chemical industry. *Lancet* 1:611–16.

Albert, R. E., et al. 1982. Gaseous formaldehyde and hydrogen chloride induction of nasal cancer in the rat. *J. Natl. Cancer Inst.* 68:597–603.

Alexandersson, R., and Hedenstierna, G. 1988. Respiratory hazards associated with exposure to formaldehyde and solvents in acid-curing plants. *Arch. Environ. Health* 43:222–27.

Alexandersson, R.; Hedenstierna, G.; and Kolmodin-Hedman, B. 1982. Exposure to formaldehyde: Effects on pulmonary function. *Arch. Environ. Health* 37:279–83.

Anonymous. 1981. The health hazards of formaldehyde (editorial). *Lancet* 1:926–27.

Ashford, N. A.; Ryan, C. W.; and Caldant, C. C. 1983. Law and science policy in federal regulation of formaldehyde. *Science* 222:894–900.

Barrow, C. S.; Steinhagen, W. H.; and Chang, J. C. F. 1983. Formaldehyde sensory irritation. In *Formaldehyde toxicity.* Ed. J. E. Gibson, 16–25. New York: Hemisphere.

Bauchinger, M., and Schmid, E. 1985. Cytogenetic effects in lymphocytes of formaldehyde workers of a paper factory. *Mutat. Res.* 158:195–99.

Bertazzi, P. A., et al. 1986. Exposure to formaldehyde and cancer mortality in a cohort of workers producing resins. *Scand. J. Work Environ. Health* 12:461–68.

Blair, A., et al. 1986. Mortality among industrial workers exposed to formaldehyde. *J. Natl. Cancer Inst.* 76:1071–84.

Blair, A., et al. 1987. Cancers of the nasopharynx and oropharynx and formaldehyde exposure (letter). *J. Natl. Cancer Inst.* 78:191.

Bolt, H. M. 1987. Experimental toxicology of formaldehyde. *J. Cancer Res. Clin. Oncol.* 113:305–9.

Breysse, P. A. 1980. *Formaldehyde exposure in mobile homes: Occupational safety and health symposia, 1979.* Washington, D.C.: Government Printing Office. DHHS Publication no. (NIOSH) 80-139.

Breysse, P. A. 1981. The health cost of "tight" homes (editorial). *JAMA* 245:267–68.

Breysse, P. A. 1985. The office environment: How dangerous? In *Indoor air, Vol. 3:*

*Sensory and hyperreactivity reactions to sick buildings.* Ed. B. Berglund, T. Lindvall, and J. Sundell, 315–20. Stockholm: Swedish Council for Building Research.

Brinton, L. A.; Blot, W. J.; and Fraumeni, J. F., Jr. 1985. Nasal cancer in the textile and clothing industries. *Br. J. Ind. Med.* 42:469–74.

Broder, I., et al. 1988a. Comparison of health of occupants and characteristics of houses among control homes and homes insulated with urea-formaldehyde foam insulation, I: Methodology. *Environ. Res.* 45:414–55.

Broder, I., et al. 1988b. Comparison of health of occupants and characteristics of houses among control homes and homes insulated with urea-formaldehyde foam insulation, II: Initial health and house variables and exposure-response relationships. *Environ. Res.* 45:156–78.

Broder, I., et al. 1988c. Comparison of health of occupants and characteristics of houses among control homes and homes insulated with urea-formaldehyde foam insulation, III: Health and house variables following remedial work. *Environ. Res.* 45:179–203.

Burge, P. S., et al. 1985. Occupational asthma due to formaldehyde. *Thorax* 40:255–60.

Connor, T. H.; Ward, J. B., Jr.; and Legator, M. S. 1985. Absence of mutagenicity in the urine of autopsy service workers exposed to formaldehyde: Factors influencing mutagenicity testing of urine. *Int. Arch. Occup. Environ. Health* 56:225–37.

Council on Scientific Affairs, American Medical Association. 1989. Formaldehyde. *JAMA* 261:1183–87.

Dallas, C. E., et al. 1985. Effects of subchronic formaldehyde inhalation on minute volume and nasal deposition in Sprague-Dawley rats. *J. Toxicol. Environ. Health* 16:553–64.

Dally, K., et al. 1981. Formaldehyde exposure in nonoccupational environments. *Arch. Environ. Health* 36:277–84.

Daugbjerg, P. 1989. Is particleboard in the home detrimental to health? *Environ. Res.* 48:154–63.

Day, J. H., et al. 1984. Respiratory responses to formaldehyde and off-gas of urea-formaldehyde foam insulation. *Can. Med. Assoc. J.* 131:1061–64.

Egle, J. L. 1972. Retention of inhaled formaldehyde, propionaldehyde, and acrolein in the dog. *Arch. Environ. Health* 25:119–24.

Fayerweather, W. E.; Pell, S.; and Bender, J. R. 1983. Case-control study of cancer deaths in Dupont workers with potential exposure to formaldehyde. In *Formaldehyde: Toxicology, epidemiology, mechanisms.* Ed. J. J. Clary, J. E. Gibson, and R. E. Waritz, 47–121. New York: Marcel Dekker.

Fleig, I., et al. 1982. Cytogenetic analyses of blood lymphocytes of workers exposed to formaldehyde in formaldehyde manufacturing and processing. *J. Occup. Med.* 24:1009–12.

Frigas, E.; Filley, W. V.; and Reed, C. E. 1981. Asthma induced by dust from urea-formaldehyde foam insulation material. *Chest* 79:706–7.

Frigas, E.; Filley, W. V.; and Reed, C. E. 1984. Bronchial challenge with formaldehyde gas: Lack of bronchoconstriction in 13 patients suspected of having formaldehyde-induced asthma. *Mayo Clin. Proc.* 59:295–99.

Gamble, J. F., et al. 1976. Respiratory function and symptoms: An environmental-epidemiological study of rubber workers exposed to a phenol-formaldehyde type resin. *Am. Ind. Hyg. Assoc. J.* 37:499–513.

Godish, T. 1985. Residential formaldehyde sampling: Current and recommended practices. *Am. Ind. Hyg. Assoc. J.* 46:105–10.

Grafstrom, R. C., et al. 1983. Formaldehyde damage to DNA and inhibition of DNA repair in human bronchial cells. *Science* 220:216–18.

Graham, J. D.; Green, L. C.; and Roberts, M. J. 1988. *In search of safety: Chemicals and cancer risk.* Cambridge, Mass.: Harvard University Press.

Green, D. J., et al. 1987. Acute response to 3.0 ppm formaldehyde in exercising healthy nonsmokers and asthmatics. *Am. Rev. Respir. Dis.* 135:1261–65.

Hanrahan, L. P., et al. 1984. Formaldehyde vapor in mobile homes: A cross-sectional survey of concentrations and irritant effects. *Am. J. Public Health* 74:1026–27.

Harrington, J. M., and Oakes, D. 1984. Mortality study of British pathologists 1974–80. *Br. J. Ind. Med.* 41:188–91.

Harrington, J. M., and Shannon, H. S. 1975. Mortality study of pathologists and medical laboratory technicians. *Br. Med. J.* 4:329–32.

Hart, R. W.; Terturro, A.; and Neimeth, L. 1984. Report of the consensus workshop on formaldehyde. *Environ. Health Perspect.* 58:323–81.

Harving, H., et al. 1986. Low concentrations of formaldehyde in bronchial asthma: A study of exposure under controlled conditions. *Br. Med. J.* 293:310.

Hayes, R. B., et al. 1986. Cancer of the nasal cavity and paranasal sinuses, and formaldehyde exposure. *Int. J. Cancer* 37:487–92.

Heck, H. d'A., et al. 1985. Formaldehyde ($CH_2O$) concentrations in the blood of humans and Fischer-344d rats exposed to $CH_2O$ under controlled conditions. *Am. Ind. Hyg. Assoc. J.* 46:1–3.

Hemminki, K., et al. 1982. Spontaneous abortions in hospital staff engaged in sterilising instruments with chemical agents. *Br. Med. J.* 285:1461–63.

Hendrick, D. J., and Lane, D. J. 1977. Occupational formalin asthma. *Br. J. Ind. Med.* 34:11–18.

Hendrick, D. J., et al. 1982. Formaldehyde asthma: Challenge exposure levels and fate after five years. *J. Occup. Med.* 24:893–97.

Hernberg, S., et al. 1983. Nasal cancer and occupational exposures: Preliminary report of a joint Nordic case-referent study. *Scand. J. Work Environ. Health* 9:208–13.

Horvath, E. P., Jr., et al. 1988. Effects of formaldehyde on the mucous membranes and lungs: A study of an industrial population. *JAMA* 259:701–7.

Imbus, H. R. 1985. Clinical evaluation of patients with complaints related to formaldehyde exposure. *J. Allergy Clin. Immunol.* 76:831–40.

Kerns, W. D.; Donofrio, D. J.; and Pavkov, K. L. 1983. The chronic effects of formaldehyde inhalation in rats and mice: A preliminary report. In *Formaldehyde toxicity.* Ed. J. E. Gibson, 111–31. New York: Hemisphere.

Kilburn, K. H.; Seidman, B. C.; and Warshaw, R. 1985. Neurobehavioral and respiratory symptoms of formaldehyde and xylene exposure in histology technicians. *Arch. Environ. Health* 40:229–33.

Kulle, T. J., et al. 1987. Formaldehyde dose-response in healthy nonsmokers. *JAPCA* 37:919–24.

Levine, R. J.; Andjelkovich, D. A.; and Shaw, L. K. 1984. The mortality of Ontario undertakers and a review of formaldehyde-related mortality studies. *J. Occup. Med.* 26:740–46.

Levine, R. J., et al. 1984. The effects of occupational exposure on the respiratory health of West Virginia morticians. *J. Occup. Med.* 26:91–98.

Mage, D. T., and Gammage, R. B. 1985. Evaluation of changes in indoor air quality occurring over the past several decades. In *Indoor air and human health*. Ed. R. B. Gammage and S. V. Kaye. Chelsea, Mich.: Lewis Publishers.

Main, D. M., and Hogan, T. J. 1983. Health effects of low-level exposure to formaldehyde. *J. Occup. Med.* 25:896–900.

Malorny, G.; Rietbrock, N.; and Scheider, M. 1965. Oxidation of formaldehyde to formic acid in blood, a contribution to the metabolism of formaldehyde. *Naunyn Schmiedebergs Arch. Exp. Pharmakol.* 250:419–36.

Marsh, G. M. 1982. Proportional mortality patterns among chemical plant workers exposed to formaldehyde. *Br. J. Ind. Med.* 39:313–22.

Marsh, G. M. 1983. Mortality among workers from a plastics producing plant: A matched case-control study nested in a retrospective cohort study. *J. Occup. Med.* 25:219–30.

Melius, J., et al. 1984. Indoor air quality: the NIOSH experience. *Ann. Am. Conf. Gov. Ind. Hyg.* 10:3–7.

Mierauskiene, J. R., and Lekevicius, R. K. 1985. Cytogenetic studies of workers occupationally exposed to phenol, styrene, and formaldehyde. *Mutat. Res.* 147:308–9.

Morgan, W. K. C. 1984. Health risks of urea-formaldehyde foam insulation (letter). *Can. Med. Assoc. J.* 130:1529.

National Research Council (Committee on Aldehydes) 1981. *Formaldehyde and other aldehydes*. Washington, D.C.: National Academy Press.

Nelson, N., et al. 1986. Contribution of formaldehyde to respiratory cancer. *Environ. Health Perspect.* 70:23–35.

Nordman, H.; Keskinen, H.; and Tuppurainen, M. 1985. Formaldehyde asthma: Rare or overlooked? *J. Allergy Clin. Immunol.* 75:91–99.

Norman, G. R., et al. 1986. Respiratory function of children in homes insulated with urea-formaldehyde foam insulation. *Can. Med. Assoc. J.* 134:1135–38.

Norsted, S. W.; Kozinetz, C. A.; and Annegers, J. F. 1985. Formaldehyde complaint investigations in mobile homes by the Texas Department of Health. *Environ. Res.* 37:93–100.

Olsen, J. H., and Dossing, M. 1982. Formaldehyde-induced symptoms in day care centers. *Am. Ind. Hyg. Assoc. J.* 43:366–70.

Olsen, J. H., et al. 1984. Occupational formaldehyde exposure and increased nasal cancer risk in man. *Int. J. Cancer* 34:639–44.

Overman, D. O. 1985. Absence of embryonic effects of formaldehyde after percutaneous exposure in hamsters. *Toxicol. Lett.* 24:107–10.

Palese, M., and Tephley, T. R. 1975. Metabolism of formate in the rat. *J. Toxicol. Environ. Health* 1:13–24.

Patterson, R., et al. 1986. Human antibodies against formaldehyde: Human serum albumin conjugates or human serum albumin in individuals exposed to formaldehyde. *Int. Arch. Allergy Appl. Immunol.* 79:53–59.

Popa, N., et al. 1969. Bronchial asthma and asthmatic bronchitis determined by simple chemicals. *Dis. Chest* 56:395–402.

Poverenny, A. M., et al. 1975. Possible mechanism of lethal and mutagenic action of formaldehyde. *Mutat. Res.* 27:123–26.

Pross, H. F., et al. 1987. Immunologic studies of subjects with asthma exposed to formaldehyde and urea-formaldehyde foam insulation (UFFI) of products. *J. Allergy Clin. Immunol.* 79:797–810.

Ritchie, I. M., and Lehnen, R. G. 1985. An analysis of formaldehyde concentration in mobile and conventional homes. *J. Environ. Health* 47:300–305.

Robbins, J. D., et al. 1984. Bioavailability in rabbits of formaldehyde from durable press textiles. *J. Toxicol. Environ. Health* 14:453–63.

Roush, G. C., et al. 1987. Nasopharyngeal cancer, sinonasal cancer, and occupations related to formaldehyde: A case-control study. *J. Natl. Cancer Inst.* 79:1221–24.

Sardinas, A. V., et al. 1979. Health effects associated with urea-formaldehyde foam insulation in Connecticut. *J. Environ. Health* 41:270–72.

Sauder, L. R., et al. 1986. Acute pulmonary response to formaldehyde exposure in healthy nonsmokers. *J. Occup. Med.* 28:420–24.

Schachter, E. N., et al. 1986. A study of respiratory effects from exposure to 2 ppm formaldehyde in healthy subjects. *Arch. Environ. Health* 41:229–39.

Schenker, M. B.; Weiss, S. T.; and Murawski, B. W. 1982. Health effects of residents in homes with urea-formaldehyde foam insulation: A pilot study. *Environ. Int.* 8:359–63.

Schoenberg, J. B., and Mitchell, C. A. 1975. Airway disease caused by phenolic (phenol-formaldehyde) resin exposure. *Arch. Environ. Health* 30:574–77.

Sexton, K.; Liu, K. S.; and Petreas, M. X. 1986. Formaldehyde concentrations inside private residences: A mail-out approach to indoor air monitoring. *J. Air Pollut. Control Assoc.* 36:698–704.

Sheppard, D.; Eschenbacker, W. L.; and Epstein, J. 1984. Lack of bronchomotor response to up to 3 ppm formaldehyde in subjects with asthma. *Environ. Res.* 35:133–39.

Starr, T. B., and Gibson, J. E. 1985. The mechanistic toxicology of formaldehyde and its implications for quantitative risk assessment. *Annu. Rev. Pharmacol. Toxicol.* 25:745–67.

Starr, T. B., et al. 1984. Estimating human cancer risk from formaldehyde: Critical issues. Research Triangle Park, N.C.: CIIT.

Stayner, L., et al. 1988. A retrospective cohort mortality study of workers exposed to formaldehyde in the garment industry. *Am. J. Ind. Med.* 13:667–81.

Stock, T. H., and Mendez, S. R. 1985. A survey of typical exposures to formaldehyde in Houston area residences. *Am. Ind. Hyg. Assoc. J.* 46:313–17.

Strittmatter, P., and Ball, E. G. 1955. Formaldehyde dehydrogenase, a glutathione-dependent enzyme system. *J. Biol. Chem.* 213:445–61.

Stroup, N. E.; Blair, A.; and Erickson, G. E. 1986. Brain cancer and other causes of death in anatomists. *J. Natl. Cancer Inst.* 77:1217–24.

Swenberg, J. A., et al. 1985. A scientific approach to formaldehyde risk assessment. In *Risk quantitation and regulatory policy.* Ed. D. G. Hoel, R. A. Merrill, and F. P. Perera, 255–67. Cold Spring Harbor, N.Y.: Cold Spring Harbor Laboratory. Banbury Report no. 19.

Thomson, E. J.; Shackleton, S.; and Harrington, J. M. 1984. Chromosome aberrations and sister-chromatid exchange frequencies in pathology staff occupationally exposed to formaldehyde. *Mutat. Res.* 141:89–93.

Thrasher, J. D., et al. 1987. Evidence for formaldehyde antibodies and altered cell immunity in subjects exposed to formaldehyde in mobile homes. *Arch. Environ. Health* 42:347–50.

Thun, M. J.; Lakat, M. F.; and Altman, R. 1982. Symptom survey of residents of homes insulated with urea-formaldehyde foam. *Environ. Res.* 29:320–34.

Tobe, M., et al. 1985. Studies of the inhalation toxicity of formaldehyde. Japan: National Sanitary and Medical Laboratory Service.

Ulsamer, A. G., et al. 1984. Overview of health effects of formaldehyde. In *Hazard assessment of chemicals: Current developments.* Ed. J. Saxena. New York: Academic Press.

U.S. Environmental Protection Agency (Office of Pesticides and Toxic Substances). 1987. *Assessment of health risks to garment workers and certain home residents from exposure to formaldehyde*. Washington, D.C.: Government Printing Office.

Vaughn, T. L., et al. 1986a. Formaldehyde and cancers of the pharynx, sinus and nasal cavity, I: Occupational exposures. *Int. J. Cancer* 38:677–83.

Vaughn, T. L., et al. 1986b. Formaldehyde and cancers of the pharynx, sinus and nasal cavity, II: Residential exposures. *Int. J. Cancer* 38:685–88.

Walker, B., et al. 1987. The Massachusetts program for reducing the risk of formaldehyde exposure. *Public Health Rep.* 102:290–94.

Walrath, J. 1983. Mortality among embalmers. *Am. J. Epidemiol.* 118:432 (abstr.).

Walrath, J., and Fraumeni, J., Jr. 1983. Mortality patterns among embalmers. *Int. J. Cancer* 31:407–11.

Ward, J. B., Jr., et al. 1984. Sperm count, morphology and fluorescent body frequency in autopsy service workers exposed to formaldehyde. *Mutat. Res.* 130:417–24.

Yager, et al. 1986. Sister-chromatid exchanges in lymphocytes of anatomy students exposed to formaldehyde embalming solution. *Mutat. Res.* 174:135–39.

# 11

# VOLATILE
# ORGANIC COMPOUNDS

Lance A. Wallace, Ph.D.

In the 1970s, a sharp increase in nonspecific complaints by office workers and schoolchildren was noted in several countries. Because the symptoms seemed to result from exposure in schools or office buildings, the term *sick-building syndrome* was applied to them. Although the cause of sick-building syndrome remains unknown, organic chemicals are highly suspect. Many chlorinated solvents, light aromatic hydrocarbons, and pesticides (Table 11.1) are known to have effects, at high concentrations, similar to sick building syndrome. Since some of the organic compounds are known or suspected human carcinogens, cancer is also a potential consequence of low-level chronic exposures to organic chemicals in indoor air. Thus, recent concern over both acute and chronic health effects has sparked interest in organics in indoor air.

During the 1970s, advances in synthetic sorbents, miniaturized pumps and data loggers, and analytical techniques facilitated the measurement of indoor concentrations and personal exposures to many organics at environmental concentrations. As a result, substantial data are now available on personal exposures and on concentrations of organics in indoor air. These data show that personal exposures are largely determined by indoor sources and that indoor air concentrations of scores of organic compounds are considerably greater than outdoor concentrations, even in urban-industrial or petrochemical manufacturing centers. Furthermore, the sources of the higher concentrations indoors are primarily consumer products, building materials, and personal activities.

These findings have profound implications for regulation and research. If indoor concentrations indeed exceed outdoor levels, then increased attention and resources should be directed to organics in indoor air. Protection of public health may require actions to reduce indoor concentrations of organics through such approaches as building codes, product labeling, component substitutions, and

Table 11.1 Common Organic Chemicals and Their Sources

| Chemicals | Measured Peak Nonoccupational Exposure ($\mu g/m^3$) | Major Sources of Exposure |
|---|---|---|
| Volatile Chemicals | | |
| Benzene | 1,000 | Smoking, auto exhaust, passive smoking, driving, pumping gas |
| Tetrachloroethylene | 1,000 | Wearing or storing dry-cleaned clothes; visiting dry cleaners |
| p-Dichlorobenzene | 1,000 | Room deodorizers, moth cakes |
| Chloroform | 250 | Showering (10-min average) |
| | 50 | Washing clothes, dishes |
| Methylene chloride | 500,000 | Paint stripping, solvent usage |
| 1,1,1-Trichloroethane | 1,000 | Wearing or storing dry-cleaned clothes, aerosol sprays, fabric protectors |
| Trichloroethylene | 100 | Unknown (cosmetics, electronic parts) |
| Carbon tetrachloride | 100 | Industrial-strength cleansers |
| Aromatic hydrocarbons (toluene, xylenes, ethylbenzene, trimethylbenzenes) | 1,000 | Paints, adhesives, gasoline, combustion sources |
| Aliphatic hydrocarbons (octane, decane, undecane) | 1,000 | Paints, adhesives, gasoline, combustion sources |
| Terpenes (limonene, $\alpha$-pinene) | 1,000 | Scented deodorizers, polishes, fabrics, fabric softeners, cigarettes, food, and beverages |
| Semivolatile Chemicals | | |
| Chlorpyrifos (Dursban), insecticides | 10 | Household |
| Chlordane, heptachlor | 100 | Termiticide |
| Diazinon | 100 | |
| Polychlorinated biphenyls (PCBs) | | Transformers, fluorescent ballasts, ceiling tiles |
| Polycyclic aromatic hydrocarbons (PAHs) | 1 | Combustion products (smoking, wood burning, kerosene heaters) |

individual consumer actions. Many questions remain concerning health effects of organics, and both laboratory and epidemiologic research are needed. Epidemiologic studies will be facilitated by the personal monitors and sensitive analytical techniques now available.

### IDENTIFICATION AND CHARACTERIZATION

Organic gases are found in all indoor locations. More than five hundred volatile organic compounds (VOCs) were identified in four buildings in Washington, D.C., and Research Triangle Park, North Carolina (Sheldon et al. 1988a). Several thousand organics have been identified in environmental tobacco smoke, which contaminates about 60 percent of all U.S. homes and workplaces (Repace and Lowrey 1980, 1985); and about 90 percent of U.S. homes use household pesticides (Immerman and Drummond 1984).

Early studies of organics indoors were carried out in the 1970s in the Scandinavian countries (Johansson 1978; Molhave and Moller 1979; Berglund, Johansson, and Lindvall 1982a, 1982b). Molhave (1982) showed that many common building materials used in Scandinavian buildings emitted organic gases. Seifert and Abraham (1982) found benzene and toluene associated with storage of magazines and newspapers in German homes. Early U.S. measurements were made in thirty-four Chicago homes (Jarke and Gordon, 1981); in nine Love Canal residences (Pellizzari, Erickson, and Zweidinger 1979); on two college campuses (Wallace et al. 1982); in twelve New Jersey and North Carolina homes (Pellizzari et al. 1981); and in several buildings (Hollowell and Miksch 1981; Miksch, Hollowell, and Schmidt 1982).

## SOURCES AND SINKS

Early studies of VOC sources concentrated on emissions from building materials (Molhave 1982) and adhesives (Girman et al. 1986). Later studies also investigated building materials (Wallace 1987a; Sheldon et al. 1988a, 1988b) but added cleaning materials and activities such as scrubbing with chlorine bleach, spraying insecticides (Wallace et al. 1987a), and using paint removers (Girman and Hodgson 1987). Knoppel and Schauenburg (1987) studied VOC emissions from ten household products (waxes, polishes, and detergents); nineteen different alkanes, alkenes, alcohols, esters, and terpenes were among the three chemicals emitted at the highest rates from the ten products. All of these studies employed either headspace analysis or chambers to measure emission rates.

Other studies estimated emission rates from measurements in homes or buildings. For example, Wallace and co-workers (1987a) estimated emissions from a number of personal activities (such as visiting a dry cleaners and pumping gas) by regressing measurements of exposure or breath levels against the specified activities. Girman and Hodgson (1987) extended their chamber studies of paint removers to a residence, finding similar concentrations of methylene chloride in this more realistic situation.

One study (Wallace et al. 1990) involved seven volunteers undertaking about twenty-five activities suspected of causing increased VOC exposures; a number of these activities (using bathroom deodorizers, washing dishes, cleaning an automobile carburetor) resulted in ten- to one-thousandfold increases in eight-hour exposures to specific VOCs.

The U.S. National Aeronautics and Space Agency (NASA) has carried out an extensive program of measuring organic emissions from materials used in space capsules and the shuttle (Nuchia 1986). Data on about five thousand materials are available; perhaps three thousand of these materials are in use in general commerce

(Ozkaynak et al. 1987). The chemicals emitted from the largest number of materials included toluene (1,896 materials), methyl ethyl ketone (1,261 materials), and xylenes (1,111 materials).

Only recently has research been directed at sinks for VOCs. It is clear from the long-lasting odor that clothes impregnated with dry-cleaning fluids or moth-control agents are capable of absorbing and reemitting these VOCs. If other household fabrics also have this property, then accurate estimates of exposure will require some knowledge of the strength of absorption. In calculating indoor concentrations, the quantitative measure of sink strength is often expressed as a *decay factor* (units of air changes per hour) to be added to the actual air exchange.

A recent forty-one-day chamber study (Berglund, Johansson, and Lindvall 1987) of aged building materials taken from a "sick" preschool more than five years old indicated clearly that the materials had absorbed about thirty VOCs, which they reemitted to the chamber during the first thirty days of the study. Only thirteen of the VOCs originally present in the first days of the study continued to be emitted in the final days, indicating that these thirteen were the only true components of the materials. This finding has significant implications for remediating sick buildings. Even if the source material is identified and removed, weeks may be needed before reemission of organics from sinks in the building stops.

Another study (Seifert and Schmahl 1987) of sorption of VOCs and semivolatile organic compounds (SVOCs) on materials such as plywood and textiles concluded that sorption was small for the VOCs studied but significant for lindane on muslin curtains and wool carpets.

## MEASUREMENT METHODS

### VOCS

For many years, the most widely used method for sampling volatile organics at *occupational* levels (ppm) was collection on activated charcoal followed by solvent ($CS_2$) desorption. However, at *environmental* levels (ppb), this method lacks sensitivity unless high volumes or long sampling times are employed.

In the mid-1970s, synthetic sorbents were developed which could be heated to high temperatures without degradation. This property permitted the use of thermal rather than solvent desorption to recover the collected organics. Thermal desorption has several advantages over solvent desorption, including fewer analytical operations, shorter operating time, and recovery of the entire collected sample for analysis rather than only the rediluted portion.

Tenax, the most popular synthetic sorbent for sampling indoor air, has a number of advantageous properties, including being hydrophobic (so that sampling under high relative humidities is possible), being stable under very high desorption temperatures, and being reusable. Its disadvantages include reduced ability to capture very volatile chemicals such as vinyl chloride and methylene chloride; formation of reaction products, including mainly acetophenone, benzaldehyde, and phenol (Pellizzari 1977, 1979); and high background levels of benzene, styrene, and possibly toluene. Since 1979, Tenax has been used widely in studies of personal exposure to organics (Pellizzari, Erickson and Zweidinger 1979; Pellizzari et al. 1984b, 1987a, 1987b; Wallace et al. 1984, 1985, 1990; Handy et al. 1987; Wallace 1987b) and of concentrations in indoor air (De Bortoli et al. 1984, 1986; Gammage, White, and Gupta 1984; Pellizzari et al. 1984a; Wallace et al. 1987b; Sheldon et al. 1988a, 1988b).

Other synthetic sorbents occasionally used to measure volatile organics in indoor air include Porapak Q (Berglund, Johannson, and Lindvall 1982a, 1982b) and XAD-2 resin. Composite sampling trains employing several different sorbents in series can be used (Hodgson, Girman, and Binenboym 1986; De Bortoli et al. 1987) to compensate for each sorbent's limitations. For example, Tenax may be used in series with activated charcoal to allow collection of very volatile compounds such as vinyl chloride.

Although activated charcoal was occasionally used in early studies of indoor air (Lebret et al. 1986) the development in the late 1970s of passive sampling devices—primarily designed for occupational sampling—permitted collection of extended-time samples without much effort or technician time (Seifert and Abraham 1983). The sampling time of one to two weeks provides enough material to overcome the twin problems of high background concentrations on the badge due to manufacturing conditions and loss of sensitivity from solvent desorption due to redilution of the collected sample. Studies of this type include a major study of VOCs in German homes (Krause et al. 1987; Mailahn, Seifert, and Ullrich 1987; Seifert et al. 1987). Passive sampling devices employing Tenax have also been developed in the United States (Coutant, Lewis, and Mulik 1985, 1986; Lewis et al. 1985) and in Europe (De Bortoli et al. 1987).

Collection of atmospheric samples in evacuated metallic containers (McClenny et al. 1986; Oliver, Pleil, and McClenny 1986) followed by direct injection into a gas chromatograph for analysis has several advantages over the sorption methods discussed previously. Since a sorption/desorption process is not involved, chemical reactions on the sorbent and low recoveries due to breakthrough or incomplete desorption can be avoided. Consequently, a wider range of compounds can be studied. Disadvantages of the method include analysis of only a small portion, about 1 ml, of the collected whole-air sample of 1–10 liters and the potential for contamination of the sample by the pump, sampling tubes, and fittings. Also, the canister may not be amenable to miniaturization to the degree necessary to provide personal air samples.

Thus, no single method of sampling VOCs in the atmosphere or indoors has become a standard or reference method. In the United States, the two preferred methods are Tenax and evacuated canisters. These two methods were compared under controlled conditions in an unoccupied house (Spicer 1986). Ten chemicals were injected at nominal levels of about 3, 9, and 27 $\mu g/m^3$. Two sets of four Tenax cartridges operating at different flow rates (Walling 1984) were compared with two evacuated canisters. The results showed that the two methods were in excellent agreement, with precisions of better than 10 percent for all chemicals at all spiked levels.

Several researchers (Gammage, White, and Gupta 1984; Sheldon et al. 1987) have attempted to use a portable gas chromatograph as a means of obtaining real-time indicators of major household sources such as gasoline fumes from attached garages. However, the sensitivity and the resolution of the instruments have limited their usefulness to date. Another approach to obtaining higher time resolution has been to use small whole-air samples collected sequentially over short (e.g., two-minute) periods. This approach has been used to study short-term peaks in automobiles and in showers (Pleil, Oliver, and McClenny 1987). Wolkoff (1987) obtained forty-minute resolution using sequential Tenax sampling in Danish town halls.

### SVOCS

Some SVOCs exist primarily in the vapor phase at room temperature whereas others are primarily bound to airborne particles. Determination of the phase is important because the appropriate method of sampling depends on whether the target compound is a gas or is bound to particles. Only recently, for example, was nicotine found to be in the vapor phase (Eudy et al. 1986; Hammond 1986), a finding that calls into question many previous studies involving quantification of nicotine on filtered samples.

Currently, the most widely used sorbent for sampling a broad spectrum of airborne pesticides is polyurethane foam (PUF) (Lewis and MacLeod 1982). Samples are usually collected at 4 liters/min for twelve to twenty-four hours. Solvent desorption (gas chromatography) followed by electron capture detection (GC-ECD) or mass spectrometry (GC-MS) analysis can detect concentrations of 10 ng/m$^3$. Approximately fifty to sixty pesticides (including organochlorines, organophosphates, and pyrethroids) have been tested successfully in laboratories using PUF.

A sorbent often used for the termiticide chlordane is Chromosorb 102 (Thomas and Seiber 1974). This sorbent was used by the U.S. armed forces in studying more than ten thousand homes on military bases (Lillie and Barnes 1987; Olds 1987).

Other SVOCs include polyaromatic hydrocarbons (PAHs), which are produced in indoor combustion processes—smoking, wood burning (Daisey, Spengler, and Kaarakka 1987), and space heating with kerosene. The mutagenic activity of PAHs is high, especially in cigarette smoke (Lewtas, Claxton, and Mumford 1987). Therefore, even though PAH concentrations are normally low (approximately 1 ng/m$^3$), it may be important to develop systems to monitor their levels in homes. At present, fully satisfactory systems do not exist. Criteria for a satisfactory indoor collection system include flow rate sufficiently low not to affect the air exchange characteristics of the home, sensitivity at the 1 ng/m$^3$ level, and separate collection of PAHs in both particle and vapor phases. This last requirement is difficult to meet because PAHs exist in both the particle and vapor phases simultaneously, in relative proportions determined by their molecular characteristics and environmental conditions. Usual methods of collection (filter followed by sorbent) may result in "blow-off" of the molecules from the material on the filter so that the vapor phase concentration is overestimated, and the particle-bound fractions are underestimated. Denuders, which collect the vapor phase *before* the particle phase, have been developed to allow better determination of the vapor particle distribution for PAHs and acid aerosols (Koutrakis, Wolfson, and Spengler 1988).

Although PUF has been used as a sorbent with good collection efficiencies and good sample recoveries for PAHs having three or more rings, side-by-side studies using XAD-2 indicate that it is preferable to PUF for PAHs with three rings or fewer (Chuang 1987).

## STUDIES OF EXPOSURE TO ORGANICS

Two types of studies involving measurement of organics indoors may be distinguished: personal exposure studies, in which subjects carry or wear personal air monitors, and indoor air studies, in which samples are taken at fixed locations within a building. Personal exposure studies require small, light, quiet personal monitors (Wallace and Ott 1982); indoor air studies can employ larger and heavier monitors.

Examples of personal exposure studies include the total exposure assessment methodology (TEAM) study of VOCs (Pellizzari et al. 1983, 1987a, 1987b; Handy et al. 1987; Wallace 1987b) and the nonoccupational pesticide exposure (NOPES) study of SVOCs (mostly pesticides) (Lewis and Bond 1987; Immerman et al. 1988).

CONCENTRATIONS

Three large studies of VOCs, involving more than one hundred homes each, have been carried out in the United States (Wallace et al. 1985, 1988), The Netherlands (Lebret et al. 1986), and West Germany (Krause, Englert, and Dube 1987). Observed concentrations were remarkably similar for most chemicals (Table 11.2), indicating similar sources in these countries. One exception is chloroform, typically present at levels of $1-4$ $\mu g/m^3$ in the United States but not found in European homes. This geographic contrast is to be expected, since the likely source is volatilization from chlorinated water (Wallace et al. 1982; Andelman 1985a, 1985b; Andelman, Wilder, and Myers 1987; McKone 1987); the two European countries do not chlorinate their water.

In the United States, indoor concentrations of many VOCs greatly exceed outdoor concentrations. Mean values of indoor levels range from two to ten times the outdoor levels. Maximum twelve-hour values indoors are often one hundred or one thousand times ambient concentrations because of personal activities.

For most organics, differences among houses are far greater than differences among cities. This observation has considerable implications for both regulatory

Table 11.2  Volatile Organic Concentrations in Indoor Air in Germany and The Netherlands Compared with Personal Exposures in the United States

| Compound/Class | Concentration (μg/m³) | | | | | |
|---|---|---|---|---|---|---|
| | Arithmetic Mean | | Median in The Netherlands[c] | Maximum | | |
| | West Germany[a] | United States[b] | | West Germany | United States[d] | The Netherlands |
| Chlorinated | | | | | | |
| Chloroform | NM[e] | 3 | NM | NM | 210 | NM |
| 1,1,1-Trichloroethane | 9 | 52 | NM | 260 | 8,300 | NM |
| Trichloroethylene | 11 | 6 | <2 | 120 | 350 | 106 |
| Tetrachloroethylene | 14 | 16 | <2 | 810 | 250 | 205 |
| p-Dichlorobenzene | 14 | 25 | 1 | 1,260 | 1,600 | 299 |
| Aromatic | | | | | | |
| Benzene | 10 | 16 | 6 | 90 | 510 | 148 |
| Styrene | 2 | 3 | NM | 41 | 76 | NM |
| Ethylbenzene | 10 | 9 | 2 | 160 | 380 | 138 |
| o-Xylene | 7 | 9 | 10[f] | 45 | 750 | 753[f] |
| m + p-Xylene | 23 | 26 | | | 300 | 3,100 |
| Toluene | 84 | NM | 35 | 1,710 | NM | 2,252 |
| Aliphatic | | | | | | |
| Octane | 5 | 4[g] | 1 | 92 | 122 | 533 |
| Nonane | 10 | 12[g] | 4 | 140 | 177 | 407 |
| Decane | 15 | 6[g] | 10 | 240 | 161 | 905 |
| Undecane | 10 | 8[g] | 6 | 120 | 385 | 445 |
| Dodecane | 6 | 4[g] | 2 | 72 | 72 | 118 |
| Terpenes | | | | | | |
| α-Pinene | 10 | 4[g] | NM | 120 | 208 | NM |
| Limonene | 28 | 43[g] | 30 | 320 | 2,530 | 773 |

[a]Seifert and Schmalhl (1987): two-week averages; 488 West German homes.
[b]Wallace (1987a): twenty-four-hour averages; 526 persons in New Jersey and California.
[c]Lebret et al. (1986): one-week averages; 319 homes in The Netherlands.
[d]Wallace (unpublished): twelve-hour averages; overnight maxima in 666 homes in New Jersey, California, and Maryland.
[e]Not measured.
[f]o + m + p-Isomers.
[g]Wallace (unpublished): twenty-four-hour averages; 315 persons in California and Maryland.

policy and scientific research. If exposure to air toxics is only weakly affected by outdoor concentrations, then the maintenance of large outdoor sampling networks and/or the establishment of outdoor ambient or emission standards will have little relevance to protecting public health. Similarly, future environmental epidemiology studies will require direct measurement of personal exposure of all study subjects and cannot rely on simply comparing a "high-exposure" geographic area with a "low-exposure" one.

SELECTED VOCS IDENTIFIED IN INDOOR AIR

Although more than five hundred VOCs have been identified in indoor air—of which approximately two dozen are carcinogenic or mutagenic (Sheldon et al. 1988a)—the list of commonly found VOCs is smaller, on the order of fifty compounds (Table 11.3). Of these, an even smaller number—perhaps ten—may have serious health effects such as cancer. These compounds are discussed individually below.

*Benzene*    Benzene ($C_6H_6$) is one of the few VOCs recognized as a human carcinogen (International Agency for Research on Cancer 1982), largely on the basis of studies of occupationally exposed persons. The main source of exposure to benzene for about fifty million American smokers has been identified recently as mainstream cigarette smoke (Higgins, Greist, and Olerich 1983). Cigarette smokers take in about 2 mg/day, compared with less than 0.2 mg for most non-smokers (Wallace et al. 1987b). Passive smokers are also exposed to higher levels of benzene (Jermini, Weber, and Grandjean 1976; Higgins 1987). Median levels in homes without smokers were 6.5 and 7.0 $\mu g/m^3$ in West Germany and the United States, respectively, compared with levels of 11 and 10.5 $\mu g/m^3$ in homes with smokers in the two countries (Krause et al. 1987; Wallace et al. 1987b). Benzene is also found in gasoline, at a concentration of about 1–2 percent; however, the total personal exposure due to driving or filling gas tanks is less than from passive smoking (Bond 1986; Wallace et al. 1990). Two recent studies (Sandler et al. 1985; Stjernfeldt et al. 1986) have shown higher mortality from leukemia in children of smoking parents compared with children of nonsmokers. This association may be attributable to the approximately tenfold increase in benzene levels in the pregnant smoker's bloodstream.

*Vinyl Chloride*    This VOC, like benzene, is a human carcinogen (International Agency for Research on Cancer 1982). Unlike benzene, however, few indoor concentrations have been measured, due in part to its low breakthrough volume on Tenax. Since vinyl chloride may be created by chemical reactions at landfills, nearby homes might be contaminated. One study of indoor air in homes near a landfill has indeed documented increased concentrations (Stephens, Ball, and Mar 1986).

*p-Dichlorobenzene*    This chemical has two main uses, as a moth-control agent and as a deodorizer. Both uses require that an elevated concentration be maintained indoors for weeks or months. Thus homes with these sources may have indoor concentrations of 10–1,000 $\mu g/m^3$ compared with typical outdoor levels of < 1 $\mu g/m^3$ (Wallace et al. 1987a). p-Dichlorobenzene was found recently to cause cancer in both rats and mice (National Toxicology Program 1987) and is thus a possible human carcinogen.

*Chloroform*    This chemical ($CHCl_3$) is created by chlorination of drinking water supplies. Despite the regulation of trihalomethanes in drinking water, levels exceed the standard (100 $\mu g/liter$ for all trihalomethanes together) in a substantial portion of drinking water supplies. The main source of airborne chloroform in homes is volatilization from household use of water, such as washing clothes or

Table 11.3  Most Common Organic Compounds
Found at Four Buildings

| Class/Compound | $N^a$ | Class/Compound | $N^b$ |
|---|---|---|---|
| Aromatic Hydrocarbons | | Aliphatics | |
|   Benzene | 16 |   Undecane | 10 |
|   Toluene | 16 |   2-Methylhexane | 9 |
|   Xylenes | 16 |   2-Methylpentane | 9 |
|   Styrene | 16 |   3-Methylhexane | 9 |
|   Ethylbenzene | 16 |   3-Methylpentane | 9 |
|   Ethylmethyl benzenes | 16 |   Octane | 9 |
|   Trimethyl benzenes | 16 |   Nonane | 9 |
|   Dimethylethyl benzenes | 15 |   Decane | 9 |
|   Naphthalene | 15 |   Dodecane | 9 |
|   Methylnaphthalenes | 15 |   Tridecane | 9 |
|   Propylmethyl benzenes | 14 |   Methylcyclohexane | 9 |
|   n-Propyl benzenes | 13 |   Heptane | 8 |
|   Diethylbenzenes | 12 |   Tetradecane | 8 |
| Halogenated Hydrocarbons | |   2-Methylheptane | 8 |
|   Tetrachloroethylene | 16 |   Cyclohexane | 8 |
|   1,1,1-Trichloroethane | 15 |   Pentadecane | 7 |
|   Trichloroethylene | 14 |   4-Methyldecane | 7 |
|   Dichlorobenzenes | 12 |   2,4-Dimethylhexane | 7 |
|   Trichlorofluoromethane | 12 |   Pentane | 6 |
|   Dichloromethane | 11 |   Hexane | 6 |
|   Chloroform | 10 |   Eicosane | 6 |
| Esters | |   3-Methylnonane | 6 |
|   Ethyl acetate | 8 |   1,3-Dimethylcyclopentane | 6 |
|   m-Hexyl butanoate | 4 | | |
| Alcohols | | | |
|   2-Ethyl-1-hexanol | 9 | | |
|   n-Hexanol | 8 | | |
|   2-Butyloctanol | 7 | | |
|   n-Dodecanol | 6 | | |
| Aldehydes | | | |
|   n-Nonanal | 13 | | |
|   n-Decanal | 10 | | |
| Miscellaneous | | | |
|   Acetone | 16 | | |
|   Acetic acid | 10 | | |
|   Dimethylphenols | 6 | | |
|   Ethylene oxide | 4 | | |

[a]Number of samples (of sixteen) with compound present.
[b]Number of samples (of ten) with compound present.

dishes. Recent studies (Andelman, Wilder, and Myers 1987; McKone 1987) indicate that exposure from inhaling chloroform volatilized from household use of water (particularly hot showers) is comparable with the exposure from ingesting household tap water.

*Tetrachloroethylene*  This chemical is used in a majority of U.S. dry-cleaning shops. The main avenue of exposure appears to be wearing or storing dry-cleaned clothes (Howie 1981; Wallace et al. 1984) although a single visit to a dry-cleaning shop can elevate body burden levels for a number of hours afterward (Wallace et al. 1984; Gordon et al. 1988). Dry-cleaning workers are exposed to ppm levels (Pellizzari et al. 1984b), and several studies (Blair, Decoufle, and Grauman 1979) have found elevated cancer mortality in laundry and dry-cleaning workers.

*Methylene Chloride*   This common solvent was found in more than 50 percent of 1,200 products tested by the U.S. Environmental Protection Agency (U.S. EPA 1987). Best known as a paint stripper, it has been measured at levels of 100 ppm in chamber and room experiments (Girman and Hodgson 1987). Normal indoor concentrations are unknown since it cannot be measured by Tenax; however, if concentrations of methylene chloride are comparable to other VOCs, a 100-ppm exposure for eight hours while stripping paint would be equivalent to a lifetime's normal exposure.

*1,1,1-Trichloroethane*   This chemical is used widely in hundreds of consumer products as a sorbent or propellant. It is also used in about 15 percent of U.S. dry-cleaning shops. It does not appear to be an animal carcinogen although few adequate animal studies have been completed.

*Aromatic Compounds (Particularly Toluene, Xylenes, Ethylbenzene, and Styrene)* These aromatic chemicals are found in gasoline, combustion products (including cigarettes), and paints, adhesives, and solvents. Concentrations in buildings may be elevated by factors of about one hundred immediately following painting or renovation (Pellizzari et al. 1984a; Sheldon et al. 1988a, 1988b). Little evidence of carcinogenicity has been noted for these compounds (National Toxicology Program 1987), although recent results indicate that toluene and xylenes may each be carcinogenic to both rats and mice (C. Maltoni, personal communication, March 1989). Neurotoxic effects have been noted at high (50–100 ppm) concentrations. As common indoor chemicals, this class of compounds may be implicated in sick-building syndrome (Molhave, Bach, and Pedersen 1986).

*Aliphatic Hydrocarbons*   Aliphatic hydrocarbons are found in petroleum products, including gasoline, paint, and adhesives. Like the aromatics mentioned above, aliphatics such as decane and undecane can be found at one hundredfold elevated concentrations in newly painted or renovated buildings (Sheldon et al. 1988a, 1988b). Little evidence of health effects is available, although some of these chemicals are classified as promoters or co-carcinogens (International Agency for Research on Cancer 1982). They may also be implicated in sick-building syndrome (Molhave, Bach, and Pedersen 1986).

*Terpenes*   This class of compounds includes several of the most popular scents used in room air fresheners, cleansers, polishes, and bathroom deodorants. Limonene (lemon scent) and α-pinene (pine scent) are emitted naturally from citrus fruit and trees but are also added to many products (including, in the case of limonene, foods and beverages). Indoor concentrations of limonene are among the highest for any VOC (Pellizzari et al. 1989).

*SVOCs*   The armed forces studies (Lillie and Barnes 1987; Olds 1987) of chlordane in more than ten thousand homes showed that 237 of 5,038 air force homes and 39 of 4,368 army homes exceeded the 5 $\mu g/m^3$ guidelines established by the National Academy of Sciences (1979).

Another large study of over two hundred homes has been carried out in the United States (Lewis and Bond 1987; Immerman et al. 1988). Preliminary results show that in the two cities studied (Jacksonville, Florida, and Springfield, Massachusetts), chlorpyrifos (Dursban) is the most frequently used pesticide and is found at the highest concentrations, with chlordane and heptachlor (termiticides) and diazinon and propoxur following (Table 11.4). Mean concentrations were below 1 $\mu g/m^3$ for most pesticides. A few homes tested for household dust accumulations showed elevated levels of pesticides. Ingestion of house dust could be an important route of exposure for toddlers (Roberts, Ruby, and Warren 1987).

European studies of SVOCs have concentrated on wood preservatives containing pentachlorophenol and lindane ($\gamma$-hexachlorocyclohexane) (Krause, Englert, and Dube 1987; Zsolnay, Gebefugi, and Korte 1987). One study of 104 West German homes (Krause, Englert, and Dube 1987) showed indoor air levels of pentachlorophenol averaging about 6 $\mu g/m^3$. Household dust had high concentrations of both lindane and pentachlorophenol. Persons reporting exposure ($N = 989$) averaged 44 $\mu g$/liter pentachlorophenol in their urine, compared with 12.7 $\mu g$/liter in controls ($N = 207$). These results led to the banning of pentachlorophenol in wood preservatives in West Germany in 1987.

A series of studies in telephone company buildings containing mostly equip-

Table 11.4   Common Pesticides Found in Indoor Air in the EPA Nonoccupational Pesticides Exposure Study $(ng/m^3)^a$

| Pesticide | Jacksonville, Florida | Springfield, Massachusetts |
|---|---|---|
| Chlorpyrifos | 230 | 7 |
| Chlordane | 260 | 120 |
| Heptachlor | 130 | 17 |
| Diazinon | 210 | 25 |
| Propoxur | 300 | 22 |
| O-Phenylphenol | 75 | 33 |
| Lindane | 13 | 5 |
| Dichlorvos | 82 | 3 |
| Bendiocarb | 32 | 0.3 |
| Aldrin | 15 | 0.2 |
| Dieldrin | 10 | 3 |

*Source*: Adapted from Immerman and Firestone (1989).
[a]Values are averages of several weighted mean concentrations.

ment showed that heavier organics ($C_{12}-C_{30}$) were present at $ng/m^3$ levels and could be traced to janitorial use of floor waxes and polishes (Weschler 1978).

CONCENTRATIONS IN THE BODY

Most of the VOCs measured in indoor air have also been identified in human exhaled breath (Krotoszynski, Gabriel, and O'Neill 1977; Krotoszynski, Bruneau, and O'Neill 1979; Wallace et al. 1986; Gordon et al. 1988). Thus, breath measurements may be used to replace or supplement indoor air measurements to determine exposure. Breath measurements of VOCs have several advantages as compared with air measurements. They represent previous exposures integrated across time and also across all routes of exposure (ingestion, inhalation, and skin absorption). For at least two common indoor air chemicals—chloroform and limonene—exposure through ingestion of food and beverages may be equally as important as inhalation. Breath measurements can detect exposures from active smoking. In fact, the finding that cigarette smoking is a major source of benzene exposure followed from the observation that the mean benzene level in the breath of smokers was nearly an order of magnitude larger than in nonsmokers (Wallace et al. 1984, 1987b). Finally, comparison of breath measurements with personal air exposures provides an indication of both body burden and metabolism of the organics. For example, breath levels of tetrachloroethylene are comparable to personal air exposures, indicating little metabolism, whereas breath levels of xylenes are only 10 percent of exposures, indicating considerable metabolism. In addition, biological half-lives of several chemicals have been measured at environmental (ppb) exposures and have been found to range between five and twenty-one hours (Gordon et al. 1988).

Organics have also been measured in other biologic samples. Brugnone and co-workers (1987) have measured benzene in the breath and blood of cigarette smokers and in occupationally exposed workers in Italy. Breast milk has also been studied extensively for SVOCs, particularly pesticides and polychlorinated biphenyls (World Health Organization 1983; Rogan et al. 1986). VOCs, especially p-dichlorobenzene and tetrachloroethylene, have also been found in mothers' milk (Sheldon et al. 1985). Adipose tissue has also been studied for both VOC and SVOC levels (U.S. EPA 1986).

## ACTIONS TO REDUCE EXPOSURES

In many cases, the major source of exposure to organic chemicals has been identified—in the words of Pogo, "We have met the enemy, and he is us." People smoke, use air deodorizers, store pesticides in their homes, and otherwise expose themselves, their spouses, and their children to a variety of toxins. The remedy is implied in identifying the source: stop smoking or limit it to a room in the house with its own ventilation system; eliminate or reduce use of air deodorizers or switch to those with less carcinogenic constituents; throw away or store outside the house unused or little-used pesticides, solvents, and spray cans. Children may be protected from ingesting house dust by having hardwood surfaces instead of carpets and by removing shoes at the front door to avoid tracking in pesticides.

Outside the home, individuals may have less control. Organics in offices and schools may be emitted by new building materials, renovations, janitorial cleaning, regular pesticide applications, and other activities. Adequate ventilation may help but cannot overcome strong intermittent sources. Cleaning, renovating, or pesticide application may be scheduled in the evenings or weekends to reduce exposure. Additional ventilation and activated charcoal filtration to supplement the building ventilation system have been implemented in a few offices although rigorous studies of the effectiveness of these measures are lacking.

Organizations such as the American Society for Testing and Materials (ASTM) may be able to establish consensus guidelines on the amount of organic emissions allowable from building materials. Manufacturers may voluntarily limit emissions or substitute less harmful chemicals on receipt of animal test data. A novel idea— "baking out" new buildings by elevating interior temperatures prior to occupancy— has been tried several times (Girman et al. 1987) with moderate success.

## SUMMARY

Organic chemicals found indoors may be implicated in either acute health effects (sick-building syndrome) or in chronic effects (cancer). However, the mechanisms of action are largely unknown and must await further research in neurobehavioral or immune system response, pharmacokinetics, and mutagenicity studies of complex mixtures.

We have good knowledge of indoor concentrations and major sources of most VOCs, particularly nonpolar VOCs that are not extremely volatile. Nearly all of these are usually at higher concentrations indoors than outdoors, with short-term indoor peaks one hundred to one thousand times greater than outdoors. Preliminary data on SVOCs indicate that 80 percent or more of personal exposure to pesticides is from indoor sources. Little is known concerning concentrations and major sources of polar organics (oxygenated compounds), high-volatility nonpolar organics (vinyl chloride, methylene chloride, and others), or particle-bound organics (PAHs, dioxin, and furans).

Major sources of indoor organics include consumer products (deodorizers, solvents, and others), personal activities (smoking, cleaning, using hot water, wearing dry-cleaned clothes, and others), and building-related products and processes (paints, adhesives, caulking, fabrics, custodial cleaning, and pest control). Few details are known regarding emission rates of organics from the myriad different consumer products.

## REFERENCES

Andelman, J. B. 1985a. Human exposures to volatile halogenated organic chemicals in indoor and outdoor air. *Environ. Health Perspect.* 62:313–18.

Andelman, J. B. 1985b. Inhalation exposure in the home to volatile organic contaminants of drinking water. *Sci. Total Environ.* 47:443–60.

Andelman, J. B.; Wilder, L. C.; and Myers, S. M. 1987. Indoor air pollution from volatile chemicals in water. In *Proceedings of the fourth international conference on indoor air quality and climate.* Ed. B. Seifert et al., Vol. 1, 37–42. Berlin: Institute for Soil, Water, and Air Hygiene.

Berglund, B.; Johansson, I.; and Lindvall, T. 1982a. A longitudinal study of air contaminants in a newly built preschool. *Environ. Int.* 8:111–15.

Berglund, B.; Johansson, I.; and Lindvall, T. 1982b. The influence of ventilation on indoor/outdoor air contaminants in an office building. *Environ. Int.* 8:395–99.

Berglund, B.; Johansson, I.; and Lindvall, T. 1987. Volatile organic compounds from building materials in a simulated chamber study. In *Proceedings of the fourth international conference on indoor air quality and climate.* Ed. B. Seifert et al., Vol. 1, 16–21. Berlin: Institute for Soil, Water, and Air Hygiene.

Blair, A.; Decoufle, P.; and Grauman, D. 1979. Causes of death among laundry and dry-cleaning workers. *Am. J. Public Health* 69:508–11.

Bond, A. E. 1986. Self-service station vehicle refueling exposure study. In *Proceedings of the 1986 EPA/APCA symposium on measurement of toxic air pollutants.* 27–30 April. Ed. S. Hochheiser and R. K. M. Jayanti, 458–66. Pittsburgh, Pa.: Air Pollution Control Association.

Brugnone, F., et al. 1987. Benzene in the breath and blood of general public. In *Proceedings of the fourth international conference on indoor air quality and climate.* Ed. B. Seifert et al., Vol. 1, 133–38. Berlin: Institute for Soil, Water, and Air Hygiene.

Chuang, J. C. 1987. Field comparison study of polyurethane foam and XAD-2 resin for air sampling of polynuclear aromatic hydrocarbons. In *Measurement of toxic and related air pollutants.* Pittsburgh, Pa.: Air Pollution Control Association.

Coutant, R. W.; Lewis, R. G.; and Mulik, J. 1985. Passive sampling devices with reversible adsorption. *Anal. Chem.* 57:219–23.

Coutant, R. W.; Lewis, R. G.; and Mulik, J. D. 1986. Modification and evaluation of a thermally desorbable passive sampler for volatile organic compounds in air. *Anal. Chem.* 58:445–48.

Daisey, J. M.; Spengler, J. D.; and Kaarakka, P. 1987. A comparison of the organic chemical composition of indoor aerosols during woodburning and non-woodburning periods. In *Proceedings of the fourth international conference on indoor air quality and climate.* Ed. B. Seifert et al., Vol. 1, 215–19. Berlin: Institute for Soil, Water, and Air Hygiene.

De Bortoli, M., et al. 1984. Integrating "real life" measurements of organic pollution in indoor and outdoor air of homes in northern Italy. In *Indoor air, Vol. 4: Chemical characterization and personal exposure.* Ed. B. Berglund, T. Lindvall, and J. Sundell, 21–26. Stockholm: Swedish Council for Building Research. NTIS PB85-104214.

De Bortoli, M., et al. 1986. Concentrations of selected organic pollutants in indoor and outdoor air in northern Italy. *Environ. Int.* 12:343–50.

De Bortoli, M., et al. 1987. Performance of a thermally desorbable diffusion sampler for personal and indoor air monitoring. In *Proceedings of the fourth international conference on indoor air quality and climate.* Ed. B. Seifert et al., Vol. 1, 139–43. Berlin: Institute for Soil, Water, and Air Hygiene.

Eudy, L. W., et al. 1986. Studies on the vapor-particulate phase distribution of environmental nicotine by selective trapping and detection methods. Paper 86-38.7. In *Proceedings* of the seventy-ninth annual meeting of the Air Pollution Control Association, 22–27 June, Minneapolis, Minn.

Gammage, R. B.; White, D. A.; and Gupta, K. C. 1984. Residential measurements of high volatility organics and their sources. In *Indoor Air*. Ed. B. Berglund, T. Lindvall, and J. Sundell, Vol. 4. 157–62. Stockholm, Sweden: Swedish Council for Building Research.

Girman, J. R., and Hodgson, A. T. 1987. Exposure to methylene chloride from controlled use of a paint remover in a residence. Presented at eightieth annual meeting of the Air Pollution Control Association, 21–26 June, New York. Berkeley, Calif.: Lawrence Berkeley Laboratory. Report LBL 23078.

Girman, J. R.; Hodgson, A. T.; and Wind, M. L. 1987. Considerations in evaluating emissions from consumer products. *Atmos. Environ.* 21:315–20.

Girman, J. R., et al. 1986. Volatile organic emissions from adhesives with indoor applications. *Environ. Int.* 12:317–21.

Girman, J. R. et al. 1987. Bake-out of an office building. In *Proceedings of the fourth international conference on indoor air quality and climate*. Ed. B. Seifert et al., Vol. 1, 22–26. Berlin: Institute for Soil, Water, and Air Hygiene.

Gordon, S., et al. 1988. Breath measurements in a clean air chamber to determine washout times for volatile organic compounds at normal environmental concentrations. *Atmos. Environ.* 22:2165–70.

Hammond, S. K. 1986. A method to measure exposure to passive smoking. In *Proceedings of the 1986 EPA/APCA symposium on measurement of toxic air pollutants*. Ed. S. Hochheiser and R. K. M. Jayanti, 16–24. Pittsburgh, Pa.: Air Pollution Control Association.

Handy, R. W., et al. 1987. *Total exposure assessment methodology (TEAM) study: Standard operating procedures, Vol. 4*. Washington, D.C.: U.S. Environmental Protection Agency.

Higgins, C. E. 1987. Organic vapor phase composition of sidestream and environmental tobacco smoke from cigarettes. In *Proceedings of the 1987 EPA/APCA symposium on measurement of toxic and related air pollutants*. Ed. S. Hochheiser and R. K. M. Jayanti, 140–51. Pittsburgh, Pa.: Air Pollution Control Association.

Higgins, C.; Greist, W. H.; and Olerich, G. 1983. Applications of Tenax trapping to cigarette smoking. *J. Assoc. Off. Anal. Chem.* 66:1074–83.

Hodgson, A. T.; Girman, J. R.; and Binenboym, J. 1986. A multisorbent sampler for volatile organic compounds in indoor air. Paper 86-37.1, presented at the seventy-ninth annual meeting of the Air Pollution Control Association, 22–27 June, Minneapolis, Minn.

Hollowell, C. D., and Miksch, R. R. 1981. Sources and concentrations of organic compounds in indoor environments. *Bull. N.Y. Acad. Med.* 57:962–77.

Howie, S. J. 1981. *Ambient perchloroethylene levels inside coin-operated laundries with dry-cleaning machines on the premises*. Research Triangle Park, N.C.: U.S. Environmental Protection Agency. Contract no. 68-02-2722.

Immerman, F. W., and Drummond, D. J. 1984. *National urban pesticide applicators survey: Overview and results*. Research Triangle Park, N.C.: Research Triangle Institute. Publication no. RTI/2764/08-01F.

Immerman, F. W., and Firestone, M. P. 1989. *Non-occupational pesticide exposure study (NOPES) summary report*. Research Triangle Park, N.C.: U.S. Environmental Protection Agency.

Immerman, F. W., et al. 1988. *Non-occupational pesticides exposure study (NOPES), phase 2 interim report, Vol. 1: Overview and results*. Research Triangle Park, N.C.: U.S. Environmental Protection Agency.

International Agency for Research on Cancer. 1982. *Evaluation of the carcinogenic risk of chemicals to humans*. Lyon, France: IARC. Monograph no. 29.

Jarke, F. H., and Gordon, S. M. 1981. Recent investigations of volatile organics in indoor air at sub-ppb levels. Paper 81-57.2 presented at the seventy-fourth annual meeting of the Air Pollution Control Association, 21–26 June, Pittsburgh, Pa.

Jermini, C; Weber, A.; and Grandjean, E. 1976. Quantitative determination of various gas-phase components of the sidestream smoke of cigarettes in room air. (In German.) *Int. Arch. Occup. Environ. Health* 36:169–81.

Johansson, I. 1978. Determination of organic compounds in indoor air with potential reference to air quality. *Atmos. Environ.* 12:1371–77.

Knoppel, H., and Schauenburg, H. 1987. Screening of household products for the emission of volatile organic compounds. In *Proceedings of the fourth international conference on indoor air quality and climate*. Ed. B. Seifert et al., Vol. 1, 27–31. Berlin: Institute for Soil, Water, and Air Hygiene.

Koutrakis, P.; Wolfson, J. M.; and Spengler, J. D. 1988. An improved method for measuring aerosol strong acidity: Results from a nine-month study in St. Louis, Missouri, and Kingston, Tennessee. *Atmos. Environ.* 22:157–62.

Krause, C.; Englert, N.; and Dube, P. 1987. Pentachlorophenol-containing wood preservatives: Analyses and evaluation. In *Proceedings of the fourth international conference on indoor air quality and climate*. Ed. B. Seifert et al., Vol. 1, 220–24. Berlin: Institute for Soil, Water, and Air Hygiene.

Krause, C., et al. 1987. Occurrence of volatile organic compounds in the air of 500 homes in the Federal Republic of Germany. In *Proceedings of the fourth international conference on indoor air quality and climate*. Ed. B. Seifert, Vol. 1, 102–6. Berlin: Institute for Soil, Water, and Air Hygiene.

Krotoszynski, B. K.; Bruneau, G. M.; and O'Neill, H. J. 1979. Measurement of chemical inhalation exposure in urban populations in the presence of endogenous effluents. *J. Anal. Toxicol.* 3:225–34.

Krotoszynski, B. K.; Gabriel, G.; and O'Neill, H. 1977. Characterization of human expired air: A promising investigation and diagnostic technique. *J. Chromatogr. Sci.* 15:239–44.

Lebret, E., et al. 1986. Volatile hydrocarbons in Dutch homes. *Environ. Int.* 12:323–32.

Lewis, R. G., and Bond, A. E. 1987. Non-occupational exposure to household pesticides. In *Proceedings of the fourth international conference on indoor air quality and climate*. Ed. B. Seifert et al., Vol. 1, 195–96. Berlin: Institute for Soil, Water, and Air Hygiene.

Lewis, R. G., and MacLeod, K. E. 1982. A portable sampler for pesticides and semivolatile industrial organic chemicals in air. *Anal. Chem.* 54:310–15.

Lewis, R. G., et al. 1985. Thermally desorbable passive sampling device for volatile organic chemicals in ambient air. *Anal. Chem.* 57:214–19.

Lewtas, J.; Claxton, L. D.; and Mumford, J. L. 1987. Human exposure to mutagens from indoor combustion sources. In *Proceedings of the fourth international conference on indoor air quality and climate*. Ed. B. Seifert et al., Vol. 1, 473–77. Berlin: Institute for Soil, Water, and Air Hygiene.

Lillie, T. H., and Barnes, E. S. 1987. Airborne termiticide levels in houses on United States Air Force installations. In *Proceedings of the fourth international conference on indoor air quality and climate*. Ed. B. Seifert et al., Vol. 1, 200–204. Berlin: Institute for Soil, Water, and Air Hygiene.

Mailahn, W.; Seifert, B.; and Ullrich, D. 1987. The use of a passive sampler for the simultaneous determination of long-term ventilation rates and VOC concentrations. In *Proceedings of the fourth international conference on indoor air quality and climate*. Ed. B. Seifert et al., Vol. 1, 149–53. Berlin: Institute for Soil, Water, and Air Hygiene.

McClenny, W. A., et al. 1986. Canister-based VOC samplers. In *Proceedings of the EPA/APCA symposium on measurement of toxic air pollutants*. Ed. S. Hochheiser and R. K. M. Jayanti. Pittsburgh, Pa.: Air Pollution Control Association.

McKone, T. E. 1987. Human exposure to VOCs in household tap water: The indoor inhalation pathway. *Environ. Sci. Technol.* 21:1194–1201.

Miksch, R. R.; Hollowell, C. D.; and Schmidt, H. E. 1982. Trace organic chemical contaminants in office spaces. *Environ. Int.* 8:129–37.

Molhave, L. 1982. Indoor air pollution due to organic gases and vapours of solvents in building materials. *Environ. Int.* 8:117–27.

Molhave, L., and Moller, J. 1979. The atmospheric environment in modern Danish dwellings: Measurements in thirty-nine flats. In *Indoor air*. Ed. B. Berglund et al., 171–86. Copenhagen: Danish Building Research Institute.

Molhave, L.; Bach, B.; and Pedersen, O. F. 1986. Human reactions to low concentrations of volatile organic compounds. *Environ. Int.* 12:167–75.

National Academy of Sciences. 1979. *An assessment of the health risks of seven pesticides used for termite control*. Washington, D.C.: National Academy of Sciences.

National Toxicology Program. 1987. *Technical report on the toxicity and carcinogenesis of 1,4-dichlorobenzene (CAS 106-46-7) in F344/n rats and B6C3F1 mice (gavage study)*. Technical Report 319. Research Triangle Park, N.C.: National Toxicology Program.

Nuchia, E. 1986. *MDAC: Houston materials testing database users' guide*. Houston, Tex.: NASA.

Olds, K. L. 1987. Indoor airborne concentrations of termiticides in department of the army family housing. In *Proceedings of the fourth international conference on indoor air quality and climate*. Ed. B. Seifert et al., Vol. 1, 205–9. Berlin: Institute for Soil, Water, and Air Hygiene.

Oliver, K. D.; Pleil, J. D.; and McClenny, W. A. 1986. Sample integrity of trace level volatile organic compounds in ambient air stored in summa polished canisters. *Atmos. Environ.* 20:1403–11.

Ozkaynak, H., et al. 1987. Sources and emission rates of organic chemical vapors in homes and buildings. In *Proceedings of the fourth international conference on indoor air quality and climate*. Ed. B. Seifert et al., Vol. 1, 3–7. Berlin: Institute for Soil, Water, and Air Hygiene.

Pellizzari, E. D. 1977. *The measurement of carcinogenic vapors in ambient atmospheres*. Research Triangle Park, N.C.: U.S. Environmental Protection Agency.

Pellizzari, E. D. 1979. Analysis of organic air pollutants by gas chromatography and mass spectroscopy. Research Triangle Park, N.C.: U.S. Environmental Protection Agency.

Pellizzari, E. D.; Erickson, M. D.; and Zweidinger, R. 1979. Formulation of a preliminary assessment of halogenated organic compounds in man and environmental media. Washington, D.C.: U.S. Environmental Protection Agency.

Pellizzari, E. D., et al. 1981. *Total exposure assessment methodology (TEAM) study, Vol. 1: Northern New Jersey; Vol. 2: Research Triangle Park; Vol. 3: Quality assurance*. Washington, D.C.: U.S. Environmental Protection Agency, Office of Research and Development. Publication no. EPA/68-01/3849. (Not available from NTIS. Project Officer Lance Wallace.)

Pellizzari, E. D., et al. 1983. Human exposure to vapor-phase halogenated hydrocarbons: Fixed-site versus personal exposure. In *Proceedings from the symposium on ambient, source, and exposure monitoring of non-criteria pollutants,* May 1982. Research Triangle Park, N.C.: Environmental Monitoring Systems Laboratory. Publication no. EPA/600/9-83/007.

Pellizzari, E. D., et al. 1984a. Sampling and analysis design for volatile halocarbons in indoor and outdoor air. In *Indoor air, Vol. 4: Chemical characterization and personal exposure.* Ed. B. Berglund, T. Lindvall, and J. Sundell, 203–8. Stockholm: Swedish Council for Building Research. NTIS PB85-104214.

Pellizzari, E. D., et al. 1984b. *Total exposure and assessment methodology (TEAM): Dry cleaners study.* Washington, D.C.: U.S. Environmental Protection Agency, Office of Research and Development. Publication no. EPA/68-02/3626. (Not available from NTIS. Project Officer Lance Wallace.)

Pellizzari, E. D., et al. 1987a. *Total exposure assessment methodology (TEAM) study: Elizabeth and Bayonne, New Jersey; Devils Lake, North Dakota; and Greensboro, North Carolina, Vol. 2.* Washington, D.C.: U.S. Environmental Protection Agency.

Pellizzari, E. D., et al. 1987b. *Total exposure assessment methodology (TEAM) study: Selected communities in northern and southern California, Vol. 3.* Washington, D.C.: U.S. Environmental Protection Agency.

Pellizzari, E. D., et al. 1989. Comparison of indoor and outdoor toxic air pollutant levels in several southern California communities. Research Triangle Park, N.C.: U.S. Environmental Protection Agency. Contract no. 68-02-4544.

Pleil, J. D.; Oliver, K. D.; and McClenny, W. A. 1987. Time-resolved measurement of indoor exposure to volatile organic compounds. In *Proceedings of the fourth international conference on indoor air quality and climate.* Ed. B. Seifert et al., Vol. 1. Berlin: Institute for Soil, Water, and Air Hygiene.

Repace, J. L., and Lowrey, A. H. 1980. Indoor air pollution, tobacco smoke, and public health. *Science* 208:464–72.

Repace, J. L., and Lowrey, A. H. 1985. A quantitative estimate of non-smokers' lung cancer risk from passive smoking. *Environ. Int.* 11:3–22.

Roberts, J. W.; Ruby, M. G.; and Warren, G. R. 1987. Mutagenic activity of house dust. In *Short-term bioassays in the analysis of complex environmental mixtures.* Ed. S. S. Sandhu et al., 355–67. New York: Plenum.

Rogan, W. J., et al. 1986. Poly-chlorinated biphenyls (PCBs) and dichlorodiphenyl dichloroethane (DDE) in human milk. *Am. J. Public Health* 76:172–77.

Sandler, D. P., et al. 1985. Cancer risk in adulthood from early life exposure to parents' smoking. *Am. J. Public Health* 75:487–92.

Seifert, B., and Abraham, H. J. 1982. Indoor air concentrations of benzene and some other aromatic hydrocarbons. *Ecotoxicol. Environ. Safety* 6:190–92.

Seifert, B., and Abraham, H. J. 1983. Use of passive samplers for the determination of gaseous organic substances in indoor air at low concentration levels. *Int. J. Environ. Anal. Chem.* 13:237–53.

Seifert, B., and Schmahl, H. J. 1987. Quantification of sorption effects for selected organic substances present in indoor air. In *Proceedings of the fourth international conference on indoor air quality and climate*. Ed. B. Seifert et al., Vol. 1, 252–56. Berlin: Institute for Soil, Water, and Air Hygiene.

Seifert, B., et al. 1987. Seasonal variation of concentrations of volatile organic compounds in selected German homes. In *Proceedings of the fourth international conference on indoor air quality and climate*. Ed. B. Seifert et al., Vol. 1, 107–11. Berlin: Institute for Soil, Water, and Air Hygiene.

Sheldon, L. S., et al. 1985. *Human exposure assessment to environmental chemicals: Nursing mothers study. Final Report*. Washington, D.C.: U.S. Environmental Protection Agency. Publication no. EPA/68-02/3679.

Sheldon, L. S., et al. 1987. Use of a portable gas chromatograph for identifying sources of volatile organics in indoor air. In *Proceedings of the fourth international conference on indoor air quality and climate*. Ed. B. Seifert et al., Vol. 1, 74–78. Berlin: Institute for Soil, Water, and Air Hygiene.

Sheldon, L. S., et al. 1988a. *Indoor air quality in public buildings, Vol. 1*. Washington, D.C.: U.S. Environmental Protection Agency. Publication no. EPA/600/6-88/09a.

Sheldon, L. S., et al. 1988b. *Indoor air quality in public buildings, Vol. 2*. Research Triangle Park, N.C.: U.S. Environmental Protection Agency. Publication no. EPA/600/6-88/09b.

Spicer, C. W. 1986. Intercomparison of sampling techniques for toxic organic compounds in indoor air. In *Proceedings of the 1986 EPA/APCA symposium on the measurement of toxic air pollutants*. Ed. S. Hochheiser and R. K. M. Jayanti, 45–60. Pittsburgh, Pa.: Air Pollution Control Association.

Stephens, R. D.; Ball, N. B.; and Mar, D. M. 1986. A multimedia study of hazardous waste landfill gas migration. In *Pollutants in a multimedia environment*. Ed. Y. Cohen, New York: Plenum.

Stjernfeldt, M., et al. 1986. Maternal smoking during pregnancy and risk of childhood cancer. *Lancet* 1:1350–52.

Thomas, T. C., and Seiber, J. 1974. Chromosorb 102: An efficient means for trapping pesticides from air. *Bull. Environ. Contam. Toxicol.* 12:17–25.

U.S. Environmental Protection Agency. 1986. *Broad scan analysis of the FY82 national human adipose tissue survey specimens, Vols. 1–5*. Washington, D.C.: Government Printing Office. Publication no. EPA/560/5-86/036.

U.S. Environmental Protection Agency. 1987. *Household solvents products: A "shelf" survey with laboratory analysis*. Washington, D.C.: Government Printing Office. Publication no. EPA/560/5/87/006.

Wallace, L. A. 1987a. Emission rates of volatile organic compounds from building materials and surface coatings. In *Proceedings of the 1987 EPA/APCA symposium on measurement of toxic and related air pollutants*. Ed. S. Hochheiser and R. K. M. Jayanti, 115–22. Pittsburgh, Pa.: Air Pollution Control Association.

Wallace, L. A. 1987b. *Total exposure assessment methodology (TEAM) study: Summary and analysis, Vol. 1*. Washington, D.C.: U.S. Environmental Protection Agency.

Wallace, L. A. 1989. Major sources of benzene exposure. *Environ. Health Perspect.* 83:165–69.

Wallace, L. A., and Ott, W. R. 1982. Personal monitors: A state-of-the-art survey. *J. Air Pollut. Control Assoc.* 32:601–10.

Wallace, L. A., et al. 1982. Monitoring individual exposure: Measurements of volatile organic compounds in breathing zone air, drinking water and exhaled breath. *Environ. Int.* 8:269–82.

Wallace, L. A., et al., 1984. Personal exposure to volatile organic compounds, I: Direct measurement in breathing-zone air, drinking water, food, and exhaled breath. *Environ. Res.* 35:293–319.

Wallace, L. A., et al. 1985. Personal exposures, indoor-outdoor relationships and breath levels of toxic air pollutants measured for 355 persons in New Jersey. *Atmos. Environ.* 19:1651–61.

Wallace, L. A., et al. 1986. Concentrations of 20 volatile organic compounds in the air and drinking water of 350 residents of New Jersey compared with concentrations in their exhaled breath. *J. Occup. Med.* 28:603–8.

Wallace, L. A., et al. 1987a. Emissions of volatile organic compounds from building materials and consumer products. *Atmos. Environ.* 21:385–93.

Wallace, L. A., et al. 1987b. Exposures to benzene and other volatile compounds from active and passive smoking. *Arch. Environ. Health* 42:272–79.

Wallace, L. A., et al. 1988. The California TEAM study: Breath concentrations and personal exposure to 26 volatile compounds in air and drinking water of 188 residents of Los Angeles, Antioch, and Pittsburg, Calif. *Atmos. Environ.* 22:2141–63.

Wallace, L. A., et al. 1990. The influence of personal activities on exposure to volatile organic compounds. *Environ. Res.,* 50:37–55.

Walling, J. F. 1984. The utility of distributed air volume sets when sampling ambient air using solid absorbents. *Atmos. Environ.* 18:855–59.

Weschler, C. J. 1978. Characterization techniques applied to indoor dust. *Environ. Sci. Technol.* 12:923–26.

Wolkoff, P. 1987. Sampling of VOC indoors under condition of high time resolution. In *Proceedings of the fourth international conference on indoor air quality and climate.* Ed. B. Seifert et al., Vol. 1, 126–30. Berlin: Institute for Soil, Water, and Air Hygiene.

World Health Organization. 1983. *Assessment of human exposure to selected organochlorine compounds through biological monitoring.* Ed. S. A. Slorach and R. Vaz. Uppsala, Sweden: Swedish National Food Association.

Zsolnay, A.; Gebefugi, I.; and Korte, F. 1987. Occurrence of lindane and PCP in Bavarian buildings. In *Proceedings of the fourth international conference on indoor air quality and climate.* Ed. B. Seifert et al., Vol. 1, 262–64. Berlin: Institute for Soil, Water, and Air Hygiene.

# 12

# INDOOR AIR POLLUTION
# AND INFECTIOUS DISEASES

Harriet A. Burge, Ph.D.
James C. Feeley, Ph.D.

## *HISTORY*

Indoor air was suspected as a potential agent for transmitting infectious disease nearly two thousand years ago by Lucretius, who saw dust motes in a sunbeam in a darkened room and considered the possibility that the motes might carry pestilences. However, many centuries passed before microorganisms were discovered and their connection to disease confirmed (Gregory 1961). It has been well documented that some diseases can be transmitted by air (National Research Council 1961, 1981; Kundsin 1980). The indoor environment can potentially place human occupants at greater risk than the outside environment because enclosed spaces can confine aerosols and allow them to build up to infectious doses (Spendlove and Fannin 1983), and ventilating systems can pick up contaminated air and distribute infectious doses of microorganisms to other parts of the building (Huddleson and Munger 1940). Components of ventilation systems can actually become contaminated with pathogenic microorganisms (e.g., *Legionella*) that are subsequently transmitted to building occupants (Glick et al. 1978; Kauffman et al. 1981).

## *MICROORGANISMS, DISEASES, AND INDOOR AIR*

Microorganisms that have been shown to cause infectious disease by transmission in indoor air include viruses, bacteria, fungi, and protozoans. Viruses are obligate parasites restricted to living cells. Most bacteria can survive on nonliving material; in other words, they are saprophytic. Some prefer the saprophytic environment whereas others can utilize both living and nonliving substrates. Only a few are obligate parasites. Fungi, in general, are saprophytic or pathogenic for plants but

273

can cause infectious disease in compromised human hosts. Only a few are primarily pathogens for vertebrate animals. Protozoa are usually free-living saprophytes although some routinely colonize vertebrates and cause disease when the host's defenses against infection are compromised by drugs, disease, or other factors (Hughes 1982).

Any respiratory pathogen that can survive aerosolization and transport in air must be considered a potential cause of airborne disease. Viruses that are known to be transmitted by the airborne route include those causing influenza, measles, chickenpox, smallpox, and the common cold (Riley 1982; Solomon and Burge 1984; Ijaz et al. 1985). Diseases caused by other viruses (e.g., rabies) have been contracted via the airborne route only under highly unusual circumstances, such as exposure in heavily contaminated bat caves (Spendlove and Fannin 1983). Theoretically, many viruses, such as hepatitis B, could be contracted through exposure to the intense aerosols that can result from laboratory accidents (Petersen 1980). Bacterial diseases that have been transmitted via indoor air are Legionnaire's disease (the only bacterial disease *primarily* transmitted via the airborne route from environmental reservoirs), tuberculosis, anthrax, and brucellosis. The fungal diseases such as histoplasmosis, cryptococcosis, blastomycosis, and coccidiodomycosis are all known to be transmitted by the airborne route although sources of these fungi are usually found outdoors, and transmission from indoor sources is not common (Solomon and Burge 1984). *Aspergillus* species and, in fact, spores of any fungus capable of growing at body temperatures under conditions present in the respiratory mucosa can cause invasive disease in compromised hosts and are routinely present in air in most environments (Rhame et al. 1984; Solomon and Burge 1984). Fungi that can grow on skin (fungal dermatophytes) can be recovered from indoor air but have not been shown to cause disease via the airborne route (Solomon and Burge 1984). Protozoans that are known to colonize human hosts via the airborne route include *Pneumocystis carinii* (Hughes 1982) and *Acanthamoeba* (Mannis et al. 1986).

## RESERVOIRS, AMPLIFIERS, DISSEMINATORS

For airborne disease transmission to occur in any environment there must be a source or reservoir for the microorganism, a means for the microorganism to multiply, particularly for a microorganism present in low numbers initially, and a mechanism for dissemination. A reservoir may serve as an amplifier and a disseminator, as in the case of many viral diseases, but reservoir, amplifier, and disseminator may be separate.

### RESERVOIRS

Common reservoirs for organisms causing airborne infectious disease include man, other vertebrates, soil, water, and air. The principal reservoir of most airborne viral diseases is man (colds, influenza, measles, chickenpox) (Muchmore et al. 1981; Spendlove and Fannin 1983). Viral diseases of other vertebrates are rarely transmitted to man through the air (e.g., rabies). Man also provides the reservoir for the organisms causing many airborne bacterial diseases including tuberculosis and most nosocomial pneumonias and staphylococcal infections (Palmer 1984). Other vertebrates serve as reservoirs for diseases such as anthrax (Brachman, Kauffman, and Dalldorf 1966) and brucellosis. Since many bacteria that can cause infectious human disease are basically saprophytic, they can be maintained in inanimate reservoirs such as soil (*Clostridium*) or water (*Pseudomonas*, *Acinetobacter*) (Solomon and Burge 1984). *Legionella* can also be maintained in wet soil and water reservoirs if suitable associate organisms are present to provide necessary amino acids (Skaliy and McEachern 1979; Wang et al. 1979; Fliermans et al. 1981; Arnow et al. 1982). These reservoirs are often outdoors but can be a part of the indoor environment. For example, any stagnant water, whether indoors or out, can provide a reservoir for a variety of potentially infectious bacteria. Soil and birds serve as reservoirs for the primarily infectious fungi such as *Histoplasma* and *Cryptococcus* (Recht et al. 1982; Williams and Moser 1987). However, the major reservoir for fungi that cause opportunistic fungal infections is dead plant material in the outdoor environment. Spores of most fungi are present in outdoor air (the disseminator) whenever snow cover is absent and are consistently present in indoor air, as a result of penetration via air intake vents or other openings, or growth on wet interior surfaces following infiltration into the building (Solomon and Burge 1984). *Aspergillus*, as well as other fungi, frequently colonizes the nose, which provides a reservoir for this potentially dangerous pathogen (Kauffman, Burge, and Solomon 1988). Reservoirs for infectious protozoa are for the most part unknown but probably include water, soil, and possibly vertebrates (Mannis et al. 1986).

AMPLIFIERS

Amplifiers enable microorganisms to multiply to concentrations sufficiently high to ensure that airborne dilution and possible injury to the organism resulting from the airborne state do not prevent transmission. In many cases the reservoir and the amplifier are the same. For viruses, which must always have a living host to grow, reservoir and amplifier are always the same; similarly, for the bacterial diseases that are primarily transferred from human to human or other vertebrate to human host, reservoir and amplifier are also the same. In contrast, any disease transmissable by a unit dose (or very low number of organisms) can be transmitted directly from the reservoir without amplification. Such transmission occurs for some of the infectious fungal diseases (*Cryptococcosis*) and for most infectious diseases that occur in immunocompromised patients (Rhame et al. 1984). Bacteria (e.g., *Legionella* and *Pseudomonas*) and fungi can survive in an outdoor reservoir, penetrate indoors via potable water, makeup air, or other routes and then increase in numbers in an interior environment. *Legionella* is an excellent example; it can contaminate and grow actively in ventilation and plumbing system components if suitable moisture and temperature conditions exist and supporting microorganisms are present (Miller 1979; Fisher-Hoch et al. 1981). *Pseudomonas* and *Legionella* frequently utilize appliances such as nebulizers and humidifiers as both reservoirs and amplifiers (Arnow et al. 1982). Fungi can grow on any surface on which adequate moisture and nutrients are present. Although most bacteria require an abundance of water, fungi are, in general, adapted for growth in relatively dry environments and can grow on apparently dry environmental surfaces (e.g., condensation on ventilation system surfaces, walls, and insulation or on scales of human skin in house dust) (Rhame et al. 1984; Solomon and Burge 1984). Requirements for amplification of protozoa are less well known. However, because protozoa are often recovered from the same environments utilized by the saprophytic bacteria, it is possible that the bacteria may serve as a food source for the protozoa (Solomon and Burge 1984). In contrast, virulent *Legionella* have been shown to infect protozoa and multiply intracellularly within food vacuoles (Fields et al. 1986).

DISSEMINATORS

Airborne transmission of infectious disease requires that the microorganism be introduced into breathing-space air in sufficient numbers for infection to occur. Although dissemination of organisms is always required to produce disease, the disseminator can be the same as the reservoir for diseases that require only a very small dose for infection (pneumonic plague, measles, chickenpox, and influenza). For example, human to human transfer of most viral and some bacterial diseases occurs through actions, often involuntary, of the human reservoir/amplifiers (e.g. sneezing, coughing, shedding of skin scales) (Letts and Doermer 1983; Spendlove and Fannin 1983). The measles virus has been shown to use both human and mechanical dissemination; the human produces the initial aerosol, but subsequent transmission to other locations takes place through mechanical ventilation systems (Riley 1982). Influenza viruses also may spread in this way. Organisms that can colonize components of building ventilation systems are growing in an environment with an inherent dissemination mechanism. Some mechanical devices, by their mode of operation, act as both amplifiers and disseminators. For example, *Legionella* grows in cooling towers, and the combined action of the water sprays and the air movement produces a droplet aerosol that contains infectious units (Miller 1979; Fisher-Hoch et al. 1981). Likewise, nebulizers and vaporizers, implicated as disseminators in other kinds of bacterial pneumonia as well as Legionnaire's disease, produce viable aerosols by their mode of operation (Arnow et al. 1982; Solomon and Burge 1984). Toilets, which are transitory reservoirs for a wide variety of human source microorganisms, can act as disseminators since aerosols are produced during flushing (Spendlove and Fannin 1983). Fortunately, few disease outbreaks, if any, have been traced to toilets. Showers, whirlpool baths, and jacuzzis have been implicated in outbreaks or single cases of infectious diseases such as legionellosis (Storch et al. 1979; Fraser 1985). All of these devices produce droplet aerosols during operation. The action of cleaning water reservoirs with vigorous mechanical agitation, such as high-power sprays, also can create a potentially dangerous aerosol if infectious microorganisms are present.

Organisms that survive and are infectious in a relatively dry state (e.g. fungus spores, bacterial spores) can be disseminated by even slight disturbance of their reservoir/amplifier. Vacuuming or walking on contaminated carpeting increases airborne levels of entrained viable particles (Rhame et al. 1984). Excavation of contaminated soil is a documented mode of dissemination for *Histoplasma*, *Blastomyces*, and *Cryptococcus*. Although initially suggested for *Legionella*, this mode is no longer considered plausible. Demolition of buildings also can produce infectious aerosols, which may be especially dangerous for immunocompromised hosts. Any aerosol, whether dry or droplet, that is produced outdoors near air intakes for ventilation systems or near open windows can enter the indoor air and cause disease among persons in the structure (Solomon and Burge 1984). Except for diseases with a very low dose requirement (e.g. cryptococcosis or any disease in a compromised host), outdoor exposure only rarely results in disease, probably because the large mass of outdoor air and its continuous movement tend to dilute aerosols rapidly.

## FACTORS INFLUENCING AIRBORNE INFECTION

### AEROSOL CHARACTERISTICS

In order to cause infectious disease through respiratory tract exposure, aerosols must be small enough to penetrate the respiratory tract ($<5$ μm) but large enough to contain the infectious agents in a viable state and in sufficient numbers to constitute an infectious dose (Knight 1973; Riley 1982; Willeke and Baron 1987). Most aerosols produced from water sources (human sneezing, coughing, water spray systems) are initially comprised of droplets too large to remain airborne, and those that do remain airborne are too large to penetrate the lower human respiratory airways. However, these large aerosols begin to desiccate immediately after generation because relative humidity in the range commonly found in most interiors is not high enough to maintain large droplet aerosols. Consequently, droplet nuclei are produced in a size range of particles that remain airborne for long periods of time and are small enough to reach the lower airways. After formation, such droplet nuclei are rapidly dispersed and become randomly distributed in the indoor air; if concentrations are sufficient, all susceptible persons inhaling the aerosol are at risk for disease. Fortunately, most droplets produced even from heavily contaminated sources carry relatively few viable agents, and dilution quickly lowers the potential dose below infective limits. If inadequate ventilation is present in an environment in which infectious aerosols are continually being produced and if the microorganism can survive aerosolization, very high rates of infection can result. For example, 72 percent of the passengers and crew of a commercial airliner that was on the ground for several hours without operating ventilation were infected with an influenza virus (Moser et al. 1979). For diseases such as measles or for highly susceptible compromised hosts for whom very small doses are effective, the risk of airborne transmission from droplet nuclei is high even in well-ventilated interiors.

Characteristics of disease agents that affect airborne transmission relate primarily to viability and virulence. Viability is influenced by the structure of the organism and its suitability for the environment. Organisms that produce spores or other resistant stages are most likely to remain viable in the aerosol state. Most fungi produce spores capable of survival during airborne travel. Desiccation, for example, has little effect on many fungal spores. In addition, many fungal spores contain melaninlike pigments that protect against damage from ultraviolet radiation. Some bacteria produce spores, bacterial endospores, that resist not only drying and ultraviolet radiation but survive at high temperatures and high atmospheric pressures and resist many biocides. Viral resistance to environmental stress appears to depend on the lipid content of the virus. In general, lipid-containing viruses tend to be more stable in air than lipid-free viruses (Loosli et al. 1943; Ijaz et al. 1985; Karim et al. 1985). However, both relative humidity and temperature have independent effects on survival of viruses, and the effects of these environmental factors differ widely for different viruses. Some of the slow viruses may be more resistant since they can survive autoclaving; however, their survival characteristics in air are unknown.

Survival of airborne bacteria is determined by equally complex interactions between structure and environment (Hambleton et al. 1983; Katz and Hammel 1987). One study indicated that *Legionella* survives best in aerosol at 65 percent relative humidity and is least stable at 55 percent relative humidity (Hambleton et al. 1983). Another study demonstrated a drop of viability by a factor of four logarithms during the first 30 seconds of aerosolization (Katz and Hammel 1987) and a similar drop of viability when growth substrate temperatures rose from 55 to 65°C. Survival of *Legionella* was also dependent upon whether the organism was in stationary or log growth phase when aerosolized. Stationary phase organisms survived at a higher rate.

The evidence indicates that infection rate varies with aerosol characteristics and viability and virulence of the organism, as well as the concentration of the virulent particles in the aerosol (Loosli et al. 1943; Arnow et al. 1982; Williams and Moser 1987). *Legionella*, for example, can be readily isolated from many sites within a hospital or an office building in which no illness has been documented. However, when amplification of *Legionella* of sufficient virulence occurs and susceptible people are exposed to the concentrated aerosols, illness results (Eickhoff 1979; Fraser 1985). A similar sequence of amplification and exposure has been demonstrated for influenza. In the influenza epidemic in an airplane, mentioned above, the virus apparently accumulated to an infectious level because of inadequate ventilation (Moser et al. 1979). The risk of such an epidemic occurring in a well-ventilated airplane, although not yet documented, is probably quite low (National Research Council 1986). On the other hand, some infectious agents can cause disease at very low concentrations. Riley (1982) has hypothesized that a single droplet nucleus containing the tuberculosis bacillus is potentially infectious. Also, as we have emphasized above, immunocompromised patients may be susceptible to serious infections from almost any agent, even when present in a unit dose. *Legionella* is no exception. Patients on corticosteroid therapy have been shown to be susceptible to legionnellosis from inhaled tap water aerosols that did not cause disease in matched patients not on immunocompromising therapy (Arnow et al. 1982).

In addition to environmental factors, virulence of most microorganisms is controlled by the genetic makeup of the organism. Strain to strain variability can occur. For example, for *Legionella*, only one of the several strains isolated from environments in which epidemics have occurred has been demonstrated to have caused infection (Fraser 1985). The effect of other indoor air pollutants on survival and virulence of microorganisms is unknown.

HOST FACTORS

Age, health, and immunity status (Centers for Disease Control 1984) are important factors in the host which determine susceptibility to infectious disease. In general, very young and very old people are at greater risk for most infectious diseases although middle-aged men appear to be at increased risk for Legionnaire's disease, possibly because of greater occupational exposure (Storch et al. 1979). Health status is by far the most powerful controlling factor in infectious disease rates. Any condition that impairs immunity or other host defenses will predispose to infectious disease (Arnow et al. 1982; Recht et al. 1982; Palmer 1984). These conditions include both intrinsic and acquired immunodeficiency syndromes, drug- or treatment-induced immunodeficiency (e.g., steroids, immunosuppressive drugs, chemotherapy, and radiation therapy), alcoholism, hematologic malignancy, and stress. Smoking, viral respiratory infections, stroke, drug overdose, and obstructive lung disease tend to impair lung defenses and increase the risk of bacterial pneumonias. Exposure to some common air pollutants may also increase the risk of infection (Melia et al. 1982). Nitrogen dioxide and ozone exposure have been shown to increase the rate of infection and decrease the survival time of mice exposed to pathogenic bacteria (Ehrlich 1980; Jakab 1987); on the other hand, sulfur dioxide does not have a similar effect in animal models of infection. The effects of nitrogen dioxide and ozone exposure on respiratory infections in humans have not yet been established and are under investigation. Mean daytime temperature appears to affect incidence of respiratory infection although the mechanism is not clear (Lidwell, Morgan, and Williams 1965). Relative humidity, although clearly affecting the disease agent, has not been documented to be related to host susceptibility to respiratory disease, in spite of widespread belief to the contrary (Anderson et al. 1974). In a study designed to test the effects of prolonged isolation on immunity to respiratory infection, a group of people who had spent six months in the Antarctic at relative humidities consistently below 25 percent showed no increased risk of infection from respiratory viruses in comparison with the general population of New Zealand, where relative humidities vary in the range common to most temperate environments (Jennings and Faoagali 1980).

Some human activities increase the risk of infection by increasing the chance of exposure to a high dose of infectious aerosol. Workers who handle organic material are inevitably exposed to biologic aerosols. Fortunately, most such aerosols are not infectious for normal people and, at worst, cause a variety of hypersensitivity diseases. However, both brucellosis and anthrax can be transmitted to workers handling infected animal materials (LaForce et al. 1969; Solomon and Burge 1984). Laboratory workers are also at greater risk of contracting infections from disease agents handled in the course of their jobs. The most common laboratory-acquired viral diseases include infectious hepatitis, Venezuelan equine encephalitis, Newcastle disease, and Epstein-Barr virus. Laboratory-acquired infection with human immunodeficiency virus, type 3, is now documented. Bacterial diseases commonly acquired in laboratory exposure include brucellosis, typhoid fever, tularemia, and tuberculosis, many of which are aerosol-transmitted diseases.

## PREVENTION OF AIRBORNE INFECTION

Airborne infection can be prevented if the organism can be removed from the environment or rendered nonviable or if susceptibility can be controlled by control of host risk factors or by immunization (Brachman, Kauffman, and Dalldorf 1966). Removal from the environment usually involves interruption of the reservoir/amplifier/disseminator sequence. If infection could result from human to human transfer, infectious individuals, both those functioning as reservoirs and those functioning as amplifiers and disseminators, can be isolated from the majority of susceptible persons. However, individuals with infectious diseases that are not considered life threatening cannot always be isolated, and in this case, dilution and filtration are the best solution. Increased ventilation has been shown to decrease rates of viral upper respiratory disease (Brundage et al. 1988). In a contaminated workplace, dilution of the air by clean-air ventilation or by removal of the organism by filtration must be done to prevent worker infection. In the case of the grounded airliner, provision of forced mechanical ventilation with no recirculation might have prevented the epidemic. In most indoor environments, ventilation rates as set out in the guidelines of the American Society of Heating, Refrigerating, and Air-Conditioning Engineers make airborne transmission of viral aerosols from human sources unlikely, providing the standards are met. However, recent efforts at energy conservation have tended to lower ventilation rates in many public buildings far below these standards, and many homes may not be adequately ventilated throughout the year.

Reduction of indoor saprophytic bioaerosols requires either preventing penetration of outdoor aerosols (either by filtration or by removing the indoor reservoir) or eliminating reservoirs and amplifiers in the indoor space. Most fungal aerosols that cause infectious disease in interiors enter from outdoors and can be kept out by adequate filtration. However, a few spores always penetrate even the best system, and prevention of amplification in the indoor environment is often necessary. The important controlling factor for indoor fungal growth is water, either as water vapor (relative humidity) or surface condensation or accumulation. In the range of 25–75 percent relative humidity, fungal spore levels are directly correlated with relative humidity. Above 75 percent relative humidity, conditions are apparently ideal for surface growth (Solomon and Burge 1984). Any standing water, especially with mineral scale or other solid substrates available, presents a suitable substrate for fungal growth. It should be noted that most fungal aerosols arising from indoor growth do not cause infectious disease except in compromised hosts. In such highly susceptible people, even very low concentrations of some fungi can present a high risk of life-threatening infection. Unfortunately, maintaining a perfectly clean environment for these people is rarely possible.

Stagnant water can also act as reservoir and amplifier for bacteria, including *Legionella*, and for protozoa. Standing water should not be permitted, especially in building ventilation systems. Cooling-coil drip pans should drain immediately, and humidification should be achieved by methods that do not allow the accumulation of microbial slimes. In general, biocides should not be added to water in ventilation systems because the biocide, like the organisms, can become aerosolized by operation of the ventilation system. When ventilation systems containing viable microorganisms are to be cleaned, the system should be turned off during cleaning, and all biocides should be removed prior to restarting. Airborne disease resulting from contaminated tap water usually results only in immunocompromised hosts (Stout, Yu, and Muraca 1987). Although disinfection of epidemiologically implicated potable water supplies as well as cooling towers is certainly necessary in epidemic situations (Soracco et al. 1983), routine disinfection (especially in nonhospital settings) to prevent disease transmission is questionable. Epidemics related to cooling towers involve direct exposure to the cooling tower aerosol (drift). Preventing exposure to this drift is a potential solution. Cooling towers should never be located in places in which the drift can enter air intakes or in which people can pass directly through the effluent; towers that are so placed should be maintained rigorously. It must be remembered that biocides added to cooling tower water will be released in the drift and may have adverse health effects.

## SUMMARY

Airborne disease transmission involves a complex sequence of events involving a reservoir, amplifier, and disseminator. The mere presence of a pathogen in the environment does not necessarily lead to human illness. For infection to occur, the pathogen must be amplified and effectively disseminated to reach a susceptible host in a condition that is adequate to cause infection. Prevention of airborne infection can be effected by source, or reservoir, removal, or by interruption of the reservoir/amplifier/disseminator sequence.

# REFERENCES

Anderson, I., et al. 1974. Human response to 78-hour exposure to dry air. *Arch. Environ. Health* 29:319–24.

Arnow, P. M., et al. 1982. Nosocomial Legionnaire's disease caused by aerosolized tap water from respiratory devices. *J. Infect. Dis.* 146:460–67.

Brachman, P. S.; Kauffman, A. F.; and Dalldorf, F. G. 1966. Industrial inhalation anthrax. *Bacteriol. Rev.* 30:646–57.

Brundage, J. F., et al. 1988. Building-associated risk of febrile acute respiratory diseases in army trainees. *JAMA* 259:2108–12.

Centers for Disease Control. 1984. Adult immunization: Recommendations of the immunization practices advisory committee. *MMWR* 33:1S–68S.

Ehrlich, R. 1980. Interaction between environmental pollutants and respiratory infections. *Environ. Health Perspect.* 35:89–100.

Eickhoff, T. C. 1979. Epidemiology of Legionnaire's disease. *Ann. Intern. Med.* 90:499–502.

Fields, B. S., et al. 1986. Comparison of guinea pig and protozoan models for determining virulence of *Legionella* species. *Infect. Immun.* 53:553–59.

Fisher-Hoch, S. P., et al. 1981. Investigation and control of an outbreak of Legionnaire's disease in a district general hospital. *Lancet* 1:932–36.

Fliermans, C. B., et al. 1981. Ecological distribution of *Legionella pneumophila*. *Appl. Environ. Microbiol.* 41:9–16.

Fraser, D. W. 1985. Potable water as a source for legionellosis. *Environ. Health Perspect.* 62:337–41.

Glick, T. H., et al. 1978. Pontiac fever, an epidemic of unknown etiology in a health department, I: Clinical and epidemiologic aspects. *Am. J. Epidemiol.* 107:149–60.

Gregory, P. H. 1961. *The microbiology of the atmosphere.* New York: Wiley Interscience.

Hambleton, P., et al. 1983. Survival of virulent *Legionella pneumophila* in aerosols. *J. Hyg.* 90:451–60.

Huddleson, I. F., and Munger, M. 1940. A study of an epidemic of brucellosis due to *Brucella melitensus*. *Am. J. Public Health* 30:944–54.

Hughes, W. T. 1982. Natural mode of acquisition for de novo infection with *Pneumocystis carinii*. *J. Infect. Dis.* 145:842–48.

Ijaz, M. K., et al. 1985. Survival characteristics of airborne human coronavirus 229E. *J. Gen. Virol.* 66:2743–48.

Jakab, G. J. 1987. Modulation of pulmonary defense mechanisms by acute exposures to nitrogen dioxide. *Environ. Res.* 42:215–28.

Jennings, L. C., and Faoagali, J. L. 1980. A study of the susceptibility of antarctic winter-over personnel to viral respiratory illness on their return to New Zealand. *Antarctic Rec.* 3:29–30.

Karim, Y. G., et al. 1985. Effect of relative humidity on the airborne survival of rhinovirus-14. *Can. J. Microbiol.* 31:1058–61.

Katz, S. M., and Hammel, J. M. 1987. The effect of drying, heat and pH on the survival of *Legionella pneumophila*. *Ann. Clin. Lab. Sci.* 17:150–56.

Kauffman, A. F., et al. 1981. Pontiac fever: Isolation of the etiologic agent (*Legionella pneumophila*) and demonstration of its mode of transmission. *Am. J. Epidemiol.* 114:337–74.

Kauffman, C.; Burge, H.; and Solomon, W. 1988. Air and human-borne *Aspergillus fumigatus* in patient care areas. *J. Allergy Clin. Immunol.* 81:273.

Knight, V. 1973. Airborne transmission and pulmonary deposition of respiratory viruses. In *Viral and mycoplasmal infections of the respiratory tract.* Ed. V. Knight. Philadelphia: Lea and Febiger.

Kundsin, R. B. 1980. Airborne contagion. *Ann. N.Y. Acad. Sci.* 353:1–341.

LaForce, F. M., et al. 1969. Epidemiologic study of a fatal case of inhalation anthrax. *Arch. Environ. Health* 18:798–805.

Letts, R. M., and Doermer, E. 1983. Conversation in the operating theater as a cause of airborne bacterial contamination. *J. Bone Joint Surg.* 65-A:357–62.

Lidwell, O. M.; Morgan, R. W.; and Williams, R. E. O. 1965. The epidemiology of the common cold, IV: The effect of weather. *J. Hyg. Camb.* 63:427–39.

Loosli, C. G., et al. 1943. Experimental airborne influenza infection, I: Influence of humidity on survival of virus in air. *Proc. Soc. Exp. Biol. Med.* 53:205–6.

Mannis, M. J., et al. 1986. Acanthamoeba sclerokeratitis: Determining diagnostic criteria. *Arch. Ophthalmol.* 104:1313–17.

Melia, R. J., et al. 1982. Childhood respiratory illness and the home environment, II: Association between respiratory illness and nitrogen dioxide, temperature and relative humidity. *Int. J. Epidemiol.* 11:164–69.

Miller, R. P. 1979. Cooling towers and evaporative condensers. *Ann. Intern. Med.* 90:667–70.

Moser, M. R., et al. 1979. An outbreak of influenza aboard a commercial airliner. *Am. J. Epidemiol.* 110:1–6.

Muchmore, H. G., et al. 1981. Persistent parainfluenza virus shedding during isolation at the South Pole. *Nature* 289:187–89.

National Research Council. 1961. Conference on airborne infection, Dec. 7–10, 1960. *Bacteriol. Rev.* 25:173–382.

National Research Council (committee on indoor pollutants) 1981. *Indoor pollutants.* Washington, D.C.: National Academy Press.

National Research Council. 1986. *Airliner cabin environment: Air quality and safety.* Washington, D.C.: National Academy Press.

Palmer, D. L. 1984. Microbiology of pneumonia in the patient at risk. *Am. J. Med.* 76:53–60.

Petersen, N. J. 1980. An assessment of the airborne route in hepatitis B transmission. *Ann. N.Y. Acad. Sci.* 353:157–66.

Recht, L. D., et al. 1982. Blastomycosis in immunosuppressed patients. *Am. Rev. Respir. Dis.* 125:359–62.

Rhame, F. S., et al. 1984. Extrinsic risk factors for pneumonia in the patient at high risk of infection. *Am. J. Med.* 76:42–52.

Riley, R. L. 1982. Indoor airborne infection. *Environ. Int.* 8:317–20.

Skaliy, P., and McEachern, H. V. 1979. Survival of the Legionnaire's disease bacterium in water. *Ann. Intern. Med.* 90:662–63.

Solomon, W. R., and Burge, H. A. 1984. Allergens and pathogens. In *Indoor air quality.* Ed. P. J. Walsh, C. Dudney, and E. D. Copenhaver. Boca Raton, Fl.: CRC Press.

Soracco, R. J., et al. 1983. Susceptibilities of algae and *Legionella pneumophila* to cooling tower biocides. *Appl. Environ. Microbiol.* 45:1254–60.

Spendlove, J. C., and Fannin, K. F. 1983. Source, significance, and control of indoor microbial aerosols: Human health aspects. *Public Health Rep.* 98:229–44.

Storch, G., et al. 1979. Sporadic community-acquired Legionnaire's disease in the United States. *Ann. Intern. Med.* 90:596–600.

Stout, J.; Yu, V.; and Muraca, P. 1987. Legionnaires' disease acquired within the homes of two patients: Link to the home water supply. *JAMA* 257:1215–17.

Wang, W. L. L., et al. 1979. Growth, survival and resistance of the Legionnaire's disease bacterium. *Ann. Intern. Med.* 90:614–18.

Willeke, K., and Baron, P. A. 1987. The size distribution of whirlpool-generated droplets, their ability to contain bacteria and their deposition potential in the human respiratory tract. In *Advances in Aerobiology.* Ed. G. Boehm, and R. Leuschner. Basel: Birkhauser.

Williams, J. E., and Moser, S. A. 1987. Chronic murine pulmonary blastomycosis induced by intratracheally inoculated *Blastomyces dermatitidis* conidia. *Am. Rev. Respir. Dis.* 135:17–25.

# 13

# BIOLOGICAL AGENTS
# AND ALLERGIC DISEASES

David N. Weissman, M.D.
Mark R. Schuyler, M.D.

Numerous inhaled biologic agents are capable of inducing immune responses that may cause respiratory disease. The type of immunologically mediated respiratory disease resulting from inhalation of a biologic agent will depend in large part on the nature of the immune response induced by the agent. Inhaled materials that trigger an immunoglobulin E (IgE) response are referred to as *allergens*; allergens frequently cause immediate reactions at the site of exposure. Thus, IgE-mediated immune reactions following exposure to allergens are important in producing attacks of asthma and allergic rhinitis (Mathison, Stevenson, and Simon 1982). In contrast, some inhaled biologic materials cause lung damage by provoking responses that involve immune cells and antibodies. The pulmonary disease hypersensitivity pneumonitis results from this type of response; if exposure persists and the disease is not treated appropriately, hypersensitivity pneumonitis can progress to irreversible fibrosis of the lung (Salvaggio 1987).

   This chapter will address the immunologically mediated respiratory diseases induced by inhalation of biologic agents commonly found in the indoor environment. We review the immune mechanisms responsible for immunologic respiratory disease, the clinical characteristics of the respiratory allergies and hypersensitivity pneumonitis, the indoor allergens responsible for respiratory allergies, the assessment of exposure and measures for controlling exposure, and hypersensitivity pneumonitis and related conditions produced by inhaled biologic agents emanating from machines that process indoor air.

*IMMUNOLOGIC MECHANISMS AND RESPIRATORY DISEASES*

The mechanisms responsible for immunologically mediated diseases have been classified into four categories (Gell and Coombs 1964; Bellanti 1985). Type I or *anaphylactic* reactions are mediated primarily by IgE antibodies. These antibodies have the characteristic property of binding to "mediator cells" such as mast cells and basophils. Following the reaction of cell-bound IgE with allergen, mediator cells release potent vasoactive substances (mediators), the actions of which produce the clinical symptoms of allergic disease. IgE-mediated respiratory allergies are the result of type I immunologic reactions. Type II or *cytolytic* (*cytotoxic*) reactions are mediated primarily by immunoglobulin G (IgG) or immunoglobulin M (IgM) antibodies. Such antibodies, after binding to a target (antigen), have the capability of binding with a series of serum proteins known collectively as *complement*. The binding of antibody and complement to a cell can result in lysis of that cell. Antibodies can also target bound antigen for ingestion and destruction by immune cells such as neutrophils, macrophages, and lymphocytes. Type III (also known as *immune complex* or *Arthus*) reactions are mediated by soluble aggregates of antibody bound to antigen (*immune complexes*). Deposition of immune complexes in tissues can result in destructive tissue inflammation.

Type IV (also known as *cell-mediated* or *delayed-type hypersensitivity* reactions) are mediated by the action of sensitized T-lymphocytes. Antibodies, which are made by B-lymphocytes, do not play a role in type IV reactions. T-lymphocytes may act through several different mechanisms to cause tissue injury: direct killing of target cells; the elaboration of immunologically active substances (*lymphokines*); or interaction with other cells, such as natural killer cells or macrophages. Immunologically mediated diseases are not necessarily due to only one of the immune mechanisms described above. For example, hypersensitivity pneumonitis shows elements of both type III and type IV immunologic reactions.

## IMMUNOLOGICALLY MEDIATED RESPIRATORY DISEASES

Immunologically mediated respiratory diseases induced by inhaled biologic indoor air pollutants include respiratory allergies (rhinitis, sinusitis, and asthma) and hypersensitivity pneumonitis. Respiratory allergies occur with increased frequency in individuals with the inherited tendency to form IgE against substances encountered in the environment. Such individuals are termed *atopic* and constitute between 5 and 22 percent of the general population (Smith 1983). Respiratory allergy is common in Western countries. For example, general population studies in Europe, the United States, Australia, and New Zealand have shown that from 2 to 6 percent of adults report ever having asthma (Smith 1983). Prevalence figures for allergic rhinitis (hay fever) in the United States have ranged between 3 percent and 19 percent (Smith 1983). In contrast to the data available for respiratory allergies, the prevalence of hypersensitivity pneumonitis in the general population has not been described (Fink 1983). However, data are available for groups exposed to inhaled biologic agents from specific occupations and hobbies. For example, in the British Isles about 7 percent of farmers develop farmer's lung disease, an example of hypersensitivity pneumonitis resulting from inhalation of moldy hay; between 6 and 21 percent of exposed pigeon breeder club members develop another example of hypersensitivity pneumonitis, pigeon breeder's disease; and in a single office, 15 percent of workers exposed to an air-conditioning system contaminated with thermophilic actinomycetes developed hypersensitivity pneumonitis (Fink 1983).

ALLERGIC RHINITIS

Clinically, allergic (IgE-mediated) respiratory disease can be recognized through characteristic symptomatology, physical signs, and laboratory findings. For example, allergic rhinitis (hay fever) manifests itself as nasal obstruction and rhinorrhea (runny nose). Patients often experience sneezing and itchy nose. Allergic rhinitis may be associated with allergic conjunctivitis (manifested as red, itchy, watery eyes) and with allergic sinusitis (manifested as a sense of fullness or pain over the sinuses and postnasal drip). IgE directed against specific allergens (specific IgE) can be demonstrated in patients with allergic rhinitis either by skin testing or by blood tests (radioallergosorbent test or RAST).

ASTHMA

Asthma refers to intermittent, reversible airway obstruction, often associated with shortness of breath and chest tightness (Reed and Townley 1983). Airways obstruction in asthma reflects the triad of mucosal edema, plugging of airways with mucus, and bronchospasm (constriction of the smooth muscles encircling the airways). Acute attacks of asthma may be triggered by either allergic mechanisms or by nonallergic mechanisms, such as exercise, respiratory infections, or exposure to irritating inhalants. Pulmonary function testing during an acute attack demonstrates an obstructive type of ventilatory impairment, but between attacks, pulmonary function may be entirely normal. However, more than 90 percent of these patients will be found to have "hyperreactive airways" when challenged by an inhaled bronchoconstrictor such as methacholine (Reed and Townley 1983). IgE-mediated allergic asthma tends to occur in atopic individuals, in whom specific IgE directed against common inhalants can be demonstrated by skin testing or RAST.

## HYPERSENSITIVITY PNEUMONITIS

Hypersensitivity pneumonitis may present clinically in either an acute or a chronic form (Fink 1983). The acute form is generally easier to recognize. Shortly after inhalation of the offending agent, the exposed person experiences fevers, chills, and shortness of breath. Chest x-ray may show radiodensities mimicking acute pneumonia. In fact, the initial episode of acute hypersensitivity pneumonitis may be confused with pneumonia, but recurring episodes after exposure to the offending antigen and the lack of evidence for infection will often lead to an accurate diagnosis.

Chronic hypersensitivity pneumonitis may be extremely difficult to diagnose. Patients do not have acute symptoms after inhalation of the offending agent, and experience a slow, insidious decline in pulmonary function that causes symptoms late in the course. Often, it is difficult to elicit a history of exposure to a causal agent. Chest x-ray shows an interstitial pattern of lung disease, and pulmonary function testing commmonly shows a restrictive pattern of ventilatory impairment. Both of these findings are nonspecific and can be seen in a number of different lung diseases. Lung biopsy may be nonspecific, especially in advanced cases associated with pulmonary fibrosis. Precipitating serum antibodies directed against offending inhalants may provide a marker for exposure in patients with hypersensitivity pneumonitis but may be present in healthy exposed individuals as well. Thus, chronic hypersensitivity pneumonitis, especially when advanced, may be a difficult diagnostic problem.

## INDOOR ALLERGENS AND ALLERGIC RESPIRATORY DISEASE

Clinicians have long appreciated the importance of the indoor environment in allergic disease. Recent studies have provided confirmation of the role of indoor allergens. For example, in a recent nationwide study, 16,204 subjects underwent skin testing with five common outdoor and three common indoor allergens. Twenty percent of the subjects had at least one positive skin test. Of those with one or more positive tests, 38 percent reacted to one or more indoor allergens (Gergen, Turkeltaub, and Kovar 1987). Indoor allergens are particularly suspect as triggers for allergic asthma or rhinitis in patients suffering from perennial symptoms, as exposure to outdoor allergens is usually seasonal in nature. House dust, animal danders, and indoor fungi have long been regarded as potent indoor allergens (Solomon and Matthews 1983).

### ASSESSMENT OF EXPOSURE TO INDOOR ALLERGENS

Measurement of indoor allergens has become increasingly sophisticated. For example, "house dust" is not a single antigen, but a complex mixture of potentially allergenic biologic materials, including human and animal hair and dander, mites, molds, textiles, food leftovers, bacteria, insect parts, and decomposed material (Lowenstein et al. 1986). Thus, the composition of house dust may vary significantly from one location to another, and techniques are now available for purification of individual allergenic molecules from crude extracts of allergenic materials (Marsh et al. 1987). The development of purified allergens and antibodies raised against those allergens has been of great practical importance. Specific antibodies can be used to detect minute quantities of allergen by powerful immunologic techniques. Such techniques have been utilized in the standardization of diagnostic and therapeutic allergenic extracts (Marsh et al. 1987), as well as in the quantitation of airborne allergens (Agarwal et al. 1981).

Techniques utilized previously to quantitate exposure to outdoor allergens are not always applicable to the indoor environment. Outdoor allergen exposures are usually quantitated by morphologic or culture techniques (Solomon and Matthews 1983). Morphology-based quantitation techniques depend upon the microscopic

288   David N. Weissman and Mark R. Schuyler

identification and counting of collected allergens. These techniques have been used widely in the identification of pollens, which can be collected, stained, and identified using microscopy because of the unique appearances of different pollen grains. Culture techniques have been used widely to quantitate exposure to fungal allergens (Salvaggio and Aukrust 1981). The use of culture techniques has been necessary because different types of fungal spores are often indistinguishable by simple microscopy. Culture-based quantitation techniques involve the collection of atmospheric allergens onto culture media. Viable agents collected on the culture media are grown into colonies that can be identified and quantified by micro-biologic techniques.

Some indoor allergens cannot be identified by either morphologic or culture techniques (Swanson, Agarwal, and Reed 1985). For example, animal danders, mite feces, or decomposed insect parts, all indoor allergens, cannot be specifically identified by these techniques. For this reason, quantification of indoor allergens by the use of antibody-based immunologic techniques has been accomplished recently by several groups (Table 13.1). These techniques have been used to detect individual allergens in dust samples (Lind et al. 1987). Immunologic identification of airborne mite, roach, cat, mouse, and guinea pig antigens has been performed using a suction technique (Swanson, Agarwal, and Reed 1985). Indoor air is suctioned through filter paper, and allergens trapped on the filter paper are then quantitated by immunologic techniques. A similar technique was used to quanti-tate the dose of the mite antigen, *Der p* I, inhaled by infants (Carswell et al. 1983). Thus, methodology now exists for the quantitation of nonviable, amorphous in-door allergens. Morphologic, culture, and immunologic techniques will all be useful in future efforts to set standards for indoor air pollution by specific indoor allergens (van Bronswijk 1987).

SPECIFIC INDOOR ALLERGENS CAUSING RESPIRATORY ALLERGY

*Dust Mites*   Mites are a major source for the allergenic content of common house dust (Platts-Mills and Chapman 1987). Of the more than fifty thousand species of mites, only a few commonly cause allergies in man. Two species of the genus *Dermatophagoides*, *D. pteronyssinus* and *D. farinae*, are of major importance throughout the world (Solomon and Matthews 1983). Dust mites thrive on shed human epidermis (Beck and Bjerring 1987). Thus, bed dust tends to be the most potent source for dust mite allergen, and the greatest exposure to airborne dust mite allergen occurs in the bedroom. High concentrations of dust mite allergen can also be found in dust from carpets, furnishings, and clothing (Swanson, Agarwal, and Reed 1985; Tovey et al. 1981). Mite allergens most often become airborne when dust deposits are disturbed, as during bedding changes or cleaning (Tovey et al. 1981; Carswell et al. 1983; Swanson, Agarwal, and Reed 1985). Thus, dust-disturbing activities within the home are one determinant of personal exposure to dust allergens. Mite population growth is fastest under conditions of high air humidity (Korsgaard 1983a). Temperature, within the range normally encountered in human habitations, does not greatly affect mite growth (Lowenstein et al. 1986).

Table 13.1  Immunochemical Quantitation of Indoor Allergens: Referenced Examples

| Allergen Measured | Assessment for Dust Contamination | Assessment for Airborne Allergen |
|---|---|---|
| Dust mite (*Der p* I) | Lind et al. (1987) | Carswell et al. (1983) |
|  | Platts-Mills et al. (1986) | Swanson, Agarwal, and Reed (1985) |
|  | Tovey et al. (1981) | Tovey et al. (1981) |
| Cat (*Fel d* I) | Lind et al. (1987) | Swanson, Agarwal, and Reed (1985) |
|  |  | Van Metre et al. (1986) |
| Dog | Lind et al. (1987) |  |
| Horse | Lind et al. (1987) |  |
| Rat | Schwartz and Lind |  |
| Mouse | (1984) | Swanson, Agarwal, and Reed (1985) |
| Guinea pig |  | Swanson, Agarwal, and Reed (1985) |
| Cockroach |  | Swanson, Agarwal, and Reed (1985) |
| Alternaria (outdoor) | Agarwal et al. (1981) |  |

Dust mite extracts have been intensively studied and characterized, particularly extracts of *D. pteronyssinus*. A major allergen, *Der p* I, has been purified from crude extracts of *D. pteronyssinus* and shown to be strongly associated with mite feces (Tovey, Chapman, and Platts-Mills 1981). Specific antibodies raised against this antigen have been utilized to quantitate mite allergen exposure in the home by immunologic techniques (Tovey et al. 1981; Carswell et al. 1983). Antibodies recognizing both *Der p* I and antigens found in extracts of *D. farinae* have been developed and used to quantitate dust contamination by both *D. farinae* and *D. pteronyssinus* (Platts-Mills et al. 1986). An international standard *D. pteronyssinus* allergen extract has been developed recently and will be an aid to future research and patient care (Ford et al. 1985).

Increased exposure to house dust mites may increase the risk of allergic respiratory disease (Korsgaard 1983b). Conversely, aggressive measures to prevent exposure have been shown to improve dust-sensitive asthmatics. Such aggressive measures have included removal from the home environment by hospital admission (Platts-Mills et al. 1982) or the creation of a dustfree bedroom by encasing mattresses, box springs, and pillows in zippered vinyl covers; laundering pillows and blankets frequently with hot water; and replacing bedroom carpets with polished floors (Murray and Ferguson 1983; Walshaw and Evans 1986). A number of other measures might be useful in controlling indoor exposures to dust mite allergen. Indoor relative humidity is by far the most important determinant of indoor mite growth, so reduction in indoor relative humidity would be expected to be the most effective means of decreasing indoor mite growth (Korsgaard 1982). Acaricides applied to areas of mite growth, such as mattresses and upholstery, may prove to be helpful in the control of indoor air pollution by mites (Bischoff 1987). Future efforts to set standards for indoor dust mite contamination will probably be based on immunochemical determinations of dust mite allergen content in representative dust samples (van Bronswijk 1987). Based on currently available data, it has been suggested that at levels above 2 μg of *Der p* I per gram of dust (equivalent to one hundred mites per gram of dust) there is an increased risk of sensitization, bronchial reactivity, and symptomatic asthma; and at levels above 10 μg of *Der p* I per gram of dust (equivalent to five hundred mites per gram of dust) the risk of acute or severe attacks of asthma is increased (Platts-Mills 1988).

*Indoor Allergens of Animal Origin*    Sensitivity to allergens of animal origin is a common problem in clinical allergy, in part because of the high prevalence of keeping furred animals as pets (Solomon and Matthews 1983). In a large Swedish epidemiologic study of 40,010 children, 52 percent of nonasthmatic children kept furred pets, and 25 percent were exposed by riding or caring for animals in barns or stables (Kjellman and Pettersson 1983). A recent epidemiologic study of 16,204 subjects in the United States showed a prevalence of 2.3 percent skin test positivity to cat or dog allergenic extracts in the general population (Gergen, Turkeltaub, and Kovar 1987). Asthmatic patients have been reported to show a 25 percent prevalence of wheal-flare cutaneous reactivity to animal proteins, indicating the presence of specific IgE directed against these allergens (Mathison, Stevenson, and Simon 1982).

Advances in the purification and standardization of allergenic materials derived from animals have paralleled those achieved for dust mites (Lowenstein et al. 1986; Marsh et al. 1987). Antibodies raised against purified animal allergens have, in turn, been used to characterize better the nature of animal allergy. The major source of allergenic material from many furred animals, such as cat, dog, horse, and cow, is dander, or shed epidermal scales (Lowenstein et al. 1986). Shed animal epidermal scales can be an important allergenic component of house dust. In a recent study of mattress dust obtained from forty-two Baltimore households, cat and dog antigens were detected in 77 and 63 percent of samples studied, respectively (Lind et al. 1987). Animals need not reside in the home in which their dander allergens are found; in the same study, horse antigens were detected in 5 percent of the homes studied. Similarly, significant amounts of dog dander have been demonstrated in homes in which dogs had never been kept (Vanto and Koivikko 1983).

Cat allergenic extracts have been particularly well characterized. *Fel d* I, the major cat allergen, is one of at least ten potentially allergenic components of cat extract (Ohman, Lowell, and Bloch 1974; Lowenstein, Lind, and Weeke 1985). It originates from salivary mucous glands and sebaceous glands in hair roots (Bartholomé et al. 1985). Immunochemical measurement of cat antigens trapped in an air filtering device has shown that airborne cat antigen levels increase markedly during periods of dust disturbance, as during bedding changes (Swanson, Agarwal, and Reed 1985). However, airborne *Fel d* I can also be demonstrated in undisturbed houses, apparently because *Fel d* I may be associated with airborne fine particles, which may remain airborne for long periods (Platts-Mills 1988).

Urine is the main source of allergen from rodents, such as guinea pigs, mice, and rats (Lowenstein et al. 1986). Measurable amounts of airborne allergen can be found in homes in which rodents are kept as pets or in tenement apartments infested by mice (Swanson, Agarwal, and Reed 1985). Allergic sensitivity to rodent allergens is primarily a problem in professional animal handlers, with up to 10 percent being affected (Taylor, Longbottom, and Pepys 1977). The role of rodent allergens in the home environment remains to be determined.

Control of indoor levels of animal allergen is accomplished by limitation of animal access to the indoor environment and by cleaning to control levels of materials brought inside by animals or by human contact with animals. Avoidance of furnishings derived from unmanufactured materials with the potential to release allergens may also be important (Lowenstein et al. 1986). Although current data do not permit the development of standards for most animal-derived allergen exposures, more information is becoming available (van Bronswijk 1987). For example, antibody-based detection techniques have been used to quantitate ambient levels of the cat allergen *Fel d* I in a room containing living cats. The levels quantitated were sufficient to induce asthma or rhinitis in ten of ten cat-allergic subjects (Van Metre et al. 1986). Another approach has been to quantitate the allergen content of dust samples. Using this technique, the amount of rat allergen in an animal laboratory was determined and expressed as allergen per square meter. An allergen elimination program was shown to cause a significant drop in rat allergen levels (Schwartz and Lind 1984).

*Cockroach-Derived Indoor Allergens*    The cockroach is increasingly recognized as a significant source of indoor allergenic material. A high prevalence of sensitivity to cockroach extract has long been documented by immediate hypersensitivity skin testing (Bernton and Brown 1964). One such study, conducted in the urban Chicago area, showed a 58 percent prevalence of cockroach hypersensitivity among asthmatic adults and a 69 percent prevalence among asthmatic children (Kang and Sulit 1978). Allergy patients with clinical dust sensitivity are much more likely to be sensitive to cockroach than are patients without clinically apparent dust sensitivity (Hulett and Dockhorn 1979). Inhalation challenge studies have documented the triggering of acute asthma in skin test-positive asthmatics following inhalation of cockroach allergen (Kang et al. 1979). Similarly, nasal provocation studies have documented the ability of cockroach allergen to trigger acute rhinitis (Steinberg et al. 1987).

As for other allergenic materials, efforts have been made to identify and characterize the individual allergens in crude cockroach extracts. Biochemical techniques have been utilized to purify three major allergens from extracts of German and American cockroaches (Twarog et al. 1977). More recent studies have demonstrated little cross-reactivity between allergens of German and American cockroaches. In the case of German cockroaches, most of the allergenic activity present can be found in cast cockroach skins. Respiratory exposure to cockroach presumably occurs through the accumulation, disintegration, and aerosolization of cast cockroach skins (Richman et al. 1984).

We do not presently have a standard for acceptable levels of indoor pollution by cockroach allergens. However, measurement of ambient levels of cockroach allergen has been accomplished recently by immunochemical techniques. Such levels were much higher in New York tenement apartments than in houses in Rochester, Minnesota, implying the importance of cockroach infestation as a source of indoor cockroach allergen (Swanson, Agarwal, and Reed 1985). Thus, control of indoor contamination by cockroach allergen would probably be best accomplished by control of cockroach infestation and cleaning of shed and disintegrated cockroach skins.

*Molds* The allergenic potential of fungal constituents has been recognized for more than one hundred years (Salvaggio and Aukrust 1981). The reported prevalence of type I allergy to molds has ranged between 2 and 30 percent of an allergic population (Lowenstein et al. 1986). Clearly, molds are capable of contaminating the indoor environment, either by entering from the outside or by local growth (Lowenstein et al. 1986). Indoor mold growth and resulting airborne spore levels depend upon the availability of an appropriate substrate for mold growth and on the relative humidity. Below a relative humidity of 30 percent, little interior mold growth occurs (except on locally wet surfaces). Conditions for mold growth are progressively more favorable up to a relative humidity of 70 percent. Above 70 percent relative humidity is optimal for mold growth. Within the range of temperatures common in human habitations, temperature is not a critical determinant of mold growth (Burge 1985). Areas in which conditions are particularly favorable for domestic mold growth include garbage containers, food storage areas, upholstery, wallpaper, and areas of increased moisture such as damp basements, shower curtains, window moldings, and portable window air-conditioning units. Improperly cleaned cold mist vaporizers may emit high levels of fungus particles (Salvaggio and Aukrust 1981). In addition to these obvious sites of potential mold growth, an important site of indoor fungal growth is house dust. Indeed, any damp, nonliving organic material can quickly become colonized by fungi (Burge 1985).

Culture studies have been performed to examine the prevalence and identity of mold contamination in the indoor environment. In one study of one hundred Danish homes, *Cladosporium, Penicillium*, and *Alternaria* were found to be the predominating airborne fungi present, each being detectable in more than 75 percent of the homes studied (Gravesen 1978). Culture of dust samples from these homes showed most frequent contamination with members of the *Mucor* genus followed by *Penicillum, Alternaria, Cladosporium*, and *Aspergillus*. The explanation offered for the predominance of *Mucor* species in dust, but not in the air, was that spores of the *Mucor* species were liberated in sticky mucilaginous droplets that did not become airborne (Gravesen 1978). Another study of cultured airborne spores from eleven Florida homes showed the presence of *Cladosporium* and *Penicillium* in all homes, the presence of *Aspergillus* in ten homes, and the presence of *Alternaria* in three homes (Binnie 1987). The airborne fungal species demonstrated in these studies are considered to be clinically important allergens (Salvaggio and Aukrust 1981).

Assessment of indoor exposure to molds has generally been accomplished by morphologic and culture techniques (Salvaggio and Aukrust 1981; Mathison,

Stevenson, and Simon 1982). Morphologic techniques, such as the rotorod technique, allow the volumetric assessment of airborne mold spore load. However, because of the often nonspecific appearance of mold spores, identification of specific fungal species must frequently be accomplished by culture. Quantitative assessment of air pollution by specific fungal species is done by volumetric air sampling utilizing a suction sampler, with culture of mold spores sucked into culture media. Improved characterization of mold allergens has created the potential for immunochemical assessment of indoor mold allergen exposure. Currently identified mold allergens include *Alt a* I (derived from *Alternaria*) and *Cla h* I and *Cla h* II (both derived from *Cladosporium*) (Marsh et al. 1987). Immunochemical techniques have already been utilized to measure outdoor levels of airborne *Alternaria* allergen (Agarwal et al. 1981).

Based on currently available data, it has been suggested that airborne levels of bacteria and fungi should not exceed a total of seven hundred colony-forming units per cubic meter of indoor air (Binnie 1987). It has been suggested further that when this level is exceeded, higher incidences of allergic reactions and eye, nose, and throat irritation are encountered. Control of indoor mold contamination is accomplished by creating an indoor environment unfavorable to mold growth. Potential substrates for mold growth should be removed or kept scrupulously clean. Indoor humidity and accumulation of indoor aeroallergens should be combated with good indoor ventilation. Building repair and the removal of cool mist humidifiers may be necessary to control indoor mold contamination. Air conditioning may act to decrease indoor exposure to mold spores from the outside (Burge 1985; Reed 1985). Thus, as standards for indoor exposure to molds become available, measures will be accessible for the control of indoor mold allergen levels.

## HYPERSENSITIVITY PNEUMONITIS AND RELATED CONDITIONS

### ANTIGENS RESPONSIBLE FOR HYPERSENSITIVITY PNEUMONITIS

A broad range of inhaled antigenic materials can cause hypersensitivity pneumonitis (Fink 1983; Salvaggio 1987). Most of these materials are complex, organic, and particulate in nature. For example, the most frequently encountered antigens causing hypersensitivity pneumonitis are the thermophilic actinomycetes. These bacteria are responsible for the form of hypersensitivity pneumonitis known as *farmer's lung disease*, mentioned earlier. Thermophilic actinomycetes, ubiquitous organisms that decompose organic matter, have been isolated from soil, manure, grain, compost, and hay. Thermophilic actinomycetes may pollute the indoor environment through contamination of forced-air heating, cooling, and humidification systems. Fungi such as *Alternaria*, *Penicillium*, and *Aspergillus* species may also contaminate the indoor environment and cause hypersensitivity pneumonitis. Avian proteins may pollute the indoor environment through the keeping of domestic birds. Avian proteins inhaled from dried excreta of parakeets, lovebirds, pigeons, or chickens may cause hypersensitivity pneumonitis. Several simple reactive chemicals, including toluene diisocyanate (TDI), diphenylmethane diisocyanate (MDI), trimellitic anhydride (TMA), and phthalic anhydride, have been documented as causing hypersensitivity pneumonitis. These chemicals are usually found in the occupational setting in paint catalysts, in the production of plastics, or through the use of heated epoxy resin, but they may enter the domestic environment through use in recreational activities or hobbies.

Inhaled organic materials causing hypersensitivity pneumonitis, such as whole microorganisms or bird excreta, are complex mixtures of many component substances. Often, the role of individual components in these complex inhaled mixtures is unclear. For example, *Micropolyspora faeni* (*M. faeni*), the bacteria that causes farmer's lung disease, is a thermophilic actinomycete with components including lipopolysaccharides, proteins (including enzymes), carbohydrates, mucopolysaccharides, and lipoproteins (Ramasamy, Khan, and Kurup 1987). Before inhalation, the responsible material is often altered by exposure to other bacterial and animal products. For example, extracellular chymotrypsin secreted by *M. faeni* changes both moldy hay, the substrate for growth of *M. faeni*, and *M. faeni* itself to produce a wide range of degradation products. These materials, in addition to the many antigens in *M. faeni*, can be inhaled and produce farmer's lung disease (Nicolet and Bannerman 1975). Regardless of the exact nature of the responsible antigens, considerable amounts of the material must be inhaled in appropriate respirable form to induce hypersensitivity pneumonitis and humidifier fever.

The material in pigeon dropping extract (PDE), which is probably responsible for pigeon breeder's disease, is known as $PDE_1$, a fragment of pigeon intestinal IgA (Fredricks and Tebo 1980). A likely source of $PDE_1$ is IgA from the pigeon gastrointestinal tract which has been enzymatically altered by exposure to gut enzymes and/or to gut bacteria (Huis and Berrens 1976).

Because exposure to these mixtures of antigens occurs in diverse settings, the specific element(s) in the complex mixtures responsible for disease have not been identified. However, inhalation exposures with soluble extracts of bacteria and pigeon droppings indicate that the responsible antigens are soluble in aqueous solvents and bind to serum antibody (Stricker et al. 1986). Another approach for identifying the specific antigens responsible for hypersensitivity pneumonitis is to screen the antibodies in the serum of affected persons. Typically, serum antibodies are present which recognize a wide variety of antigens in the inhaled material. For example, careful separation of PDE indicates that at least twenty-five different antigens can elicit antibodies in exposed individuals (McCormick et al. 1982). Thus, there are many possible antigens that could be important in the pathogenesis of hypersensitivity pneumonitis.

IMMUNOPATHOGENESIS OF HYPERSENSITIVITY PNEUMONITIS

The presence of multiple immunologic markers in persons with hypersensitivity pneumonitis indicates the importance of immune factors in the pathogenesis of this syndrome. Since Pepys' redescription of hypersensitivity pneumonitis in the 1950s, various types of immune reactions have been implicated as causes of lung damage in hypersensitivity pneumonitis. Initially, hypersensitivity pneumonitis was thought to result from a type III immunologic reaction involving the combination of inhaled antigen and antibody present in the serum into inflammatory antigen-antibody complexes (Pepys 1969). This hypothesis was suggested by the clinical features of the disease and the presence of serum antibodies against the causative antigen. More recent hypotheses have emphasized the role of type IV immunologic reactions, cell-mediated immunity, in the immunopathogenesis of hypersensitivity pneumonitis (Fink 1983; Salvaggio 1987).

The agents that cause hypersensitivity pneumonitis may be directly toxic but also directly activate complement and cause macrophages to secrete complement components and proteolytic enzymes. The inflammation resulting from the direct injury and the indirect injury modulated by complement and macrophages probably has an important role in the immunopathogenesis of hypersensitivity pneumonitis. The injury itself might enhance exposure to inhaled antigen by reducing the integrity of surface barriers and thereby promote immunologic sensitization and subsequent lung damage. Many of the agents responsible for hypersensitivity pneumonitis can act as adjuvants and thus promote the development of heightened humoral and cell-mediated immunity. In addition, the particulate nature of the inciting antigen would tend to cause retention of antigen within the lung for prolonged periods of time.

Figure 13.1 represents mechanisms that may be important in lung injury in hypersensitivity pneumonitis. The agents are particulate, persistent, and nondegradable. They interact with humoral mediators, complement and antibody, and cells in the lung to produce inflammation. The agents can induce injury by causing polymorphonuclear leukocytes and macrophages to release phlogistic substances such as reactive oxygen compounds, proteolytic enzymes, and products of arachidonic acid metabolism such as prostaglandins and leukotrienes. The agents can also cause the production and release of interleukin–1 from macrophages and soluble mediators called lymphokines (IL–2, $\gamma$-interferon, and B-cell growth and differentiation factors) from lymphocytes. These mediators promote pulmonary inflammation. This conceptual model, as depicted in Figure 13.1, must be incomplete because it does not include any mechanisms for opposing inflammation.

Any scheme for the pathogenesis of hypersensitivity pneumonitis must explain the wide range of susceptibility among the exposed population and the apparent resistance to illness of most exposed individuals. The apparent variation in susceptibility could reflect differences in exposure. Although personal exposures to antigen have not been assessed in naturally occurring hypersensitivity pneumonitis, the exposures of symptomatic and asymptomatic subjects are similar (Fink et al. 1972). However, individual to individual variation in doses to target tissues in the lung, for the same exposure, might explain variation in susceptibility. In this regard, particle deposition and clearance material vary considerably among individuals. Cigarette smoking affects particle handling in the lungs and might be expected to influence susceptibility to hypersensitivity pneumonitis. Smokers have a reduced risk for hypersensitivity pneumonitis, but the mechanism for the

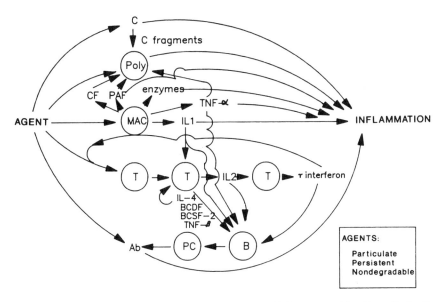

Figure 13.1. Possible mechanisms responsible for hypersensitivity pneumonitis. Ab, antibody; B, B-cell; BCDF, B-cell differentiation factor; BCSF-2, B-cell stimulatory factor-2; C, complement; CF, chemotactic factor(s); IL-1, interleukin-1; IL-2, interleukin-2; IL-3, interleukin-3; IL-4, interleukin-4; MAC, macrophage; PAF, platelet-activating factor; PC, plasma cell; Poly, polymorphonuclear leukocyte; T, T-cell; TNF-α, tumor necrosis factor-α; TNF-β, tumor necrosis factor-β.

altered risk is unknown. Susceptibility to hypersensitivity pneumonitis might also reflect the immune response mounted by the host. Immune responses are tightly modulated by helper and suppressor influences, and the immune system is under genetic control.

HUMIDIFIER-ASSOCIATED DISEASES

Air in both the workplace and home is frequently conditioned thermally and for moisture content in order to optimize industrial processes or to promote comfort. Adverse effects on health may result inadvertently. Respiratory infections are a well-known consequence of problems with air conditioning systems. Humidifier lung and humidifier fever are also caused by inhalation of air contaminated by these systems. In this instance, lung injury is not caused by infection but by pulmonary inflammation resulting from immune responses to the inhalation of antigenic material. The relevant antigens, typically baffle plate slime, may be found in those parts of contaminated air-processing machines designed to alter the attributes of indoor air by heating, cooling, humidification, or dehumidification. Such air-processing units usually introduce water into a moving current of air, eliminate large water droplets by a system of baffle plates, and often recirculate unused water. The baffle plates and/or water reservoir can become contaminated with a multitude of microorganisms, including bacteria, protozoa (Friend et al.

1977), thermophilic actinomycetes, and fungi. The units linked to humidifier lung and humidifier fever include air conditioners (Banaszak, Thiede, and Fink 1970), humidified heating units (Fink et al. 1976), cool mist vaporizers (Hodges, Fink, and Schlueter 1974), humidifiers (Tourville et al. 1972; Miller et al. 1976; Burke et al. 1977), and evaporative air coolers (Metzger et al. 1976). Most episodes of illness occur when subjects are exposed to conditioned air. However, humidifier-associated lung disease occasionally occurs when natural conditions permit growth of organisms, aerosolization, and subsequent inhalation of antigenic material. For example, sauna lung results from inhalation of aerosolized fungi that grow on the handles of ladles used to store water (Jacobs et al. 1986).

Despite the diverse environments that allow growth of microorganisms and facilitate inhalation, the terms *humidifier lung* and *humidifier fever* are firmly entrenched and will be used in this discussion, although many devices other than humidifiers may be responsible for these syndromes. Inhalational exposure to contaminated ventilation units causes these two closely related clinical syndromes (Table 13.2). The predominant form of disease which results from exposure to contaminated ventilation units seems to differ in North America and Europe, as reflected by the use of the term *humidifier lung* in North America and of *humidifier fever* in Europe. In North America, *humidifier lung* refers to hypersensitivity pneumonitis that is usually caused by inhalation of thermophilic actinomycetes. In Europe, *humidifier fever* has some similarity to hypersensitivity pneumonitis, but is clearly a different clinical entity. It is caused by inhalation of water contaminated by a wide variety of microorganisms including ameba, Gram-negative bacteria, and thermophilic actinomycetes. Endotoxin, a large molecular weight lipopoly-saccharide constituent of the cell wall of most bacteria, may also be important in causing humidifier fever.

These different manifestations of illness caused by inhalation of apparently similar material on either side of the Atlantic might be caused by differing flora and

Table 13.2   Comparison of Humidifier Lung and Humidifier Fever

|  | Humidifier Lung | Humidifier Fever |
|---|---|---|
| Symptoms | F, D, M, M[a] | F, D, M, M[a] |
| Latency period | 4–12 h | 4–12 h |
| Monday illness[b] | Yes | No |
| Hypoxemia | Yes | Yes |
| Lung volumes | Decreased | ?Decreased |
| Diffusing capacity | Decreased | ?Decreased |
| Responsible material | Thermophilic ac-tinomycetes | Bacteria, ameba, fungi, ?endotoxin |
| Chest roentgenogram | Often abnormal | Normal |
| Geographic predominance | North America | Europe |

[a]F, D, M, M = fever and chills, dyspnea, myalgias, malaise.
[b]Symptoms are prominent following the first exposure after a period of nonexposure (Monday morning after a weekend or vacation). Symptoms become less prominent during the remainder of the work week despite continued exposure ("tolerance").

fauna within the humidifiers or by differing perceptions of humidifier-induced disease by physicians. In fact, humidifier fever has been described in the North American literature but designated as *humidifier lung* (Ganier et al. 1980). Conversely, humidifier lung has also been described in Europe (Van Assendelft et al. 1979).

The North American and European forms of humidifier-induced disease are similar in several respects. Both are more common in nonsmokers than smokers (Parrott and Blyth 1980; Hodgson et al. 1987); serum antibodies against relevant antigens are often present in exposed asymptomatic subjects (Banaszak, Thiede, and Fink 1970; Fink et al. 1976; Pickering et al. 1976; Friend et al. 1977; Medical Research Council 1977; Reed et al. 1983); and the disease is not related to the presence of IgE mediated "allergic" diseases (Banaszak, Thiede, and Fink 1970). There is some evidence that both forms of humidifier-induced disease may occur after the same exposure (Solley and Hyatt 1980).

*Humidifier Lung*   The North American form (humidifier lung), an example of hypersensitivity pneumonitis, is characterized by fever, chills, myalgias, cough, dyspnea, leukocytosis, arterial hypoxemia, reduction of lung volumes, and of diffusing capacity, and roentgenologic changes four to twelve hours after exposure. Symptoms are not exaggerated after a period of not being exposed. Prolonged exposure can cause chronic pulmonary roentgenologic and physiologic changes similar to other types of hypersensitivity pneumonitis (Banaszak, Thiede, and Fink 1970; Fink et al. 1971; Tourville et al. 1972; Burke et al. 1977; Arnow et al. 1978). Most patients have serum antibodies to thermophilic microorganisms (Banaszak, Thiede, and Fink 1970; Fink et al. 1971, 1976; Tourville et al. 1972; Burke et al. 1977), but antibodies to other microorganisms such as fungi (*Penicillium, Cephalosporium, Pullularia, Hormodendrum, Aspergillus*) and bacteria (*Cytophagia*) may be present (Hodges, Fink, and Schlueter 1974; Metzger et al. 1976; Solley and Hyatt 1980; Patterson et al. 1981; Flaherty et al. 1984; Jacobs et al. 1986).

Acute disease is characterized by chest x-ray changes and pulmonary function abnormalities. The chest x-ray may show small nodules located predominantly in the lower lung zones, or diffuse patchy radiodensities, also with a predilection for the lower lobes. Resolution of acute disease is often followed by complete radiologic resolution. Chronic humidifier lung can result in the development of interstitial fibrosis with nodular and streaky densities, often with upper lobe predominance, which may progress to a radiologic picture of end-stage disease. During an acute episode of humidifier lung, lung volumes, diffusing capacity, pulmonary compliance, and arterial $Po_2$ are generally decreased. Chronic disease is usually associated with a "restrictive" pattern, with decreased lung volumes and diffusing capacity. Pulmonary function tests may be completely normal if performed after resolution of acute disease but before the development of chronic interstitial fibrosis.

The prognosis in humidifier lung depends on the extent of permanent pulmonary histologic changes at the time of diagnosis and removal from exposure. If exposure is stopped before there are permanent radiologic or pulmonary function test abnormalities, the prognosis is excellent. However, advanced abnormalities may not completely reverse and can lead to disability and death. Cases of significant pulmonary interstitial fibrosis resulting from humidifier lung have been described (Banaszak, Thiede, and Fink 1970; Fink et al. 1971; Fink et al. 1976). Corticosteroids are often administered, but the efficacy of this therapy is not established.

*Humidifier Fever*    The European form of humidifier-associated diseases (humidifier fever) is characterized by fever, chills, myalgias, arthralgias, headache, malaise, cough, dyspnea, leukocytosis, and arterial hypoxemia beginning four to twelve hours after exposure. Some investigators report decreased lung volumes with normal flow rates (restrictive pattern) and decreased diffusing capacity (Friend et al. 1977; Newman Taylor et al. 1978) whereas others report normal lung volumes and diffusing capacity (Solley and Hyatt 1980; Edwards and Cockcroft 1981). The clinical syndrome remits after twelve to twenty-four hours without specific therapy. Symptoms and signs are exaggerated after an exposure that occurs following a period of nonexposure (such as a vacation or a weekend) but then becomes blunted despite continued exposure (Monday illness). All signs and symptoms of humidifier fever remit after cessation of exposure, and permanent physiologic and roentgenologic changes do not occur. Serum antibodies to thermophilic organisms are rarely present, but antibodies are often present to extracts of humidifier water or slime, Gram-negative and -positive bacteria, fungi, or ameba (Edwards, Griffiths, and Mullins 1976; Pickering et al. 1976; Newman Taylor et al. 1978; Parrott and Blyth 1980; Cockcroft et al. 1981; Edwards and Cockcroft 1981).

Some cases of humidifier fever may be caused by endotoxin; many of the symptoms of humidifier fever can be reproduced by exposure to endotoxin. Rylander and Haglind (1984) described a printing factory in which twenty of fifty workers developed symptoms of humidifier fever. The humidifier water was heavily contaminated with *Pseudomonas* and endotoxin, and airborne endotoxin was detected in the factory atmosphere when the humidifier was operating. However, other investigations of the etiology of humidifier fever, using pyrogen assay, have not detected endotoxin in humidifier water (Edwards and Cockcroft 1981), so that the role of endotoxin in humidifier fever is uncertain.

Treatment requires elimination of contaminated humidifier water by frequent cleaning of the humidifiers or by removing affected workers from exposure. Permanent cleaning of the humidifier may be difficult; any cleansing agent added to the water must be removed before the humidifier can be put back in use, to avoid worker exposure to the cleansing agent. Prognosis in humidifier fever after removal from exposure seems to be excellent, as there are no permanent physiologic or roentgenologic changes.

## SUMMARY

Indoor air may be contaminated by diverse organic and inorganic antigenic materials that can produce or exacerbate respiratory disease through immune mechanisms. Some of the disorders such as hay fever and asthma are common whereas others such as humidifier lung and humidifier fever are uncommon. Increasingly sensitive and specific methods to measure biologic antigens in the indoor environment are providing data on human exposures and on levels of exposure associated with disease. However, substantially more information is needed before exposure guidelines can be set to prevent the diseases caused by the myriad biologic agents. The control of humidity in indoor environments and proper maintenance of humidifying equipment are both important preventive strategies. Clinicians must consider the role of biologic agents in the indoor environment as causes of diverse respiratory and nonrespiratory diseases.

## REFERENCES

Agarwal, M. K., et al. 1981. An immunochemical method to measure atmospheric allergens. *J. Allergy Clin. Immunol.* 68:194–200.

Arnow, P. M., et al. 1978. Early detection of hypersensitivity pneumonitis in office workers. *Am. J. Med.* 64:236–41.

Banaszak, E.; Thiede, W.; and Fink, J. 1970. Hypersensitivity pneumonitis due to contamination of an air conditioner. *N. Engl. J. Med.* 283:271–76.

Bartholomé, K., et al. 1985. Where does cat allergen 1 come from? *J. Allergy Clin. Immunol.* 76:503–6.

Beck, H. I., and Bjerring, P. 1987. House dust mites and human dander. *Allergy* 42:471–72.

Bellanti, J. A. 1985. Immunologically mediated diseases. In *Immunology III*. Ed. J. A. Bellanti, 346–408. Philadelphia: W. B. Saunders.

Bernton, H. S., and Brown, H. 1964. Insect allergy: Preliminary studies of the cockroach. *J. Allergy* 35:506–13.

Binnie, P. W. H. 1987. Airborne microbial flora in Florida homes. In *Indoor air: Proceedings of the fourth international conference on indoor air quality and climate*. Ed. B. Seifert et al., Vol. 1, 660–64. Berlin: Institute for Water, Soil and Air Hygiene.

Bischoff, E. 1987. Sources of pollution of indoor air by mite allergen containing house dust. In *Indoor air: Proceedings of the fourth international conference on indoor air quality and climate*. Ed. B. Seifert et al., Vol. 2, 742–46. Berlin: Institute for Water, Soil, and Air Hygiene.

Burge, H. A. 1985. Fungus allergens. *Clin. Rev. Allergy* 3:319–29.

Burke, G. W., et al. 1977. Allergic alveolitis caused by home humidifiers. *JAMA* 238:2705–8.

Carswell, F., et al. 1983. The dose of house dust mite antigen ($P_1$) inhaled by infants aged one month. *Ann. Allergy* 51:539–42.

Cockcroft, A., et al. 1981. An investigation of operating theatre staff exposed to humidifier fever antigens. *Br. J. Ind. Med.* 38:144–51.

Edwards, J., and Cockcroft, A. 1981. Inhalation challenge in humidifier fever. *Clin. Allergy* 11:227–35.

Edwards, J.; Griffiths, A.; and Mullins, J. 1976. Protozoa as sources of antigen in "humidifier fever." *Nature* 264:438–39.

Fink, J. N. 1983. Hypersensitivity pneumonitis. In *Allergy principles and practice*. Ed. E. Middleton, C. E. Reed, and E. F. Ellis, 1085–1100. St. Louis: C. V. Mosby.

Fink, J. N., et al. 1971. Interstitial pneumonitis due to hypersensitivity to an organism contaminating a heating system. *Ann. Int. Med.* 74:80–83.

Fink, J. N., et al. 1972. Clinical survey of pigeon breeders. *Chest* 62:277–81.

Fink, J. N., et al. 1976. Interstitial lung disease due to contamination of forced air systems. *Ann. Int. Med.* 84:406–13.

Flaherty, D., et al. 1984. A *Cytophaga* species endotoxin as a putative agent of occupation related lung disease. *Infect. Immun.* 43:213–16.

Ford, A., et al. 1985. A collaborative study on the first international standard of *Dermatophagoides pteronyssinus* (house dust mite) extract. *J. Allergy Clin. Immunol.* 75:676–86.

Fredricks, W., and Tebo, T. 1980. The antigens of pigeon breeder's disease. *Int. Arch. Allergy Appl. Immunol.* 61:65–74.

Friend, J., et al. 1977. Extrinsic allergic alveolitis and contaminated cooling water in a factory machine. *Lancet* 1:297–300.

Ganier, M., et al. 1980. Humidifier lung: An outbreak in office workers. *Chest* 77:183–87.

Gell, P. G. H., and Coombs, R. R. A. 1964. *Clinical aspects of immunology*. Philadelphia: F. A. Davis.

Gergen, P. J.; Turkeltaub, P. C.; and Kovar, M. G. 1987. The prevalence of allergic skin test reactivity to eight common aeroallergens in the U.S. population: Results from the second national health and nutrition examination survey. *J. Allergy Clin. Immunol.* 80:669–79.

Gravesen, S. 1978. Identification and prevalence of culturable mesophilic microfungi in house dust from 100 Danish homes. *Allergy* 33:268–72.

Hodges, G.; Fink, J.; and Schlueter, D. 1974. Hypersensitivity pneumonitis caused by a contaminated cool-mist vaporizer. *Ann. Int. Med.* 80:501–4.

Hodgson, M. J., et al. 1987. An outbreak of recurrent acute and chronic hypersensitivity pneumonitis in office workers. *Am. J. Epidemiol.* 125:631–38.

Huis, J., and Berrens, L. 1976. Inactivation of hemolytic complement in human serum by an acylated polysaccharide from a gram-positive rod: Possible significance in pigeon-breeder's disease. *Infect. Immun.* 13:1619–25.

Hulett, A. C., and Dockhorn, R. J. 1979. House dust, mite (*D. farinae*), and cockroach allergy in a midwestern population. *Ann. Allergy* 42:160–65.

Jacobs, R. L., et al. 1986. Hypersensitivity pneumonitis caused by *Cladosporium* in an enclosed hot tub area. *Ann. Int. Med.* 105:204–6.

Kang, B., and Sulit, N. 1978. A comparative study of prevalence of skin hypersensitivity to cockroach and house dust antigens. *Ann. Allergy* 41:333–36.

Kang, B., et al. 1979. Cockroach cause of allergic asthma: Its specificity and immunologic profile. *J. Allergy Clin. Immunol.* 63:80–86.

Kjellman, B., and Pettersson, R. 1983. The problem of furred pets in childhood atopic disease. *Allergy* 38:65–73.

Korsgaard, J. 1982. Preventive measures in house-dust allergy. *Am. Rev. Respir. Dis.* 125:80–84.

Korsgaard, J. 1983a. House-dust mites and absolute indoor humidity. *Allergy* 38:85–92.

Korsgaard, J. 1983b. Mite asthma and residency: A case-control study on the impact of exposure to house-dust mites in dwellings. *Am. Rev. Respir. Dis.* 128:231–35.

Lind, P., et al. 1987. The prevalence of indoor allergens in the Baltimore area: House dust-mite and animal-dander antigens measured by immunochemical techniques. *J. Allergy Clin. Immunol.* 80:541–47.

Lowenstein, H.; Lind, P.; and Weeke, B. 1985. Identification and clinical significance of allergenic molecules of cat origin: Part of the DAS 76 study. *Allergy* 40:430–41.

Lowenstein, H., et al. 1986. Indoor allergens. *J. Allergy Clin. Immunol.* 78:1035–39.

Marsh, D. G., et al. 1987. Allergen nomenclature. *J. Allergy Clin. Immunol.* 80:639–45.

Mathison, D. A.; Stevenson, D. D.; and Simon, R. A. 1982. Asthma and the home environment. *Ann. Int. Med.* 97:128–30.

McCormick, D., et al. 1982. The antigens of pigeon breeder's disease, VII: Isoelectric focusing studies on unfractioned pigeon dropping extract. *J. Immunol.* 129:1493–98.

Medical Research Council. 1977. Humidifier fever: Report of a symposium held 14 and 15 of December 1976 at the MRC Pneumoconiosis Unit, Cardiff. *Thorax* 32:653–63.

Metzger, W., et al. 1976. Sauna-takers disease: Hypersensitivity pneumonitis due to contaminated water in a home sauna. *JAMA* 236:2209–11.

Miller, M., et al. 1976. Chronic hypersensitivity lung disease with recurrent episodes of hypersensitivity pneumonitis due to contaminated central humidifier. *Clin. Allergy* 6:451–62.

Murray, A. B., and Ferguson, A. C. 1983. Dust-free bedrooms in the treatment of asthmatic children with house-dust mite allergy: A controlled trial. *Pediatrics* 71:418–22.

Newman Taylor, A., et al. 1978. Respiratory allergy to a factory humidifier contaminant presenting as pyrexia of undetermined origin. *Br. Med. J.* 2:94–95.

Nicolet, J., and Bannerman, E. 1975. Extracellular enzymes of *Micropolyspora faeni* found in moldy hay. *Infect. Immun.* 12:7–12.

Ohman, J. L.; Lowell, F. C.; and Bloch, K. J. 1974. Allergens of mammalian origin, III: Properties of a major feline allergen. *J. Immunol.* 113:1668–77.

Parrott, W., and Blyth, W. 1980. Another causal factor in the production of humidifier fever. *J. Soc. Occup. Med.* 30:63–68.

Patterson, R., et al. 1981. Hypersensitivity lung disease presumptively due to *Cephalosporium* in homes contaminated by sewage flooding or by humidifier water. *J. Allergy Clin. Immunol.* 68:128–32.

Pepys, J. 1969. Hypersensitivity diseases of the lung due to fungi and organic dusts. *Monogr. Allergy* 4:1–145.

Pickering, C. A. C., et al. 1976. Investigation of a respiratory disease associated with an air-conditioning system. *Clin. Allergy* 6:109–18.

Platts-Mills, T. A. E. 1988. The importance of indoor allergens in the treatment of asthma. In *The American Academy of Allergy and Immunology postgraduate course syllabus, forty-fourth annual meeting,* 158–75. Milwaukee: The American Academy of Allergy and Immunology.

Platts-Mills, T. A. E., and Chapman, M. D. 1987. Dust mites: Immunology, allergic disease, and environmental control. *J. Allergy Clin. Immunol.* 80:755–75.

Platts-Mills, T. A. E., et al. 1982. Reduction of bronchial hyperreactivity during prolonged allergen avoidance. *Lancet* 2:675–78.

Platts-Mills, T. A. E., et al. 1986. Cross-reacting and species-specific determinants on a major allergen from *Dermatophagoides pteronyssinus* and *D. farinae:* Development of a radioimmunoassay for antigen $P_1$ equivalent in house dust and dust mite extracts. *J. Allergy Clin. Immunol.* 78:398–407.

Ramasamy, M.; Khan, Z.; and Kurup, V. 1987. A partially purified antigen from *Faeni rectivirgula* in the diagnosis of farmer's lung disease. *Microbios* 49:171–82.

Reed, C. E. 1985. What we do and do not know about mold allergy and asthma. *J. Allergy Clin. Immunol.* 76:773–75.

Reed, C. E., and Townley, R. G. 1983. Asthma: Classification and pathogenesis. In *Allergy: Principles and practice.* Ed. E. Middleton, Jr., C. E. Reed, and E. F. Ellis, 811–31. St. Louis: C. V. Mosby.

Reed. C. E., et al. 1983. Measurement of IgG antibody and airborne antigen to control an industrial outbreak of hypersensitivity pneumonitis. *J. Occup. Med.* 25:207–10.

Richman, P. G., et al. 1984. The important sources of German cockroach allergens as determined by RAST analyses. *J. Allergy Clin. Immunol.* 73:590–95.

Rylander, R., and Haglind, P. 1984. Airborne endotoxins and humidifier disease. *Clin. Allergy* 14:109–12.

Salvaggio, J. E. 1987. Hypersensitivity pneumonitis. *J. Allergy Clin. Immunol.* 79:558–71.

Salvaggio, J., and Aukrust, L. 1981. Mold-induced asthma. *J. Allergy Clin. Immunol.* 68:327–46.

Schwartz, B., and Lind, P. 1984. Immunochemical method for investigations of allergic patients' environment: Results of elimination treatment of the allergen source. *J. Allergy Clin. Immunol.* 73:156.

Smith, J. M. 1983. Epidemiology and natural history of asthma, allergic rhinitis, and atopic dermatitis (eczema). In *Allergy: Principles and practice.* Ed. E. Middleton, Jr., C. E. Reed, and E. F. Ellis, 771–803. St. Louis: C. V. Mosby.

Solley, G., and Hyatt, R. 1980. Hypersensitivity pneumonitis induced by *Penicillium* species. *J. Allergy Clin. Immunol.* 65:65–70.

Solomon, W. R., and Matthews, K. P. 1983. Aerobiology and inhalant allergens. In *Allergy: Principles and practice.* Ed. E. Middleton, Jr., C. E. Reed, and E. F. Ellis, 1143–1202. St. Louis: C. V. Mosby.

Steinberg, D. R., et al. 1987. Cockroach sensitization in laboratory workers. *J. Allergy Clin. Immunol.* 80:586–90.

Stricker, W. E., et al. 1986. Immunologic response to aerosols of affinity purified antigen in hypersensitivity pneumonitis. *J. Allergy Clin. Immunol.* 78:411–16.

Swanson, M. C.; Agarwal, M. K.; and Reed, C. E. 1985. An immunochemical approach to indoor aeroallergen quantitation with a new volumetric air sampler: Studies with mite, roach, cat, mouse, and guinea pig antigens. *J. Allergy Clin. Immunol.* 76:724–29.

Taylor, A. N.; Longbottom, J. L.; and Pepys, J. 1977. Respiratory allergy to urine proteins of rats and mice. *Lancet* 2:847–49.

Tourville, D., et al. 1972. Hypersensitivity pneumonitis due to contamination of home humidifier. *J. Allergy Clin. Immunol.* 49:245–51.

Tovey, E. R.; Chapman, M. D.; and Platts-Mills, T. A. E. 1981. Mite faeces are a major source of house dust allergens. *Nature* 289:592–93.

Tovey, E. R., et al. 1981. The distribution of dust mite allergen in the houses of patients with asthma. *Am. Rev. Respir. Dis.* 124:630–35.

Twarog, F. J., et al. 1977. Immediate hypersensitivity to cockroach: Isolation and purification of the major antigens. *J. Allergy Clin. Immunol.* 59:154–60.

Van Assendelft, A., et al. 1979. Humidifier associated extrinsic allergic alveolitis. *Scand. J. Work Environ. Health* 5:35–41.

van Bronswijk, J. E. M. H. 1987. Towards hygienic standards for the allergenicity of the indoor environment. In *Indoor air: Proceedings of the fourth international conference on indoor air quality and climate.* Ed. B. Seifert et al., Vol. 2, 747–51. Berlin: Institute for Water, Soil, and Air Hygiene.

Van Metre, T. E., et al. 1986. Dose of cat (*Felis domesticus*) allergen 1 (*Fel d* 1) that induces asthma. *J. Allergy Clin. Immunol.* 78:62–75.

Vanto, T., and Koivikko, A. 1983. Dog hypersensitivity in asthmatic children. *Acta Paediatr. Scand.* 72:571–75.

Walshaw, M. J., and Evans, C. C. 1986. Allergen avoidance in house dust mite-sensitive adult asthma. *Q. J. Med.* 58:199–215.

# 14

# BUILDING-RELATED ILLNESSES

Marian C. Marbury, Sc.D.
James E. Woods, Jr., Ph.D.

Since the early 1970s, outbreaks of work-related health complaints have occurred in large numbers in a wide variety of nonindustrial workplaces such as hospitals, schools, and office buildings. In some cases, careful evaluation of the building or the affected population has revealed an agent responsible for the outbreak. In most cases, however, no specific etiologic agent can be identified as its cause.

The investigation described by Turiel and colleagues (Turiel et al. 1983) of an outbreak of health complaints in an office building exemplifies the type of problem occurring in buildings and the difficulty of investigating such problems. This investigation was initiated because of health complaints, primarily eye, nose, and throat irritation, registered by employees in the building. After documentation showed the prevalence of these health complaints to be significantly higher than in a nearby comparison building, the investigators evaluated the outside airflow rates; the indoor air temperature and relative humidity; the microbial burden and particulate mass; the concentrations of formaldehyde and other organics of carbon dioxide, carbon monoxide, and nitrogen dioxide; and the odor perception. Measurements were made with the ventilation system operating in a mode that brought in outside air exclusively and in a recirculation mode that brought in 15 percent outside air and 85 percent inside air. Although concentrations of all contaminants were lower when the ventilation system used outside air exclusively, concentrations of these contaminants were still well below current health standards when the ventilation system was recirculating 85 percent of the air. The investigators concluded that although contaminant concentrations were low, a synergistic effect of the various contaminants could account for the problems experienced by the building occupants.

This outbreak of work-related health complaints and the resulting investigation exemplify the emerging problem of building-related sickness. Although the number of such episodes nationally is not known, there may be hundreds of occurrences annually. Outside experts, either from private firms or from federal, state, or local agencies, are often consulted by management because of persistent health complaints from employees. Through 1985, the National Institute for Occupational Safety and Health alone conducted 356 health hazard evaluations for building-related complaints, and the number of such investigations increases each year (Samet, Marbury, and Spengler 1988). Typically, symptom questionnaires used in the investigations document a high prevalence of nonspecific symptoms that appear to be work related, and industrial hygiene monitoring reveals the presence of a number of contaminants. The contaminants are at such low concentrations, however, that the reported symptoms cannot plausibly be related to them. In some investigations, a walk-through inspection of the building may suggest one or more specific factors as the cause of the problem, and remedial actions may be advised. However, since the efficacy of the recommended changes is rarely evaluated by follow-up, the relationship between the presumed etiologic factors and the outbreak may not be established.

At present, we understand little about building-related health problems. Research has been hampered by the lack of definitions and standardized terminology for describing the health problems, the failure to evaluate outbreaks according to a comprehensive and standardized protocol, and the intrinsic limitation of the cross-sectional epidemiologic approach that has generally been used to evaluate outbreaks. Investigations have been limited mostly to buildings with identified problems, and evaluation of a random sample of buildings has been performed only rarely. In addition, the results of investigations conducted by private firms are usually maintained in confidence to protect management and building operators; this prevents characterization of the nationwide frequency of building-related problems and the types of outbreak which occur.

The lack of standardized nomenclature merits emphasis as a barrier in understanding building-related problems. In the past, diverse health problems in nonindustrial buildings have frequently been grouped together in spite of the heterogeneity of the specific etiologic agents. Outbreaks were frequently labeled as *sick-building syndrome* or *tight-building syndrome* even though a specific etiologic agent had been identified or the affected building was not "tight."

To clarify the terminology, a committee of the National Research Council (NRC) has proposed two distinct categories of illness associated with problem buildings: building-related illness, and sick building syndrome (NRC 1987). Building-related illness comprises illnesses arising from exposure to indoor contaminants that cause a specific clinical syndrome. The most commonly identified forms of building-related illness include nosocomial infections, humidifier fever, and hypersensitivity pneumonitis, all from exposure to bioaerosols (e.g., fungi and bacteria); Legionnaires' disease from exposure to bacteria; and the symptoms and signs characteristic of exposure to chemical or biologic substances such as carbon monoxide, formaldehyde, chlordane, endotoxins, or mycotoxins. The symptoms of building-related illness frequently do not disappear on exit from the building and often affect only a few workers. Successful mitigation of building-related illness requires identification and removal of the source.

In contrast, sick-building syndrome is characterized by an increased prevalence of certain nonspecific symptoms in more than 20 percent of the work force. The most common symptoms are eye irritation, irritation of the mucous membranes of the nose and throat, and lethargy and headache. Relief of these symptoms usually occurs almost immediately on leaving the building. In outbreaks of sick-building syndrome, conventional industrial hygiene monitoring generally does not show individual pollutants to be at unsafe levels. Modification of the ventilation system often eliminates the symptoms of sick-building syndrome.

This dichotomous classification has potential limitations. Building-related illness and sick-building syndrome may occur simultaneously within a building. Furthermore, some cases of building-related illness may have the characteristics of apparent sick-building syndrome. For example, elevated carbon monoxide levels caused an episode of building-related illness in a school when an exhaust fan was accidently reversed and functioned as an intake fan. The fan was situated only a few feet from a boiler stack (Kreiss and Hodgson 1984). Many of the characteristics of sick-building syndrome were present in this episode: a high percentage of teachers and students experienced the symptoms of headache and nausea, but they experienced relief from symptoms soon after leaving the building, and modification of the ventilation system ended the problem. Nonetheless, since the problem could be traced to a specific source and agent, this episode should be classified as a building-related illness.

Outbreaks of building-related illness have been more readily recognized and controlled than outbreaks of sick building syndrome. The frank clinical symptoms usually associated with building-related illness demand the attention of building management and may readily indicate the source of the problem. For example, in one outbreak, cases of allergic alveolitis among office workers led to the identification of contaminated humidifiers as the source of the problem (Banaszak, Thiede, and Fink 1970). Many of the etiologic agents that cause building-related illness and the associated illnesses are described in other chapters of this book and in other published papers (Kreiss and Hodgson 1984; Finnegan and Pickering 1986); this chapter concentrates upon a discussion of sick-building syndrome.

## THE OFFICE BUILDING ENVIRONMENT

We describe the complex environment of the modern office building because most outbreaks of sick building syndrome have occurred in such structures. Most contaminants in ambient air can be brought indoors; for example, improperly placed air intake vents may entrain vehicle exhaust or vented air from nearby exhaust systems and plumbing vents. Cigarette smoking and unvented combustion emissions may add particles and gases to the air in an office. Volatile organic compounds (VOCs), including formaldehyde, may be released from adhesives, tiles, vinyl wall coverings, rugs, office furniture, and wet-process copying machines. Ozone and carbon particulates can be emitted from copying machines, and carbonless copy paper has been shown to cause skin and mucous membrane irritation, although the specific etiologic agent has not been identified (Scansetti 1984). Solvents, cleansers, pesticides, and fibers may also contaminate the air in an office. Microbial contaminants, including fungi and bacteria, may be harbored in niches throughout the building, including heating, ventilating, and air-conditioning (HVAC) systems, carpets, books, floors, and ceiling spaces. Bio-effluents such as butyric acid, an odiferous compound, are contributed by building occupants.

In addition to chemical and biologic contaminants, occupant perceptions of indoor air quality may be affected by other aspects of the environment including temperature, humidity, and lighting. Temperature and humidity are closely related. A building's thermal environment depends on the air temperature and also on the radiant temperature of the surrounding environment, determined by the air velocity and the humidity. Since these other factors vary within a building and as there are individual differences in metabolic rate and clothing styles, satisfying the thermal preferences of more than about 80–90 percent of building occupants can be difficult (NRC 1987). An environment that is too warm creates a perception of stuffiness and inadequate airflow; these environmental conditions can lead to lethargy and fatigue whereas an environment that is too cool can lead to discomfort and inattentiveness. Furthermore, elevated temperatures can lead to increased offgasing of VOCs, and insufficient humidity can cause drying and irritation of the mucous membranes.

Complaints about lighting are common. Satisfaction with artificial lighting depends on both its quantity and quality. The quantity of light is related to the strength of the light source and the distance of the source from the work surface. The quality of light refers to the absence of glare, reflections, and flicker. Inadequate lighting may lead to eyestrain, and glare can cause headaches.

Other aspects of the environment can also alter perceptions of environmental acceptability: the quality and comfort of the furniture, the availability of privacy and adequate personal workspace, the degree of control over the environment and the work pace, and the harmony of relationships among management, supervisors, and the work force (NRC 1987).

## EPIDEMIOLOGY OF SICK-BUILDING SYNDROME

The descriptive epidemiology of the sick building syndrome has not yet been well characterized. The incidence and prevalence of the syndrome are unknown although more than 20 percent of office workers have been estimated to be affected (Woods, Drewry, and Morey 1987a). Most investigations have been directed toward identifying risk factors for the sick-building syndrome. These investigations have often been cross-sectional studies of the occupants of a number of randomly chosen buildings with health information collected by a standardized questionnaire. Another approach has been to investigate the role of specific factors considered to be plausible etiologic agents.

In England, Finnegan, Pickering, and Burge (1984) performed one of the first comprehensive epidemiologic studies of sick-building syndrome. These investigators administered questionnaires to the occupants of nine buildings, only two of which had been selected because of employee complaints. Of these nine buildings, three had natural ventilation, one had mechanical ventilation but no conditioning (humidification) of the air, two had air conditioning with no air recirculation, and three had air conditioning with air recirculation. The prevalences of nasal and mucous membrane irritation, headache, and lethargy were all markedly elevated in occupants of the buildings without natural ventilation (Table 14.1). Eye irritation, tight chest, and dry and itchy skin were also reported in excess by occupants of buildings with air humidification in comparison with occupants of buildings with natural ventilation.

In a subsequent study, these investigators ascertained symptom prevalence and performed extensive environmental measurements in two buildings, one with natural and one with mechanical ventilation (Robertson et al. 1985). Rhinitis, nasal blockage, dry throat, lethargy, and headache were again significantly elevated among occupants of the building with mechanical ventilation. However, temperature, relative humidity, moisture content, air velocity, positive and negative ions, and carbon monoxide, ozone, and formaldehyde concentrations were similar in the two buildings.

These cross-sectional studies have provided comprehensive descriptions of the symptoms that most commonly occur in sick-building syndrome and have documented the potentially widespread nature of sick-building syndrome. The comparability of the environmental measurements in the two intensively studied buildings (Robertson et al. 1985) suggests that differences in symptom prevalence cannot be attributed to easily identified environmental factors, a finding consistent with other investigations. However, although these studies suggest strongly that sick-building syndrome is a problem of the modern, sealed office building with its environment controlled by a HVAC system, the cause or causes of sick-building syndrome remain elusive.

A recent large investigation in the United Kingdom demonstrates that the occurrence of sick-building syndrome is not associated directly with the type of ventilation system. Burge and co-workers (Burge et al. 1987) studied 4,373 office workers in forty-two different office buildings with forty-seven different ventilation systems. These systems included natural ventilation ($n$ = eleven), mechanical ventilation without air conditioning ($n$ = seven), local induction units that carried out heating and cooling locally (n = six), central induction/fan coil units ($n$ = ten), and "all air" variable or constant air volume systems that carried out all heating and cooling centrally ($n$ = ten). Similar to previous studies, symptom prevalence was higher in women than in men and, independently of gender, in clerical and secretarial workers than in managers and professionals. As in the study by Finnegan and

Table 14.1    Prevalence (%) of Symptoms in British Workers in Relationship
to the Air Supply in Their Office Buildings

| | Type of Air Supply | | | |
| Symptom | Natural Ventilation ($n = 259$) | No Humidification or Air Recirculation ($n = 73$) | Humidification, no Air Recirculation ($n = 354$) | Humidification, Air Recirculation ($n = 477$) |
|---|---|---|---|---|
| Nasal | 5.8 | 13.7 | 22.4 | 17.2 |
| Eye | 5.8 | 8.2 | 28.3 | 17.6 |
| Mucous membrane | 8.1 | 17.8 | 37.9 | 32.6 |
| Tight chest | 2.3 | 1.1 | 9.6 | 7.8 |
| Shortness of breath | 1.6 | | 4.3 | 2.9 |
| Wheeze | 3.1 | | 5.1 | 4.4 |
| Headache | 15.7 | 37.0 | 34.7 | 39.5 |
| Nosebleed | 0.5 | | 1.4 | 2.2 |
| Dry skin | 5.7 | 5.5 | 16.2 | 14.9 |
| Rash | 1.9 | 2.7 | 3.1 | 2.9 |
| Itchy skin | 2.9 | 2.7 | 7.4 | 7.2 |
| Lethargy | 13.8 | 45.2 | 49.9 | 52.5 |

*Source*: Adapted from Table II in Finnegan, Pickering, and Burge (1984), with permission.

co-workers (1984), symptom prevalence was highest in buildings with local or centrally supplied induction/fan coil units, which treat air from a room either locally or centrally; intermediate in buildings with all-air variable or constant air volume systems, which treat the air centrally and do not permit local adjustment; and lowest in buildings with natural or mechanical ventilation.

Caution is warranted in interpreting the results of this study. Although Burge and colleagues (1987) reported that their findings are generally consistent with those of Finnegan and Pickering (1986) and Robertson et al. (1985), the symptom prevalences in the report by Burge and colleagues are much higher than in the other studies; for example, in naturally ventilated buildings, the prevalence rates were 40, 50, and 39 percent for blocked nose, headache, and lethargy, respectively. Furthermore, additional analyis showed that the prevalence of symptoms was substantially higher in public sector than in private sector buildings in the study (Hedge et al. 1987). In fact, the prevalence rates of most symptoms in naturally ventilated public sector buildings were comparable to the prevalence rates found in private sector buildings with local or centrally supplied induction/fan coil units. These findings suggest strongly that sick-building syndrome cannot be linked in a simple fashion to the type of ventilation system. In addition, the data demonstrate the need for consideration of potential confounding factors, including gender and job classification, in assessing environmental factors.

The Danish town hall study, a cross-sectional study of more than four thousand workers in fourteen town halls and fourteen affiliated buildings in Copenhagen, represents the largest and most ambitious investigation of sick-building syndrome performed to date (Skov and Valbjørn 1987; Valbjørn and Skov 1987). In addition to the administration of detailed questionnaires concerning work-related symptoms and other factors, the investigators measured environmental factors in one representative office in each of the halls. Preliminary results suggest that a number of work force characteristics are associated with symptom prevalence (Table 14.2) in addition to the "building factor," which appears to represent environmental characteristics (Skov and Valbjørn 1987).

As part of the environmental evaluation in the Danish town hall study, the investigators measured temperature, humidity, air exchange, air velocity, static electricity, airborne particulates, VOCs, formaldehyde, lighting conditions, acoustic conditions, microorganisms, the number of open filled-up shelves, and the amount of fleecy surfaces, including textile floorings, curtains, and seats (Valbjørn and Skov 1987). The investigators calculated a *fleece factor*, the area of all fleecy materials divided by the room volume, and a *shelf factor*, the length of all open shelves and cupboards divided by the room volume. The potentially allergenic part of floor dust, total floor dust weight, the fleece factor, and the shelf factor were found to be associated with both mucosal irritation and headache and fatigue. In addition, the air temperature and the number of workplaces, considered an index of activity, were also associated with headache and fatigue. Although six of the town halls had natural ventilation and eight had varying forms of mechanical ventilation, the type of ventilation system and symptom prevalence were not associated after taking other environmental factors into account.

The investigators hypothesized that the fleece and shelf factors were significantly associated with sick-building syndrome symptoms because both fleecy material and shelves act as sinks for pollutants, which are then released back into the room. This hypothesis is consistent with other Danish data showing a higher prevalence of complaints by occupants of rooms with carpets, which have higher microbial and dust levels, than by occupants of carpetless rooms (Gravesen et al. 1986).

Although the Danish town hall study should provide valuable information on the occurrence and causes of sick-building syndrome, the available reports are too preliminary to allow a complete assessment of either the methods or the data. Although the early results suggest that dust and microbial agents may play an etiologic role, generalization of these results should be cautious. When Harrison and co-workers (1987) studied "clean rooms" in two buildings, that is, rooms with high-efficiency filters, they found that in one room the symptom prevalence was higher than in other parts of the building, whereas in the other room the symptom prevalence was the same as in other parts. In both rooms, however, the levels of particulates, fungi, and bacteria were significantly lower.

These cross-sectional studies have been limited by inadequate characterization of the buildings, including age and size, and the maintenance procedures employed for the HVAC system. Although the type of ventilation system has generally been described, published reports rarely document appropriate assessment of the system's design and operation. For example, the difference in symptom prevalence between occupants of public and private sector buildings with the same type of ventilation in the Hedge study (Hedge et al. 1987) might reflect differences in

Table 14.2   Adjusted[a] Odds Ratios (OR) and 95% Confidence Limits (CL) of the Associations Between Work-Related Symptoms in Office Workers and Personal and Job-Related Characteristics, Danish Town Hall Study (Skov and Valbjørn 1987)

| | Work-Related Symptoms | |
|---|---|---|
| Characteristics | Mucous Membrane Irritation OR (95% CL) | Headache, Fatigue, Malaise OR (95% CL) |
| Female gender | 1.6 (1.3–2.1) | 1.8 (1.5–2.3) |
| History of hay fever | 1.6 (1.2–2.1) | NS[b] |
| History of migraines | NS | 1.8 (1.4–2.2) |
| Smoking ≥10 grams/day | NS | 1.3 (1.1–1.6) |
| Residential air quality problems | NS | 1.6 (1.3–2.2) |
| Job category | | |
|     Principal | 2.5 (1.0–6.1) | 1.1 (0.5–2.1) |
|     Head clerk | 2.5 (1.1–5.8) | 1.2 (0.6–2.3) |
|     Clerk | 3.1 (1.4–7.3) | 1.6 (0.8–3.0) |
|     Social worker | 1.8 (0.7–4.5) | 2.1 (1.0–4.3) |
| Handling carbonless copy paper | 1.3 (1.1–1.6) | 1.4 (1.1–1.7) |
| Photocopying >25 sheets per day | 1.5 (1.2–2.0) | NS |
| VDT work >1 h per day | 1.5 (1.2–2.0) | NS |
| Work not varied | NS | 1.3 (1.1–1.6) |
| Dissatisfied with supervisor | 1.7 (1.4–2.0) | NS |
| Dissatisfied with colleagues | NS | 2.0 (1.6–2.6) |
| Job satisfaction inhibited by work quantity | 1.4 (1.1–1.7) | 1.7 (1.4–2.1) |
| Little influence, high work speed | NS | 1.4 (1.1–1.7) |

[a]Odds ratios adjusted for "building factor."
[b]NS, not significant in the final multivariate analysis.

maintenance or in office crowding. This information is needed to understand the contributions of system design and of system maintenance to the sick-building syndrome.

In another set of investigations, the role of specific agents in causing the sick-building syndrome has been assessed. The suspect agents have included VOCs, "photochemical smog," inadequate concentrations of negative ions, excessive or insufficient relative humidity, and psychological factors, including stress. Although the results of these studies have not been definitive, the findings demonstrate the diversity of agents that may play a role in sick-building syndrome.

VOCs have been considered a potential cause of sick-building syndrome. With new analytical methods, hundreds of VOCs have been found in indoor air (Wallace, Pellizzari, and Gordon 1985). A comprehensive investigation of sick-building syndrome in a San Francisco office building documented the presence of more than forty VOCs, with indoor concentrations sixfold higher than outdoor concentrations (Turiel et al. 1983). Although concentrations of individual VOCs measured in buildings are nearly always substantially below workplace standards, the complex mixtures of VOCs found in indoor air may produce effects that would not be anticipated on the basis of individual concentrations. Further, many of the VOCs have irritant effects and could plausibly contribute to the eye, mucous membrane, and respiratory tract irritation common in sick-building syndrome.

Data from experimental investigations lend support to this hypothesized role of VOCs. Ahlstrom and colleagues (Ahlstrom et al. 1984) exposed healthy volunteers to 0.82 ppm formaldehyde in a chamber. Varying percentages of air from a building in which sick-building syndrome had occurred were added to the chamber. Symptoms of mucous membrane irritation were four times more common when the percentage of air from the office building was increased from 10 to 100 percent.

Molhave and co-workers (1984) exposed sixty-two healthy volunteers, all of whom suffered from sick-building syndrome, to a mixture of twenty-two VOCs commonly found in indoor air. The exposure concentrations of 0, 5, and 25 mg/$m^3$ corresponded to concentrations found in clean air, in air normally present in new houses, and in very contaminated indoor air, respectively. In a double-blind design each subject was exposed to a concentration of 0 mg/$m^3$ and to a concentration of either 5 or 25 mg/$m^3$ mixed VOCs. Subjects rated the air quality unacceptable and reported symptoms of nose and throat irritation and inability to concentrate significantly more often when exposed to VOCs at either 5 or 25 mg/$m^3$. Additionally, the investigators evaluated objectively the participants' responses to different exposure levels using the digit span test, the graphic continuous performance test, and a trigeminal nerve irritation test (Bach, Molhave, and Pedersen 1984). Performance on the digit span test, which measures the ability to concentrate and short-term memory, was impaired at both exposure levels; the results of other tests were normal.

Kjaergaard and colleagues (1987) studied the response of sixty-three healthy volunteers to n-decane at concentrations of 1, 10, 35, or 100 ppm in a controlled double-blind study. This VOC is commonly found in residential and workplace environments although concentrations in office buildings are generally below 10 ppm (Wallace et al. 1987). A dose-response relationship was found between n-decane and irritation of the mucous membranes with the increase beginning at the lowest concentration. Tear film stability was decreased in all exposure groups in comparison with the control.

Field investigations of the relationship of VOCs to sick-building syndrome have not confirmed these experimental studies. VOCs were measured in the Danish town hall study (Valbjørn and Skov 1987). Indoor VOC concentrations were low (mean = 1.56 mg/$m^3$) and not related to symptom prevalence. In another study, Sterling and co-workers (1987) investigated areas with and without complaining workers in an eight-story office building. The two sets of work areas did not differ in the presence of detectable odor, formaldehyde concentrations, temperature, or relative humidity. Although the air changes per hour were lower in the affected as compared with the control areas (0.4 versus 0.1 air exchanges per hour), the concentrations of VOCs were higher on average in the control areas.

These findings do not rule out a causative role for VOCs in some cases of sick-building syndrome, but they suggest that the role of VOCs may be limited. In new buildings, where VOC concentrations tend to be higher, these compounds may produce sick-building syndrome more often. Wallace and co-workers (1987) found that the concentrations of most VOCs were an order of magnitude higher in three newly constructed buildings when compared with seven buildings that were one to thirteen years in age.

Sterling and Sterling (1983) suggested that the action of ultraviolet radiation from fluorescent lights on VOCs may produce a photochemical smog that is responsible for the symptoms found in sick-building syndrome. To test this hypothesis, the investigators studied the occupants of two buildings, one mechanically ventilated and the other naturally ventilated. On the initial survey of symptoms, the investigators documented a higher prevalence of eye irritation, headaches, dizziness, nausea, sleepiness, and poor concentration in workers in the mechanically ventilated building. Subsequently, the employees completed a questionnaire on symptoms and environmental quality twice a week during the ten-week study period.

Without the employees' knowledge, the investigators varied the percentage of fresh air entering the mechanically ventilated building and replaced the lights with standard cool white fluorescent lights. During the period that a greater percentage of fresh air was circulated, the employees reported an improvement in environmental quality, including better air movement, decreased stuffiness, and more comfortable temperatures. Symptoms of eye irritation decreased 6.8 percent when the ventilation was changed, 8 percent when the lighting was changed, and 31.2 percent when both were changed simultaneously. Reporting of other symptoms also decreased although the changes were not statistically significant. Negative perceptions of environmental quality and reports of eye irritation rose to the levels documented at the start of the experiment when the ventilation and lighting were restored to their original state.

A deficiency of negative air ions has also been postulated to cause sick-building syndrome (Hawkins and Morris 1984). Clinical studies have suggested that excess negative ions can improve concentration and reaction times whereas a deficiency of negative ions (or an excess of positive ions) can cause upper respiratory tract and eye irritation, dizziness, and headaches (Hawkins and Barker 1978; Tom et al. 1981). To evaluate this hypothesis, Hawkins (1981) studied 106 workers over a twelve week period in a double-blind study. He found that increasing the negative ion concentration led to an increased feeling of alertness and reduced complaints of headache, nausea, and dizziness. However, a subsequent study by the same investigators, using a similar design, was not confirmatory (Hawkins and Morris 1984).

Studies by other investigators have also failed to find a beneficial effect of excess negative ions. Finnegan and colleagues (1987) studied twenty-six workers in five different rooms in a building in which occupants had a high prevalence of typical complaints of sick-building syndrome. A negative ion generator was placed in each room for twelve weeks. An on/off switch on the generator indicated that the generator was on for the entire twelve weeks whereas in actuality the generator was turned on in three rooms after four weeks and in the other two rooms after six weeks. The study subjects filled out a daily questionnaire on the environment and their symptoms. Symptom rates did not drop when the generator was on. These investigators also measured the positive and negative ion concentrations in two buildings, one with workers affected by sick-building syndrome and one with unaffected workers, and found no differences in concentrations of ions (Robertson et al. 1985).

Low relative humidity, which has been reported to increase the incidence of upper respiratory infections and to cause dryness and irritation of the eyes and mucous membranes (Arundel et al. 1986), could also plausibly cause sick-building syndrome. Prevalence studies of sick-building syndrome have suggested that occupants of buildings with humidification systems have higher symptom prevalence rates than those in buildings with mechanical ventilation without humidification (Hedge et al. 1987). However, several studies that measured the relative humidity in buildings with and without sick-building syndrome did not show any difference in the humidity level between the two groups of buildings (Robertson et al. 1985; Sterling, Moschandreas, and Relwani 1987).

Several investigators have also suggested that high stress levels, precipitated by the inability to control environmental conditions in a sealed building, poor labor-management relationships, or other human factors may contribute to sick-building syndrome (Breysse 1984; Waller, Atkins, and Partners 1984; Morris and Hawkins 1987). For example, Morris and Hawkins (1987) administered questionnaires concerning symptoms and perceptions of the environment to workers in three buildings in which occupants had previously had high complaint rates. Questionnaires were administered daily to occupants in two buildings for a period of two to four weeks and on one occasion only to occupants of the third building. Little correlation was shown between symptoms and reported environmental conditions that might cause those symptoms (e.g., nasal congestion and low humidity). In addition, daily fluctuations in the prevalence of symptoms were not correlated with temperature and humidity. However, in all three buildings, a higher percentage of people with health complaints complained of stress than did people without complaints.

The studies on psychological factors and sick-building syndrome are inherently limited by use of the cross-sectional design. The temporal relationship between the occurrence of stress and the onset of sick-building syndrome must be described but cannot be addressed in a cross-sectional study. A report of psychological stress could plausibly antedate or follow the occurrence of sick-building syndrome. Longitudinal studies will be needed to investigate the relationship between stress and sick-building syndrome.

The available evidence suggests the improbability of a single cause of sick-building syndrome; instead, the symptoms commonly found in sick-building syndrome are most likely to represent a nonspecific response to an array of environmental stimuli, the particular components of which vary from office to office. For example, in one office, nose and throat irritation might be caused by exposure to irritant chemicals such as VOCs whereas in another these same symptoms might be due to low relative humidity. By the same token, a ventilation system alone does not cause sick-building syndrome, but when the ventilation is inadequate, regardless of cause, the concentration of pollutants may exceed threshold levels and so produce symptoms. Future research must be directed toward a more complete characterization of the pollutants and environmental conditions most likely to cause sick-building syndrome if the syndrome is to be prevented.

## THE ROLE OF HEATING, VENTILATION, AND AIR-CONDITIONING SYSTEMS

HVAC systems probably contribute to the onset of sick-building syndrome by allowing a buildup of pollutants when the capacity of the HVAC system is inadequate. Although an understanding of the pollutants or conditions directly responsible for sick-building syndrome is essential to developing strategies for prevention, a thorough analysis of the HVAC system is often the key to mitigating the problem in a particular problem building.

In a recent paper, Woods (1988) summarized the experience of more than thirty investigations of problem buildings. Although these buildings are probably not representative of all office buildings, the types of problems found are illustrative and will be described in some detail. Woods classified HVAC deficiencies as reflecting operational problems, inadequate system design, or both.

Operational problems can occur even though the system was adequately designed at installation. For example, failure to maintain the HVAC system adequately, exceeding the original design load, and changes in the original control strategies may all render the HVAC's functioning inadequate. Inadequate maintenance may result in the removal or inadequate servicing of air filters, dirty makeup air intakes, fouled and contaminated heating and cooling coils, and contaminated supply air ducts.

The characteristics of a building and the patterns of building use often change during the lifetime of a building. Occupant density frequently becomes higher than initially planned; unanticipated thermal loads, such as lighting and computers, may be added; and new sources of contaminants, such as copy machines and printers, may be installed. The interior of the building may be redesigned, with, for example, partitions erected in an open bay or the sizes of private offices altered. Because of such changes, the total system capacity may no longer be sufficient to meet demands, or the total system capacity may remain adequate for the whole building but with a load imbalance in certain areas which causes locally inadequate ventilation.

Deviations from the original control strategies are probably one of the most common problems. As energy costs increased over the last decade, many building managers sought to economize by reducing the amount of ventilation with outdoor air and increasing the amount of air that was recirculated; by reducing the temperature differentials between supply and return air systems; and by reducing airflow rates to occupied spaces. This approach to energy management was encouraged by a standard promulgated by the American Society of Heating, Refrigerating, and Air-Conditioning Engineers (ASHRAE). This standard, originally known as ASHRAE 90-75, suggested that the previous standard, set in 1973, for the minimum acceptable ventilation rate (ASHRAE 62-73, 5 cubic feet per minute (cfm) per person), should now be used for design purposes (NRC 1981). The subsequent decrease in air quality in buildings prompted a revision of the ventilation standard, ASHRAE 62–1981, which specified the required outdoor air ventilation rate for smoking and nonsmoking spaces (20–30 cfm and 10 cfm/per person, respectively) (ASHRAE 1981).

Inadequate design of HVAC systems has been implicated in many investigations of sick-building syndrome. Some systems lack adequate makeup air for ventilation, particularly those designed to use fixed minimum amounts of outdoor air. HVAC systems may also be supplied with contaminated makeup air from an intake located at ground level, where it may entrain soil or vehicle exhaust, or from a roof intake that entrains air that is cross-contaminated with discharges from cooling towers, plumbing vents, and toilet or other exhaust fans. Poor air distribution may also result from inadequate design, particularly in unducted ceiling return systems, variable air volume systems, and distributed heat pump systems. In addition, inadequate design may result in unbalanced exhaust air, particularly if a central exhaust air system is not in place. Airflow imbalances result from short-circuiting of the supply air.

Many of these problems can be identified during a walk-through investigation involving the gathering of complaint information from office managers, affected employees, and facility engineers, and an examination of the HVAC system and the control strategies in use. A smoke pencil, a complete set of mechanical plans and specifications, and the availability of the facility engineer along with direct-reading instruments for measuring temperature, humidity, and $CO_2$ levels are usually essential for the initial assessment. More detailed aspects of HVAC system analysis, system performance simulations, air sampling, and questionnaire assessment should be deferred until a later stage of evaluation, which is frequently not necessary.

## FUTURE DIRECTIONS

In the past five years, the concept of sick-building syndrome as a distinct phenomenon, albeit one with diverse and poorly understood etiologies, has received increasing scientific and lay acceptance. Growing understanding that sick-building syndrome and building-related illness are related but fundamentally different problems has also helped focus scientific effort. We anticipate better understanding of the causes and prevention of sick-building syndrome in the next decade from more refined epidemiologic approaches and the use of multidisciplinary investigative teams. To be more informative, the new epidemiologic studies must assess a sample of buildings, and not only buildings with identified problems. The new studies must incorporate objective measures of health outcomes rather than relying solely on questionnaire assessments of symptoms. High response rates must be achieved to reduce selection bias, and confounding variables must be considered and their effects controlled. Appropriate control populations must be selected.

The use of multidisciplinary teams to investigate outbreaks should also improve our understanding of sick-building syndrome. Typically, the protocol for the evaluation of a building varies with the expertise of the lead investigator. Building engineers focus on the HVAC system; industrial hygienists measure chemical contaminants; ergonomic specialists address lighting, acoustics, and furniture design; architects evaluate workplace design; and physicians are generally concerned with microbial agents. Consequently, understanding of what sick-building syndrome is and what causes it has varied with the investigator. It is clear, however, that sick-building syndrome is multifactorial in nature, and the physical, psychological, and biologic factors must all be considered.

## SUMMARY

Although scientific uncertainties remain, the cost of sick-building syndrome has become increasingly apparent. Sick-building syndrome was initially considered to be a comfort problem that was perhaps less important than the money saved by

Table 14.3   Criteria for Characterization of Healthy Buildings

| | |
|---|---|
| Human responses<br>  Criteria must be met for<br>  building to be characterized<br>  as healthy | No known clinical signs of building-related illness among<br>  any building occupants<br>Frequency of reported sick-building syndrome symptoms<br>  and complaints of discomfort should be below 20 percent |
| System performance<br>  Criteria must be met for<br>  building to be characterized<br>  as healthy | Compliance with environmental criteria<br>Ventilation efficiencies for each space should exceed 80%<br>Energy management strategies should not compromise en-<br>  vironmental acceptability<br>Outdoor air for ventilation should not be contaminated by<br>  exogenous or endogenous sources (e.g., combustion prod-<br>  ucts or cross-contamination for exhaust air)<br>Supply and return air ductwork should not be conducive to<br>  contaminant accumulation<br>Exhaust air systems should be balanced with makeup air<br>  systems to assure acceptable ventilation in all occupied<br>  spaces<br>Systems should be designed for ease of maintenance |
| Service factors<br>  Criteria should be met to<br>  assure continued acceptable<br>  building performance | Records should be established to document occupant com-<br>  plaints and symptoms; structured preventive maintenance<br>  should be instituted to include:<br>• Periodic inspections and routine procedures for all compo-<br>  nents comprising the HVAC system<br>• Scheduled filter changing or cleaning<br>• Scheduled control calibration<br>• Scheduled air and hydronic balancing of systems |

emphasizing energy efficiency. More recently, however, the high dollar costs of sick-building syndrome in terms of employee productivity and morale have been recognized (Woods et al. 1987).

Recognition of the cost of sick-building syndrome has prompted attention to the conditions necessary to keep buildings "healthy," that is, free of problems. Woods (1988) suggested recently that healthy buildings can be characterized in terms of three sets of criteria: human responses, system performance, and service factors (Table 14.3). Although the proposed criteria will undoubtedly undergo refinement and expansion, they nonetheless provide guidance to the individuals responsible for the design, construction, and maintenance of buildings. This new emphasis on the conditions necessary to create an acceptable environment should help to prevent future cases of sick-building syndrome.

## *REFERENCES*

Ahlstrom, R., et al. 1984. Odor interaction between formaldehyde and indoor air of a sick building. In *Proceedings of the third international conference on indoor air quality and climate.* Ed. B. Berglund, T. Lindvall, and J. Sundell, Vol. 3, 349–53. Stockholm: Swedish Council for Building Research.

American Society of Heating, Refrigerating, and Air-Conditioning Engineers, and American National Standards Institute. 1981. *ASHRAE/ANSI standard 62-1981: Ventilation for acceptable indoor air quality.* Atlanta, Ga.: ASHRAE.

Arundel, A. V., et al. 1986. Indirect health effects of relative humidity in indoor environments. *Environ. Health Perspect.* 65:351–61.

Bach, B.; Molhave, L.; and Pedersen, O. F. 1984. Human reactions during controlled exposures to low concentrations of organic gases and vapors known as normal indoor air pollutants: Performance tests. In *Proceedings of the third international conference on indoor air quality and climate.* Ed. B. Berglund, T. Lindvall, and J. Sundell, Vol. 3, 397–402. Stockholm: Swedish Council for Building Research.

Banaszak, E. F.; Thiede, W. H.; and Fink, J. N. 1970. Hypersensitivity pneumonitis due to contamination of an air conditioner. *N. Engl. J. Med.* 283:271–76.

Breysse, P. A. 1984. The Office environment: How dangerous? In *Proceedings of the third international conference on indoor air quality and climate.* Ed. B. Berglund, T. Lindvall, and J. Sundell, Vol. 3, 315–20. Stockholm: Swedish Council for Building Research.

Burge, S., et al. 1987. Sick-building syndrome: A study of 4373 office workers. *Ann. Occup. Hyg.* 31:493–504.

Finnegan, M. J., and Pickering, C. A. C. 1986. Building-related illness. *Clin. Allergy* 6:389–405.

Finnegan, M. J.; Pickering, C. A.; and Burge, P. S. 1984. The sick-building syndrome: Prevalence studies. *Br. Med. J.* 289:1573–75.

Finnegan, M. J., et al. 1987. Effect of negative ion generators in a sick building. *Br. Med. J.* 295:1195–96.

Gravesen, S., et al. 1986. Demonstration of microorganisms and dust in schools and offices. *Allergy* 41:520–25.

Harrison, J., et al. 1987. The sick-building syndrome: Further prevalence studies and investigations of possible causes. In *Proceedings of the fourth international conference on indoor air quality and climate.* Ed. B. Seifert et al., Vol. 2, 487–91. Berlin: Institute for Water, Soil, and Air Hygiene.

Hawkins, L. H. 1981. The influence of air ions, temperature and humidity on subjective well-being and comfort. *J. Environ. Psychol.* 1:279–92.

Hawkins, L. H., and Barker, T. 1978. Air ions and human performance. *Ergonomics* 21:273–78.

Hawkins, L. H., and Morris, L. 1984. Air ions and the sick-building syndrome. In *Proceedings of the third international conference on indoor air quality and climate.* Ed. B. Berglund, T. Lindvall, and J. Sundell, Vol. 3, 197–200. Stockholm: Swedish Council for Building Research.

Hedge, A., et al. 1987. Indoor climate and employee health in offices. In *Proceedings of the fourth international conference on indoor air quality and climate.* Ed. B. Seifert et al., Vol. 2, 492–96. Berlin: Institute for Water, Soil, and Air Hygiene.

Kjaergaard, S.; Molhave, L.; and Pedersen, O. F. 1987. Human reactions to indoor air pollution: *n*-Decane. In *Proceedings of the fourth international conference on indoor air quality and climate.* Ed. B. Seifert et al., Vol. 1, 97–101. Berlin: Institute for Water, Soil, and Air Hygiene.

Kreiss, K., and Hodgson, M. J. 1984. Building-associated epidemics. In *Indoor air quality.* Ed. P. J. Walsh et al., 87–106. Boca Raton, Fla.: CRC Press.

Molhave, L.; Bach, B.; and Pedersen, O. F. 1984. Human reactions during controlled exposures to low concentrations of organic gases and vapors known as normal indoor air pollutants. In *Proceedings of the third international conference on indoor air quality and climate.* Ed. B. Berglund, T. Lindvall, and J. Sundell, Vol. 3, 431–36. Stockholm: Swedish Council for Building Research.

Morris, L., and Hawkins, L. 1987. The role of stress in the sick-building syndrome. In *Proceedings of the fourth international conference on indoor air quality and climate.* Ed. B. Seifert et al., Vol. 2, 566–71. Berlin: Institute for Water, Soil, and Air Hygiene.

National Research Council (committee on indoor pollutants). 1981. *Indoor pollutants.* Washington, D.C.: National Academy Press.

National Research Council (committee on indoor air quality). 1987. *Policies and procedures for control of indoor air quality.* Washington, D.C.: National Academy Press.

Robertson, A. S., et al. 1985. Comparison of health problems related to work and environmental measurements in two office buildings with different ventilation systems. *Br. Med. J.* 291:373–76.

Samet, J. M.; Marbury, M. C.; and Spengler, J. D. 1988. Health effects and sources of indoor air pollution, part 2. *Am. Rev. Respir. Dis.* 137:221–42.

Scansetti, G. 1984. Toxic agents emitted from office machines and materials. In *Ergonomics and health in modern offices.* Ed. E. Grandjean, 1–18. London: Taylor and Francis.

Skov, P., and Valbjørn, O. 1987. The sick-building syndrome in the office environment: The Danish town hall study. In *Proceedings of the fourth international conference on indoor air quality and climate.* Ed. B. Seifert et al., Vol. 2, 439–43. Berlin: Institute for Water, Soil, and Air Hygiene.

Sterling, D. A.; Moschandreas, D. J.; and Relwani, S. M. 1987. Office building investigation. In *Proceedings of the fourth international conference on indoor air quality and climate.* Ed. B. Seifert et al., Vol. 2, 444–48. Berlin: Institute for Water, Soil, and Air Hygiene.

Sterling, E., and Sterling, T. 1983. The impact of different ventilation levels and fluorescent lighting types on building illness: An experimental study. *Can. J. Public Health* 74:385–92.

Tom, G., et al. 1981. The influence of negative air ions on human performance and mood. *Hum. Factors* 23:633–36.

Turiel, I., et al. 1983. The effects of reduced ventilation on indoor air quality in an office building. *Atmos. Environ.* 17:51–64.

Valbjørn, O., and Skov, P. 1987. Influence of indoor climate on the sick-building syndrome prevalence. In *Proceedings of the fourth international conference on indoor air quality and climate.* Ed. B. Seifert et al., Vol. 2, 593–97. Berlin: Institute for Water, Soil, and Air Hygiene.

Wallace, L. A.; Pellizzari, E. D.; and Gordon, S. M. 1985. Organic chemicals in indoor air: A review of human exposure studies and indoor air quality studies. In *Indoor air and human health.* Ed. R. B. Gammage and S. V. Kaye, 361–78. Chelsea, Mich.: Lewis Publishers.

Wallace, L. A., et al. 1987. The influence of personal activities on exposure to volatile organic compounds. In *Proceedings of the fourth international conference on indoor air quality and climate.* Ed. B. Seifert et al., Vol. 1, 117–21. Berlin: Institute for Water, Soil, and Air Hygiene.

Waller, R. A.; Atkins, W. S.; and Partners, U. K. 1984. Case study of a sick building. In *Proceedings of the third international conference on indoor air quality and climate.* Ed. B. Berglund, T. Lindvall, and J. Sundell, Vol. 3, 349–53. Stockholm: Swedish Council for Building Research.

Woods, J. E. 1988. Recent developments for heating, cooling, and ventilating buildings: Trends for assuring healthy buildings. In *Proceedings of the CIB conference "healthy buildings '88."* Stockholm, Sweden.

Woods, J. E.; Drewry, G. M.; and Morey, P. R. 1987a. Office worker perceptions of indoor air quality effects on discomfort and performance. In *Proceedings of the fourth international conference on indoor air quality and climate.* Ed. B. Seifert et al., Vol. 2, 464–68. Berlin: Institute for Water, Soil, and Air Hygiene.

Woods, J. E., et al. 1987b. Relationships between building energy management and indoor air quality: Perceptions of conflict and opportunity in the United States and Europe. In *Proceedings of the third international conference on building energy management,* 49–70. Lausanne, Switzerland: Presses Polytechniques Romandes.

# 15

# RADON

Jonathan M. Samet, M.D., M.S.

Radon (radon-222), an inert gas at usual temperatures, is a naturally occurring decay product of radium-226, the fifth daughter of uranium-238. Both uranium-238 and radium-226 are present in most soils and rocks although the concentrations vary widely (National Council on Radiation Protection and Measurements [NCRP] 1984a). As radon forms from the decay of radium-226, some of the molecules leave the soil or rock and enter the surrounding air or water. As a result, radon is ubiquitous in indoor and outdoor air, and its concentration is increased by the presence of a rich source and by low ventilation of the air in contact with that source.

Radon decays with a half-life of 3.82 days into a series of solid, short-lived radioisotopes that are collectively referred to as *radon daughters*, *radon progeny*, or *radon decay products* (Figure 15.1). Two of the decay products, polonium-218 and polonium-214, emit α-particles, high-energy and high-mass particles consisting of two protons and two neutrons. When these emissions take place within the lung as inhaled radon progeny decay, the cells lining the airways may be damaged, and lung cancer may ultimately result.

The mining of radioactive ores that release radon was the first occupation to be associated with an increased risk of lung cancer. More than one hundred years ago, Harting and Hesse (1879) described autopsy findings in Eastern European miners which documented an occupational hazard of lung cancer. Excess occurrences of lung cancer have subsequently been found in uranium miners in the United States, Czechoslovakia, France, and Canada, and in other underground miners exposed to radon progeny, including Newfoundland fluorspar miners, Swedish and U.S. metal miners, British and French iron miners, and Chinese and British tin miners (National Research Council [NRC] 1988). In recent years, the exposure of animals

323

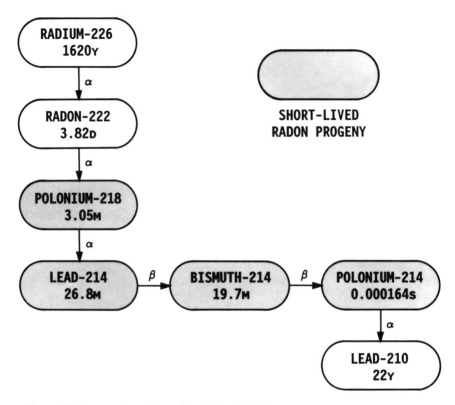

Figure 15.1. Decay pathway from radium-226 to lead-210. y, year; d, day; m, minute; s, second.

to radon and its progeny has confirmed that radon progeny cause lung cancer (Cross 1988; NRC 1988).

As information on air quality in indoor environments accumulated in the late 1970s, it became apparent that radon and its decay products are invariably present in indoor environments and that concentrations may reach unacceptably high levels in some dwellings. The well-documented excess of lung cancer among underground miners exposed to radon progeny raised concern that exposure to radon progeny might also be a cause of lung cancer in smokers and nonsmokers in the general population. During the 1970s, the Scandinavian and other European countries and the United States developed research programs on radon in homes. However, the problem of radon in indoor environments did not receive great attention in the United States until a widely publicized incident in 1984. During routine monitoring, a Pennsylvania nuclear power plant worker was found to be contaminated with radioactivity. This contamination was subsequently traced to a high concentration of radon in his home, which was located on a geologic formation named the Reading Prong. High levels of radon have now been documented in numerous homes on the Reading Prong (Logue and Fox 1985) and in other locations throughout the United States.

This dramatic incident and the subsequent finding of high levels of radon in many homes have resulted in substantial media coverage of radon in the indoor environment and intense public concern about the problem. Several books on radon have been published for the general public (Cohen and Nelson 1987; Lafavore 1987), and the subject has been covered in numerous magazine articles. The Environmental Protection Agency (U.S. EPA), although without direct authority to regulate indoor air quality, has published "action guidelines" for acceptable levels of radon indoors in its pamphlet "A Citizen's Guide to Radon" (U.S. EPA 1986). In September 1988 the EPA and the Centers for Disease Control issued an advisory urging that most houses in the United States be tested for radon. A 1988 amendment to the Toxic Substances Control Act sets a national long-term goal of making the air in buildings "as free of radon as the ambient air outside of buildings."

New research initiatives on radon have been implemented in the United States by the Department of Energy, the EPA, and the National Institutes of Health, by state agencies, and by other governments throughout the world. This research addresses not only biologic aspects of radon exposure, but also geologic aspects, the movement of radon into homes, and control measures. Recent monographs (Cothern and Smith 1987; Nazaroff and Nero 1988) cover these areas comprehensively.

Other isotopes of radon, radon-219 (actinon) and radon-220 (thoron), occur naturally, and their progeny also include $\alpha$-emitters. Radon-219, which has a half-life of only 3.9 seconds, is present in extremely low concentrations and contributes little to human exposure. Because of its short half-life (56 seconds), the concentration of radon-220 is also usually low. Further, the dosimetry of thoron progeny in the respiratory tract implies much lower doses to the target tissues from thoron daughters than from radon daughters. Accordingly, this chapter does not consider either radon-219 or radon-220.

## EXPOSURE TO RADON

For historical reasons, the concentration of radon progeny is generally expressed as working levels (WL), where 1 WL is any combination of radon progeny in 1 liter of air which ultimately releases $1.3 \times 10^5$ MeV of $\alpha$-energy during decay (Holaday et al. 1957). Concentrations of radon are also frequently expressed as picocuries (pCi) per liter; a concentration of 1 pCi/liter translates to about 0.005 WL under usual conditions in a home. Exposure to 1 WL for 170 hours equals one working level month (WLM) of exposure. The WLM was developed to describe exposure sustained by miners during the average number of hours spent underground. Because most persons spend much more than 170 hours in their home each month, a concentration of 1 WL in a residence results in an exposure much greater than 1 WLM on a monthly basis. Thus, if one assumes that 70 percent of one's time is spent at home, a 1-WL concentration (200 pCi/liter at 50 percent equilibrium) would yield an exposure of 3.0 WLM monthly or 36 WLM annually. The approximate average concentration in U.S. homes (1.5 pCi/liter) (Nero 1988), under the same occupancy assumptions, results in an exposure of about 0.02 WLM monthly, about 0.3 WLM annually, and about 20 WLM over a seventy-year lifetime.

These units are now frequently replaced by Système International (SI) units. In SI units, the concentration of radon in air is expressed as Becquerels per cubic meter $(Bq/m^3)$; at radioactive equilibrium between radon and its decay products, 1 WL corresponds to $3.7 \times 10^3 Bq/m^3$. Cumulative exposure in SI units is expressed in Joule-hours per cubic meter $(Jh/m^3)$, and 1 WLM is $3.5 \times 10^{-3} Jh/m^3$.

The predominant source of radon in indoor air is the soil beneath structures, but building materials, water used within the home, and utility natural gas may also contribute (NCRP 1984a; Nero and Nazaroff 1984; Nazaroff, Moed, and Sextro 1988; Nazaroff et al. 1988; Stranden 1988) (Figure 15.2). The concentrations of radium in soil and in rock vary over several orders of magnitude; this variation in source strength, rather than a variation in ventilation rate, underlies most of the variation in radon concentration among dwellings (Nero and Nazaroff 1984; Nazaroff, Moed, and Sextro 1988). The rate of exchange of indoor air with outdoor air, the "tightness" of the home, also determines the indoor radon concentration. However, air exchange rate is a less important determinant of variation of radon concentrations among homes than is the source strength of the soil (Nero and Nazaroff 1984; Nero 1988).

For the most part, building materials make only a small contribution to indoor radon. Certain materials, however, have high concentrations of radium and are strong sources of radon: granites, Swedish concrete made with alum shale, and building materials made with wastes from industrial processes, such as phosphogypsum, phosphate slag, and fly ash (Nero and Nazaroff 1984; Stranden 1988). Drinking water from most sources contributes little to indoor radon, but water from some private wells may add significant amounts of radon to indoor air (Nazaroff et al. 1988).

The movement of radon through building materials and soil is a complex process that involves molecular diffusion, gas flow, and transport via water (Nero and Nazaroff 1984; Nazaroff, Moed, and Sextro 1988). The entry of radon into a building is determined by the structural characteristics and the flow of radon-containing air into the building, as the flow is influenced by wind, temperature, barometric pressure, and soil moisture (see Chapter 3). Portals of entry include cracks and sump holes in basements, crawlspaces, and cracks in concrete slabs. Short-term variation in the concentration of radon within a home results from changes in air exchange rates, varying meteorologic conditions, and the use of water and natural gas.

Radon concentrations have not yet been measured within a large random sample of U.S. homes although surveys have been undertaken in other countries (see

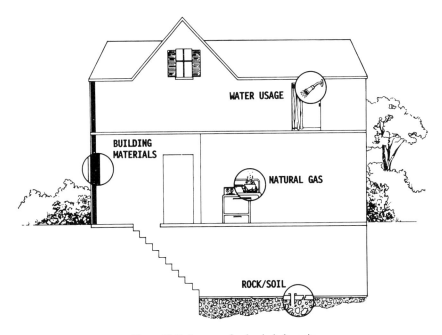

Figure 15.2. Sources of radon in indoor air.

Nazaroff and Nero [1988] for a review of these data). Three nationwide data bases and surveys of states conducted by the EPA provide descriptions of concentrations within U.S. homes. Nero and colleagues (1986) examined thirty-five data sets of radon measurements taken in the United States and identified twenty-two considered to provide unbiased data on concentrations in single-family homes. The data followed a log normal distribution (Figure 15.3). The average concentration was approximately 1.5 pCi/liter; 1–3 percent of the homes exceeded 8 pCi/liter. Based on this analysis, Nero et al. (1986) suggested that more than one million U.S. homes may have annual average radon concentrations exceeding 8 pCi/liter.

Cohen (1986) conducted a survey of radon levels in homes of 453 physics professors from forty-two states. One-year measurements were made with nuclear track detectors. The distribution of the measurements was log normal, with a geometric mean of 1.0 pCi/liter and an arithmetic mean of 1.5 pCi/liter.

Alter and Oswald (1987) reported the results of more than sixty thousand indoor radon measurements made with Track Etch radon detectors. The data are limited because the dwellings do not represent a random sample, and measurement values rather than concentrations within individual residences were reported. The measurements document that most states have homes with concentrations above the action limit of 8 pCi/liter set by the EPA. After the removal of the measurements most likely to introduce bias, the geometric mean concentration was approxi-

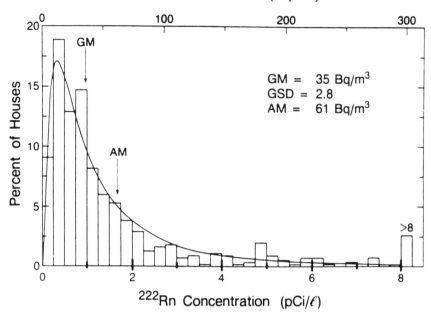

Figure 15.3. Probability distribution of radon in U.S. homes. The distribution represents data from 552 U.S. homes taken from nineteen sets of data. GM, geometric mean; GSD, geometric standard deviation; AM, arithmetic mean. *Source:* Nazaroff W. W. and Nero A. V. Jr., *Radon and Its Decay Products in Indoor Air* (New York: John Wiley and Sons, 1988). Reprinted with permission.

mately 1.5 pCi/liter and the arithmetic mean concentration about 4 pCi/liter. However, as pointed out by Nero et al. (1986), this result may be misleading since approximate adjustment of the average to take account of the sampling protocols yields a result similar to the 1.5 pCi/liter cited above.

Through 1988, the EPA had surveyed homes in seventeen states with the use of charcoal canisters to make short-term measurements. The measurement protocol used by the EPA for screening homes specifies conditions that tend to bias concentrations upward in relation to the annual average concentration (Samet and Nero 1989); the agency's protocol specifies that measurements should be made in the lowest potentially habitable space under closed-house conditions. In the initial survey of ten states, more than one-fifth of the homes tested had levels above the action guideline of 4 pCi/liter. In a September 1988 press conference, the agency reported that nearly one in three homes surveyed in seven additional states had a concentration above the guideline, as assessed with the screening protocol. The EPA projected that more than three million homes in the seventeen states surveyed have screening concentrations above 4 pCi/liter.

Although radon measurements have not yet been made within a nationwide sample of homes, the available data provide important insights into the population's exposure. Most of the collective exposure results from homes with low concentrations, well below the action limit of 4 pCi/liter set by the EPA (Figure 15.3). Thus, the population's total burden of exposure and of radon-related lung cancer reflects primarily the average concentration in all homes rather than in the small proportion of homes with extremely high levels. Such homes, however, place long-term occupants at particularly high risk.

## RESPIRATORY DOSIMETRY OF RADON PROGENY

OVERVIEW

The relationship between exposure to radon decay products, measured as WLM or $Jh/m^3$, and dose to target tissues in the respiratory tract is extremely complex and is dependent on both biologic and nonbiologic factors, including the physical characteristics of the inhaled air, the amount of air inhaled, breathing patterns, and the biologic characteristics of the lung (Table 15.1) (NCRP 1984b; James 1988). The factors influencing the relation between exposure and dose could plausibly differ for the circumstances of exposure in homes and in mines; it cannot be assumed that the same exposures in a home and in a mine lead to the same doses of α-radiation to target cells in the lung and hence to the same lung cancer risk. Thus, if the epidemiologic evidence from studies of miners is to be used to estimate the risk of indoor radon, the comparative dosimetry of radon decay products in the mining and indoor environments must be assessed.

Certain aspects of lung structure and function are important determinants of the dosimetry of radon decay products (Murray 1986; James 1988). Inhaled air flows through the nasal and oral airways to the trachea; at rest, the nasal route predominates, but flow through the oral route increases with exercise. The lung comprises the airways, a dichotomously branching system of tubes, and the alveoli, the saccular structures in which gas exchange takes place. Gas flow is turbulent in

Table 15.1  Physical and Biologic Factors Influencing the Dose to Target Cells in the Respiratory Tract from Radon Exposure

Physical Factors
Fraction of daughters unattached to particles
Aerosol size distribution
Equilibrium of radon with its progeny

Biologic Factors
Tidal volume and respiratory frequency
Partitioning of breathing between the oral and nasal routes
Bronchial morphometry
Mucociliary clearance rate
Mucus thickness
Location of target cells

the larger airways and laminar in the smaller airways; gases move by diffusion in the alveolar spaces. The respiratory system has multiple defense mechanisms for handling inhaled particles such as radon decay products and gases. The nose efficiently removes soluble gases, large particles, and charged particles, such as the unattached fraction of radon decay products. In the lung, particles in the size range of 2–10 μm tend to deposit in the airways and are cleared by the mucociliary apparatus, which moves mucus toward the larynx, where it is coughed or swallowed. Submicron particles also deposit in the airways with increasingly high deposition fractions as the particle diameter decreases.

Most human lung cancers arise at the level of segmental and subsegmental airways, at about the third through the fifth airways generations (Fraser et al. 1989). Relatively few human lung cancers occur peripherally. The airways where most lung cancers develop have a cartilaginous structure and are lined by a pseudostratified ciliated columnar epithelium; that is, the superficial layer includes cells with cilia, which beat in an organized fashion to propel mucus toward the trachea, and the cells appear to be in multiple strata although only one layer is present (Murray 1986). The cellular components of the airways epithelium include the ciliated epithelial cells, mucus-secreting cells, basal reserve cells, and other types. Although the cellular origins of human lung cancer are controversial, all of the principal cell types of the airways epithelium are considered to have the potential to undergo malignant transformation (McDowell and Trump 1983). The relevant target for carcinogenesis by α-particles is assumed to be the entire epithelium and not just the basal cells.

The dose of α-energy delivered to target cells in the lungs cannot be measured directly; modeling approaches are used to simulate the complex sequence of events from inhalation of radon decay products to cellular injury by α-particles. The models incorporate the biologic processes that follow inhalation as well as the physical state of the inhaled radon decay products, also an important determinant of the exposure-dose relationship for radon decay products.

Radon is an inert gas, but its decay products are solid, charged particles. Although most of the decay products attach to aerosols immediately after formation, a variable proportion of the atoms remains unattached and is referred to as the *unattached fraction* (Phillips, Khan, and Leung 1988). The fraction of unattached radon decay products in inhaled air is an important determinant of the dose received by target cells at a particular concentration in inhaled air; as the unattached fraction increases, the dose also increases because of the efficient deposition of the unattached decay products in the larger airways (James 1988). The size distribution of particles in the inhaled air also influences the dose to the airways because particles of different sizes deposit preferentially in different generations of airways (James 1988). The specific mixture of radon decay products also affects the dose to target cells, although to a lesser extent.

The amount of inhaled radon decay products varies directly with the minute ventilation, the total volume of air inhaled each minute. The increased ventilation associated with activity increases the inhaled burden of radon decay products. The deposition of radon decay products within the lung, however, does not vary in a simple fashion with the minute ventilation but varies with the flow rates in each airway generation (James 1988). The dose changes approximately with the square root of the breathing rate. The proportions of oral and of nasal breathing also influence the relationship between exposure and dose (James 1988). A substantial proportion of the unattached radon decay products deposits in the nose with nasal breathing whereas unattached decay products do not deposit in the mouth with oral breathing but rather on the bronchial epithelium, where target cells are located.

Characteristics of the lung also influence the relationship between exposure and dose (Table 15.1). The sizes and branching patterns of the airways affect deposition, and these aspects of airways configuration may differ between children and adults and between males and females. At a given level of exposure, the dose to target cells may be higher for children (International Commission on Radiological Protection [ICRP] 1987; James 1988). Once deposited in the airways, radon decay products are cleared by the mucociliary apparatus. Thus, the rate of mucociliary clearance and the thickness of the mucous layer in the airways also enter into dose calculations. The dose increases as the mucociliary clearance slows and diminishes with increasing thickness of the mucous layer. Cigarette smoking tends to reduce the rate of clearance and to increase the thickness of the mucous layer.

The cells of the airways absorb $\alpha$-energy as $\alpha$-particles released in the decay of polonium-218 and polonium-214 on the epithelium's surface move through the epithelial layer. These particles have a short range in tissue but can penetrate to the basal layer. Cellular doses can be calculated (James 1988).

Computer models have been developed to describe the relationship between exposure to radon decay products and the dose of $\alpha$-radiation to target tissues and to assess the consequences on this relationship of the physical and biologic factors listed in Table 15.1. These complex models generally incorporate biologic factors including airways geometry, mucociliary deposition, particle deposition, ventilation pattern, and location of the target cells, and physical factors including the unattached fraction and the aerosol size distribution (Nuclear Energy Agency 1983; NCRP 1984b; James 1988). Using such models, factors for converting exposure to an absorbed radiation dose can be calculated, but the range of published dose conversion factors is wide (James 1988). As summarized by James (1988), the values span from 0.8 rad/WLM (0.8 mGy/WLM) to about 10 rad/WLM (100 mGy/WLM). For the attached and unattached fractions specifically, the dose conversion factors cover a narrower range. Recent estimates for the attached fraction are about 0.2–1.3 rad/WLM (2–13 mGy/WLM); and for the unattached fraction, from about 10 to 20 rad/WLM (100–200 mGy/WLM). To convert absorbed dose to tissue dose equivalent in units of rem or sieverts in the SI system, the absorbed dose in rads or grays is multiplied by twenty, the quality factor for $\alpha$-radiation.

Dosimetric models have proved useful for evaluation of uncertainties in extrapolating from the mining to the general indoor environment. Using dosimetry models, the $\alpha$-dose to the respiratory tract has been compared under the circumstances of exposure in homes and in mines (James 1988). In comparison with mines, the unattached fraction is higher in homes, and the aerosol size distributions may differ in the two environments. The ventilation rates of working miners are higher on average than those of the general population during usual home activities. In addition, the airways geometry of children differs from that of adults. These comparative analyses indicate that exposures to radon decay products in homes and in mines yield essentially comparable doses of $\alpha$-energy to the respiratory tracts of adults (NCRP 1984b; James 1988); for children, the estimated doses are higher than for adult miners and nonminers because of the morphometric differences between the lungs of children and adults. For adults, the equivalence of the exposure-dose relationship holds in each of the currently prominent dosimetric models (James 1984).

The Committee on the Biological Effects of Ionizing Radiation (BEIR IV) (NRC 1988) used a descriptive approach and also concluded that exposure-dose relationships were similar for exposure in homes and in mines. The committee reviewed the likely range dose conversion factors for particle size, unattached fraction, equilibrium factor, and minute ventilation in homes and in mines. The committee's estimates for the ratios of these factors in homes to mines were 1.4, 1.2, 1, and 0.56, respectively. When considered together, the product of these ratios is near unity. The committee's approach assumed that the remaining biologic determinants of the exposure-dose relationship were comparable in miners and in the general population. A separate analysis was not performed for children.

## RADON AND LUNG CANCER

INTRODUCTION

The causal association of exposure to radon and decay products with lung cancer has been amply documented through epidemiologic investigations of underground miners (NRC 1988). Studies of miners have shown rising lung cancer risk as cumulative exposure to radon decay products increases and have provided some insights into the combined effects of cigarette smoking and exposure to radon decay products. Quantitative exposure-response relationships have been described with the use of data from several of the cohort studies (Lubin 1988; Samet 1989). The range of excess relative risk coefficients, from 0.5 to 3.0/100 WLM, is remarkably narrow in view of the differing assessments of exposure and analytic methods among the investigations. These studies have been less informative concerning the temporal expression of the excess risk and the effect of varying exposure rates.

Animal experiments have also provided data on exposure-response relationships and on the modifying effects of exposure rate and the physical characteristics of the inhaled radon decay products (NRC 1988). Animal models have proved less useful for studying the interaction of radon decay products with cigarette smoking because of the difficulties of replicating smoking patterns of humans with animals.

The lung cancer risk associated with exposure to radon decay products must be considered in the context of the extensive literature on cigarette smoking and lung cancer. This malignancy, uncommon at the start of the century, has become the leading cause of cancer death in the United States (U.S. Department of Health and Human Services [DHHS] 1982). Most lung cancers are caused by cigarette smoking, and only 5–10 percent of the total occurs in lifelong nonsmokers (U.S. DHHS 1982; World Health Organization 1986). In cigarette smokers, the risk of developing lung cancer increases with the number of cigarettes smoked daily and with the number of years smoked (U.S. DHHS 1982; Doll and Peto 1978). The risk of lung cancer for a smoker compared with a nonsmoker is increased approximately tenfold on average but reaches twentyfold or higher in heavier smokers.

Because cigarette smoking predominates as the cause of lung cancer, the risk from exposure to radon decay products must be addressed separately for smokers and for nonsmokers. When one agent (cigarette smoke, for example) modifies the effect of another (radon, for example), interaction is present. Interactions between two agents may be either synergistic or antagonistic; *synergism* refers to an increased effect of the independent exposures when both are present whereas *antagonism* refers to a reduced effect. Synergism is considered to be present if the joint effect of the two exposures exceeds the sum of the independent effects. If the combined effect equals the product of the independent risks, then the interaction is considered to be multiplicative; the interaction is considered additive if the combined effect equals the sum of the independent risks.

If two agents interact in a synergistic fashion, then some cases can be attributed to the two factors acting alone and some to their joint action. The cases having shared causation can in theory be prevented by removing either of the two interacting agents. Estimates of the numbers or proportions of preventable cases may thus exceed the total number of cases or 100 percent. For agents interacting synergistically with cigarette smoking, the cases attributable to the agent are not only those in never smokers, but those in smokers that are caused by the interaction. For radon decay products, which appear to interact synergistically with cigarette smoking, the proportion or number of attributable lung cancer cases exceeds the approximately 10 percent or fifteen thousand cases estimated to occur in never smokers.

Cigarette smoking has well-described effects on both the airways and the lung parenchyma (U.S. DHHS 1984); these effects may plausibly modify the relationship between exposure to radon and dose of $\alpha$-energy to cells. In comparison with that in nonsmokers, the dose in smokers might be increased by the greater central deposition, the increased airways permeability, and the slowed mucociliary transport that have been demonstrated to result from smoking. The dose in smokers might be reduced by mucosal edema and by the increased mucus thickness, on average, secondary to the heightened mucus production in the airways of smokers.

Components of tobacco smoke might also interact with α-particles in the process of carcinogenesis itself. At present, a conclusion cannot be reached through biologically based arguments alone concerning the net consequence of interaction between cigarette smoking and exposure to radon decay products. Thus, the determination of the form of interaction between exposure to radon decay products and cigarette smoking has been based primarily on the epidemiologic studies of underground miners.

Additional insight into the interaction between exposure to radon and cigarette smoking can be gained from those epidemiologic studies of miners which documented both of these exposures; unfortunately, such information is not available for all of the study groups. Small case numbers in some of the studies also limit the statistical precision with which the interaction can be described. Although the smaller investigations have yielded inconsistent results, the largest investigation, that of Colorado Plateau uranium miners, indicates a multiplicative or somewhat submultiplicative interaction (Whittemore and McMillan 1983; Hornung and Meinhardt 1987; NRC 1988). Analyses of data from the New Mexico uranium miners, at present the only other large cohort with smoking information for all cohort members, also indicate a multiplicative interaction (Samet et al. 1989). A multiplicative interaction yields the same level of relative risk in smokers and nonsmokers for a particular exposure, but the higher background risk of the smokers is multiplied by that resulting from radon.

EPIDEMIOLOGIC INVESTIGATIONS

To date, epidemiologic investigations of indoor exposure to radon as a risk factor for lung cancer have been limited by the methodologic difficulties of studying this exposure. Both descriptive and analytical approaches have been used to examine the association between exposure to radon in the home and lung cancer. Techniques for accurately estimating lifetime exposure of individuals to radon in indoor air are not yet available, and surrogates for exposure based on residence type, geology, or limited measurements have of necessity been used in the case-control and cohort studies. The principal published reports are reviewed; Borak and Johnson (1988) summarized the relevant literature, including several unpublished investigations.

In the descriptive studies, incidence or mortality rates for lung cancer within geographic units were correlated with measures of exposure for inhabitants of these units (Table 15.2). In spite of crude exposure measures, most of these studies showed associations between exposure to radon and incidence or mortality from lung cancer. Two studies of counties in the Reading Prong are of particular interest because of the number of homes in this region with high radon concentrations (Fleischer 1986; Archer 1987). Both studies indicated increased mortality from lung cancer in residents of the counties with the highest exposures. However, these descriptive studies, which did not consider the exposures of individuals to radon decay products and other agents, can provide only suggestive evidence that exposure to radon in the home increases the risk of lung cancer.

Table 15.2 Descriptive Studies of Exposure to Radon and Lung Cancer

| Location (Reference) | Outcome Measure | Exposure Measure | Findings |
|---|---|---|---|
| U.S. (Fleischer 1981) | Lung cancer mortality for U.S. counties, 1950–69 | Presence of a phosphate deposit, mine, or processing plant in the county | Significant excess of high lung cancer rates in counties with phosphate mills |
| Iowa, U.S. (Bean et al. 1982) | Lung cancer incidence for municipalities of 1,000–10,000 residents for years 1969–79 | Mean level of radium-226 in the water supply | Significantly increasing cancer incidence for males with exposure; increase not significant for females |
| Sweden (Edling et al. 1982) | Lung cancer mortality rates by county, 1969–78 | Estimated background γ-radiation, assumed to correlate with radon | Significant correlations for lung cancer rates in males and females with exposure |
| Canada (Letourneau et al. 1983) | Lung cancer mortality rates for 18 cities for 1966–79 | Geometric mean WL from a survey of 14,000 homes done 1978–80 | No association of lung cancer mortality rates with radon daughter levels |
| Maine, U.S. (Hess, Weiffenbach, and Norton 1983) | Lung cancer mortality rates by county, 1950–69 | Estimated county average for radon concentration in water | Significant associations in males and females of lung cancer mortality with exposure |
| Central Italy (Forastiere et al. 1985) | Lung cancer mortality rates for 31 towns, 1969–78 | Soil geologic features | Nonsignificant increase for males and females in higher exposure area |
| Guangdong Province, China (Hofmann, Katz, and Zhang 1985) | Lung cancer mortality rates for two areas, 1970–83 | By area: "control" and "high background" | Similar lung cancer mortality rates in the two areas |
| Limousin and Poitou-Charentes, France (Dousset and Jammet 1985) | Lung cancer mortality rates for the two regions, 1968–75 | By area: from geology indoor radon estimated three to four times higher in Limousin region | Similar lung cancer mortality rates in the two regions |
| Reading Prong, U.S. (Fleischer 1986) | Lung cancer mortality rates by county, 1950–69) | By county, based on the proportion within the Reading Prong | For the three counties mostly within the Reading Prong, lung cancer mortality significantly elevated in all three for men and in two for women |
| Reading Prong, U.S. (Archer 1987) | Lung cancer mortality rates by county, 1950–79 | By county, based on geology; three levels of exposure | For both sexes combined, lung cancer mortality follows a gradient consistent with exposure |
| U.S. (Cohen 1988) | Lung cancer mortality rates for 411 U.S. counties, 1950–69 | By county, geometric mean concentration measured in 10 or more homes | For males and females, lung cancer mortality rates were inversely associated with county-average radon levels |

The association of exposure to radon and lung cancer has been more directly tested in case-control and cohort studies (Table 15.3). In the first of these investigations, Axelson, Edling, and Kling (1979) conducted a case-control study in a rural area of Sweden. Those subjects who lived in stone houses were assumed to be most exposed, and those who lived in wooden houses were assumed to be least exposed; other types of dwellings were considered to be a source of intermediate exposure. In spite of this crude exposure classification, the study showed that residence in stone houses was associated with a significantly increased relative risk compared with residency in wooden houses (age- and sex-adjusted relative risk = 5.4). The study did not consider data on cigarette smoking or lifetime residence history.

In several later case-control studies performed in Sweden (Table 15.3), surrogate exposure indexes were validated against measurements of radon with satisfactory agreement (Edling, Kling, and Axelson 1984; Edling, Wingren, and Axelson 1984; Svensson, Eklund, and Pershagen 1987). The findings of these case-control studies were mixed; some showed significantly increased risk associated with exposure whereas others did not. However, this may be due to the small number of cases in several of the studies and the general use of surrogate measures of exposure. Reliance on surrogate measures may introduce misclassification; that is, some subjects may be assigned higher or lower exposures than they actually received. If misclassification occurs randomly in cases and controls alike, the relative risk estimates will be biased toward unity, and an effect of exposure may not be found.

The more recent studies in Sweden have included larger numbers of cases and controls than those reported initially, and some have incorporated measurement of radon for large numbers of dwellings (Axelson et al. 1988; Svensson, Pershagen, and Klominek 1989). Two investigations in Stockholm have shown approximately doubled lung cancer risk for more exposed compared with less exposed subjects (Svensson, Eklund, and Pershagen 1987; Svensson, Pershagen, and Klominek 1989). A study in northern Sweden which assumed exposure from type of residence found no increased risk overall (Damber and Larsson 1987). In a study in southern Sweden, Axelson and colleagues (1988) used measurement data and information on residence type and geology to estimate exposure to radon; association was found in rural but not urban dwellers. This variation in the effect of exposure to radon with residence location could not be readily explained by the investigators.

In the United States, Simpson and Comstock (1983) examined the relationship between the incidence of lung cancer and housing characteristics. During a twelve-year period in Washington County, Maryland, the incidence of lung cancer in the county's residents was not significantly affected by the type of basement construction or building materials. Without specific validation, the dwelling characteristics were assumed to be surrogates for exposure to radon.

In New Jersey, Klotz and colleagues (Klotz, Petix, and Zagraniski 1989) evaluated mortality of 752 persons who had resided in forty-five homes contaminated by radon from radium processing waste. Overall, lung cancer mortality was not elevated. The standardized mortality ratio for white males was increased, but the excess was not statistically significant. In another recent study in New Jersey, radon exposures for the ten to thirty years before diagnosis were estimated for 433 cases and 402 controls drawn from a previously completed study of 994 cases and 995 controls (New Jersey State Department of Health 1989). Overall, the risk of lung cancer tended to increase at higher exposures, but the association of radon with lung cancer was not statistically significant in most analyses. Inexplicably, the risk from radon exposure was less among heavier cigarette smokers.

More recently, a case-control study was conducted in Port Hope, Ontario, where some homes had been constructed with contaminated building materials (Lees, Steele, and Roberts 1987). Exposures were estimated for the period of residence in Port Hope on the basis of earlier measurement data. The analyses indicated an increased risk for subjects with higher exposure, which persisted when cigarette smoking was controlled. However, the number of subjects was small, and the results were not statistically significant.

Many new case-control studies are now in progress throughout the world. Most incorporate measurement of radon concentrations in current and former residences. The sample sizes of most of the investigations are substantially greater than many of the completed studies (Table 15.3). Results of most of the newer studies will not be forthcoming for several years, however.

RISK ASSESSMENTS

Because only scant epidemiologic data on domestic exposure are available, the hazard posed by exposure to radon in indoor air has been addressed primarily with risk assessment procedures (Table 15.4). Information on the population distribution of exposure in dwellings is used in a risk-projection equation or "model" that describes the increment in the occurrence of lung cancer per unit of exposure. For the United States, however, the needed data on the concentrations of radon in homes have not yet been collected from large population samples. The selection of risk coefficients to describe the excess lung cancer risk associated with exposure to radon decay products is also problematic; the studies of miners include only males, much of the exposure of miners was at concentrations higher than generally occur in homes, and none of the miner populations has yet been followed throughout the full lifetime of the subjects. Furthermore, the various factors that affect the dosimetry of radon decay products may differ substantially in homes and in mines (Table 15.1). As discussed previously, analyses based on dosimetric models of the respiratory tract suggest, however, that exposures to radon decay products in homes and in mines have approximately equivalent potency in causing lung cancer.

To accomplish the risk estimation, a mathematical model is used to project the occurrence of cases of lung cancer caused by exposure. These risk projection models require assumptions concerning the temporal pattern of the occurrence of lung cancer after exposure and the effects of such potentially important cofactors as age at exposure, age at risk, and cigarette smoking. The two most widely

Table 15.3  Epidemiologic Studies of Domestic Exposure to Radon and Lung Cancer

| Location (Reference) | Study Design | Subjects | Exposure Measure | Findings |
|---|---|---|---|---|
| Southern Sweden (Axelson, Edling, and Kling 1979) | Case-control | 37 cases and 178 controls | Residence type: wood, "mixed," or stone | $RR^a$ = 1.8 ($p < .05$) for stone and mixed versus wood |
| Oeland, Sweden (Edling, Kling, and Axelson 1984) | Case-control | 23 cases and 202 controls | Residence type and 4 months' measurements | RR = 4.3 (90% $CI^b$ 1.7–10.6) for low versus high by home type; RR = 2.7 (90% CI 1.4–18.5) low versus high by measurement |
| Southern Sweden (Edling, Wingren, and Axelson 1984) | Case-control | 23 cases and 202 controls | Measurement with $\alpha$-sensitive film | RR increased for higher versus lowest exposure categories; multiplicative interaction with smoking |
| Northern Sweden (Pershagen, Damber, and Falk 1984) | Case-control | 15 nonsmoker and 15 smoker case-control pairs | Construction characteristics | Estimated mean exposure significantly higher for smoking cases than controls; exposure not different for nonsmokers |
| Sweden (Pershagen, Damber, and Falk 1984) | Case-control | 11 nonsmoker and 12 smoker case-control pairs | Construction characteristics | Estimated mean exposures comparable for cases and controls regardless of smoking |
| Northern Sweden (Damber and Larsson 1986, 1987) | Case-control | 589 male cases, 582 deceased controls, 453 living controls | Residence type: wood or nonwood | RR not increased, with or without smoking adjustment; RR increased for those never employed in occupations not associated with lung cancer |

| Location (Reference) | Study type | Sample | Exposure assessment | Results |
|---|---|---|---|---|
| Stockholm, Sweden (Svensson, Eklund, and Pershagen 1987) | Case-control | 292 female cases and 584 controls | Geology and living near ground level | RR = 2.2 (95% CI 1.2–4.0) for exposed versus nonexposed; exposure-response relationship not found |
| Southern Sweden (Axelson et al. 1988) | Case-control | 177 cases and 677 controls | Residence type and geology, all homes; 2-month measurement, some homes | Exposure associated with increased risk for rural but not urban dwellers |
| Stockholm, Sweden (Svensson, Pershagen, and Klominek 1989) | Case-control | 210 female cases, and 209 population and 191 hospital | 2-week measurement and assumed values | RR = 1.8 (95% CI 1.2–2.9) comparing high and intermediate with low; RR highest for small-cell cancer |
| Maryland, U.S. (Simpson and Comstock 1983) | Cohort | 298 cases over a 12-year period | Housing characteristics | No associations of incidence rates with housing characteristics |
| New Jersey, U.S. (Klotz, Petix, and Zagraniski 1989) | Cohort | 752 persons who had resided in 45 homes contaminated by radium waste | Residence for at least 1 year in one of the homes | SMR[c] = 1.7 (95% CI 0.8–3.2) for lung cancer in white males; no excess for females |
| New Jersey, U.S. (N.J. State Dept. of Health 1989) | Case-control | 433 female cases and 402 controls | Year-long α-track measurements, some estimates | RR = 1.9 (95% CI 1.0–3.4) comparing ≥2 pCi/liter with lower values |
| Ontario, Canada (Lees, Steele, and Roberts 1987) | Case-control | 27 cases and 49 controls | Reconstructed exposures based on measurements | RR = 2.4 (95% CI 0.8–7.1) with smoking adjustment for exposed versus nonexposed |

[a]RR, relative risk.
[b]CI, confidence interval.
[c]SMR, standardized mortality ratio.

Table 15.4   Recent Risk Projection Models for Radon and Lung Cancer

| Agency | Type of Model | Source of Risk Estimate |
|---|---|---|
| National Council on Radiation Protection and Measurements (NCRP 1984b) | Attributable risk, time dependent | Average risk coefficient from principal studies of miners |
| International Commission on Radiological Protection (ICRP 1987) | Constant relative risk | Adjusted risk coefficient from three studies of miners |
| Environmental Protection Agency (U.S. EPA 1987) | Constant relative risk | Range of coefficients based on studies of miners |
| National Institute for Occupational Safety and Health (NIOSH 1987) | Relative risk, time dependent | Risk based on Colorado Plateau uranium miners |
| National Research Council, Biological Effects of Ionizing Radiation (BEIR) IV Committee (NRC 1988) | Relative risk, time dependent | Risk based on analysis of four studies of miners |
| Environmental Protection Agency (Puskin and Nelson 1989) | Relative risk, time dependent | Combines the ICRP and BEIR IV models |

applied models are the relative risk and attributable risk models; the relative risk model assumes that the background risk is multiplied by the risk from radon decay products whereas the attributable risk model assumes that the excess risk is additive to the background risk. Two models, those of the BEIR IV committee (NRC 1988) and of the (NCRP 1984b), describe the risk as varying with the time since the exposure.

The manner in which exposure to radon decay products and cigarette smoking are assumed to interact strongly influences the results of risk estimation models for radon-associated lung cancer. If a multiplicative interaction is assumed, then the risk for smokers, already much greater than that for nonsmokers, is multiplied by the risk from exposure to radon decay products. If an additive interaction is assumed, then the same excess risk is added to the background rates for smokers and for nonsmokers. The interaction between the two agents might plausibly take some form other than purely additive or purely multiplicative.

Diverse risk projection models have been developed; Table 15.4 describes the most recent and widely used models (see NRC [1988] for a review of earlier models). Each of the recent models estimates lung cancer risk on the basis of the epidemiologic evidence from underground miners, but the biologic assumptions underlying the models and their resulting risk projections differ substantially. Table 15.5 provides additional description of the most prominent risk models: those of the NCRP (1984b), the ICRP (1987), and the BEIR IV committee of the NRC (1988).

The NCRP model generally projects the lowest excess risk because it is an additive model, and the radon-associated excess declines over time (Table 15.6). The ICRP model, a constant relative risk model, projects the highest risks. Exposures received by age twenty years lead to a particularly large excess because of

Table 15.5   Features of Selected Risk Projection Models for Radon and Lung Cancer

| | NCRP | ICRP | BEIR IV |
|---|---|---|---|
| Form of model | Attributable risk | Relative risk | Relative risk |
| Time dependent | Yes; risk declines exponentially after exposure | No | Yes; risk declines as time since exposure lengthens |
| Lag interval | 5 years | 10 years | 5 years |
| Age at exposure | No effect of age at exposure | Three-fold increased risk for exposures before age 20 years | No effect of age at exposure |
| Age at risk | Risk commences at age 40 years | Constant relative risk with age | Lower risks for ages 55 years and older |
| Dosimetry adjustment | Increased risk for indoor exposure | Decreased risk for indoor exposure | No adjustment |
| Risk coefficient | $10 \times 10^{-6}$/year/WLM | Excess relative risks: 1.9%/WLM at ages 0–20 years and 0.64%/WLM for ages 21 years and above | Excess relative risk of 2.5%/WLM but modified by time since exposure |

*Source*: Data from Samet and Hornung (1990).

Table 15.6   Increments in Lung Cancer Risks for One WLM[a], Projected by *NCRP, ICRP,* and *BEIR IV* Models

| Increment at Age (years) | Exposure at Age 15 Years (%) | | | |
|---|---|---|---|---|
| | NCRP[b] | | ICRP | BEIR IV |
| | Male | Female | | |
| 35 | 0 | 0 | 1.9 | 1.5 |
| 50 | 0.3 | 0.7 | 1.9 | 1.5 |
| 65 | 0.05 | 0.2 | 1.9 | 0.5 |
| 85 | 0.02 | 0.1 | 1.9 | 0.5 |
| | Exposure at Age 35 Years (%) | | | |
| 50 | 0.6 | 1.4 | 0.6 | 3.0 |
| 65 | 0.1 | 0.4 | 0.6 | 0.5 |
| 85 | 0.05 | 0.2 | 0.6 | 0.5 |

*Source*: Data from Samet and Hornung (1990).

[a]An annual exposure of 1 WLM would be received in a home with a concentration of 6 pCi/liter, assuming 70 percent occupancy.

[b]The excess is additive for the NCRP model. The percent excess relative risk was calculated for illustration using sex-specific lung cancer mortality rates for the United States, 1980–84. The additive increments are $3.0 \times 10^{-6}$, $1.8 \times 10^{-6}$ and $0.9 \times 10^{-6}$ for ages 50, 65, and 85 years, respectively, for exposure at age 15 years; and $6.0 \times 10^{-6}$, $3.5 \times 10^{-6}$, and $1.8 \times 10^{-6}$, respectively, for exposure at age 35 years.

Table 15.7 Lung Cancer Mortality Rates Per 100,000 Projected for Nonsmoking and Smoking Males at Age 65 Years by *NCRP, ICRP,* and *BEIR IV* Models[a]

|  | NCRP | ICRP | BEIR IV |
|---|---|---|---|
| Exposure to 10 WLM at age 15 years |  |  |  |
| Nonsmoking | 59.8 | 69.0 | 60.9 |
| Smoking | 698.3 | 828.8 | 731.3 |
| Exposure to 10 WLM at age 35 years |  |  |  |
| Nonsmoking | 61.5 | 61.5 | 60.9 |
| Smoking | 700.0 | 738.3 | 731.3 |

*Source*: Data from Samet and Hornung (1990).
[a]Background lung cancer mortality rates estimated as $58.0 \times 10^{-5}$ for nonsmokers and $696.5 \times 10^{-5}$ for smokers (NRC 1988).

the threefold higher risk assumed up to age twenty years than at subsequent ages. In the BEIR IV model, the percent of excess risk varies with both age and time since exposure.

When smokers and nonsmokers are considered separately, the substantial difference between assuming an additive or a multiplicative interaction between smoking and radon exposure is evident (Table 15.7). The additive NCRP model projects small increments for smokers in comparison with the multiplicative ICRP and BEIR IV models. Lifetime excess lung cancer risks for smokers estimated by the three models are markedly different. Land (1988) has calculated the excess lung cancer risk per one hundred thousand smokers exposed to 1 WLM at age fifteen as follows: NCRP, 7.4; ICRP, 278.7; BEIR IV, 114.5; for exposure to 1 WLM at age thirty-five, the corresponding projections are 15.5, 94.3, and 129.4, respectively.

These models have been used to project the lung cancer burden associated with exposure to indoor radon. For exposure at 0.2 WLM/year (approximately equivalent to residence in a home at 1.5 pCi/liter), the approximate average annual exposure, the NCRP model projects lifetime lung cancer risk as 0.18 percent; the NCRP report estimates that nine thousand lung cancer deaths annually in the United States can be attributed to indoor radon. For an annual exposure of about 0.16 WLM, the ICRP model estimates lifetime risk of lung cancer as 0.42 percent for males and as 0.09 percent for females. The BEIR IV report describes risk for exposures received above background; for an exposure rate of 0.20 WLM/year, the model projects attributable lifetime risks of 0.7 percent for males and 0.3 percent for females. Using the BEIR IV model, Lubin and Boice (1989) estimated that approximately 13,300 lung cancer deaths annually can be attributed to indoor radon exposure. Using the current model of the EPA, Puskin and Nelson (1989) calculated that radon exposure in single-family homes may cause twenty thousand lung cancer deaths annually in the United States.

Thus, in spite of the differing underlying assumptions and risk projections, each of the models indicates that radon must be considered as an important cause of lung

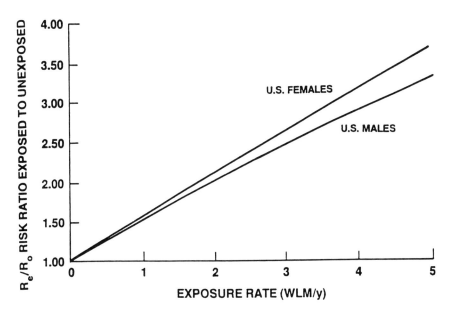

Figure 15.4. Risk ratio ($R_e/R_o$) of lung cancer mortality for lifetime exposure to radon decay products at constant rates of annual exposure, as estimated by the BEIR IV committee model. *Source: Health Risks of Radon and Other Internally Deposited Alpha-Emitters,* ©1988, by the National Academy of Sciences, National Academy Press, Washington, D.C. Reprinted with permission.

cancer for the general population. Each also demonstrates that unacceptable levels of risk are associated with higher levels of exposure. For example, in the BEIR IV model, exposure at 4 WLM/year above background leads to a tripling of the lifetime risk of lung cancer for males and females (Figure 15.4); this level of exposure would be received from residing in a home with a concentration of about 25 pCi/liter. As a basis for policy decisions, these risk projection models can be used to estimate the risks associated with levels of exposure that might be designated as guidelines or standards. The models can also be used to estimate the reduction in lung cancer occurrence which would follow reduction of exposure.

## SUMMARY

Radon and its decay products are invariably present in indoor environments; most homes have concentrations of only a few pCi/liter, but concentrations in some homes are as high as those measured in uranium and other underground mines. Exposure to radon decay products has been shown to increase the mortality from lung cancer of underground miners working in mines with high concentrations. An increased risk of lung cancer must also be presumed to result from domestic exposure although the epidemiologic data are scant and preliminary at present. Risk assessments have been performed to evaluate the magnitude of the problem of lung cancer associated with domestic exposure to radon. The most recent, by the BEIR IV committee, showed a doubling exposure rate of 2.0 WLM/year for males and 1.8 WLM/year for females.

## REFERENCES

Alter, H. W., and Oswald, R. A. 1987. Nationwide distribution of indoor radon measurements: A preliminary data base. *J. Air Pollut. Control Assoc.* 37:227–31.

Archer, V. E. 1987. Association of lung cancer mortality with precambrian granite. *Arch. Environ. Health* 42:87–91.

Axelson, O.; Edling, C.; and Kling, H. 1979. Lung cancer and residency: A case-referent study on the possible impact of exposure to radon and its daughters in dwellings. *Scand. J. Work Environ. Health* 5:10–15.

Axelson, O., et al. 1988. Indoor radon exposure and active and passive smoking in relation to the occurrence of cancer. *Scand. J. Work Environ. Health* 14:286–92.

Bean, J. A., et al. 1982. Drinking water and cancer incidence in Iowa, II: Radioactivity in drinking water. *Am. J. Epidemiol.* 116:924–32.

Borak, T. D., and Johnson, J. A. 1988. Estimating the risk of lung cancer from inhalation of radon daughters indoors: Review and evaluation. Las Vegas, Nev.: EPA Publication no. EPA/600/6-88/008.

Cohen, B. L. 1986. A national survey of $^{222}$Rn in U.S. homes and correlating factors. *Health Phys.* 51:175–83.

Cohen, B. L. 1988. An experimental test of the linear–no threshold theory of radiation carcinogenesis. Presented at the U.S. Environmental Protection Agency 1988 symposium on radon and radon reduction technology, October, Denver, Colo.

Cohen, B. L., and Nelson, D. 1987. Radon, a homeowner's guide to detection and control: A consumer report book. Mount Vernon, N.Y.: Consumers' Union.

Cothern, C. R., and Smith, J. E., Jr., eds. 1987. *Environmental radon.* New York: Plenum.

Cross, F. T. 1988. Evidence of lung cancer from animal studies. In *Radon and its decay products in indoor air.* Ed. W. W. Nazaroff and A. V. Nero, Jr., 373–406. New York: John Wiley & Sons.

Damber, L., and Larsson, L.-G. 1986. Lung cancer in males: An epidemiological study in northern Sweden with special regard to smoking and occupation. Umeå University medical dissertation, Department of Oncology. Umeå, Sweden.

Damber, L. A., and Larsson, L.-G. 1987. Lung cancer in males and type of dwelling: An epidemiologic pilot study. *Acta Oncol.* 26:211–15.

Doll, R., and Peto, R. 1978. Cigarette smoking and bronchial carcinoma: Dose and time relationships among regular smokers and life-long non-smokers. *J. Epidemiol. Community Health* 32:303–13.

Dousset, M., and Jammet, H. 1985. Comparaison de la mortalite par cancer dans la Limousin et le Poitou-Charentes: (Etude preliminaire 1968–1975). *Radioprotection GEDIM* 20:61–67.

Edling, C.; Kling, H.; and Axelson, O. 1984. Radon in homes: A possible cause of lung cancer. *Scand. J. Work Environ. Health* 10:25–34.

Edling, C.; Wingren, G.; and Axelson, O. 1984. Radon daughter exposure in dwellings and lung cancer. In *Indoor air, Vol. 2: Radon, passive smoking, particulates and housing epidemiology.* Ed. B. Berglund, T. Lindvall, and J. Sundell, 29–34. Stockholm: Swedish Council for Building Research.

Edling, C. et al. 1982. Effects of low-dose radiation: A correlation study. *Scand. J. Work Environ. Health* 8(Suppl. 1):59–64.

Fleischer, R. L. 1981. A possible association between lung cancer and phosphate mining and processing. *Health Phys.* 41:171–75.

Fleischer, R. L. 1986. A possible association between lung cancer and a geological outcrop. *Health Phys.* 50:823–27.

Forastiere, F., et al. 1985. Lung cancer and natural radiation in an Italian province. *Sci. Total Environ.* 45:519–26.

Fraser, R. G., et al. 1989. *Diagnosis of diseases of the chest,* Vol. 2, 1367–68. Philadelphia: W. B. Saunders.

Harting, F. H., and Hesse, W. 1879. Der lungenkrebs, die bergkrankheit in den Schneeberger gruben. *Vjschr. Gerichtl. Med. Offentl. Gesundheitswesen* 31:102–32, 313–37.

Hess, C. T.; Weiffenbach, C. V.; and Norton, S. A. 1983. Environmental radon and cancer correlations in Maine. *Health Phys.* 45:339–48.

Hofmann, W.; Katz, R.; and Zhang, C. X. 1985. Lung cancer in a Chinese high background area: Epidemiological results and theoretical interpretation. *Sci. Total Environ.* 45:527–34.

Holaday, D. A., et al. 1957. *Control of radon and daughters in uranium mines and calculations on biologic effects.* Washington, D.C.: Government Printing Office. Public Health Service Publication no. 494.

Hornung, R. W. and Meinhardt, T. J. 1987. Quantitative risk assessment of lung cancer in U.S. uranium miners. *Health Phys.* 52:417–30.

International Commission on Radiological Protection. 1987. *Lung cancer risk from indoor exposures to radon daughters.* Oxford, England: Pergamon Press. ICRP Publication no. 50.

James, A. C. 1984. Dosimetric approaches to risk assessment for indoor exposure to radon daughters. *Radiat. Prot. Dosim.* 7:353–56.

James, A. C. 1988. Lung dosimetry. In *Radon and its decay products in indoor air.* Ed. W. W. Nazaroff and A. V. Nero, Jr., 259–309. New York: John Wiley & Sons.

Klotz, J. B.; Petix, J. R.; and Zagraniski, R. T. 1989. Mortality of a residential cohort exposed to radon from industrially contaminated soil. *Am. J. Epidemiol.* 129:1179–86.

Lafavore, M. 1987. Radon: The invisible threat. Emmaus, Pa.: Rodale Press.

Land, C. E. 1988. The ICRP 50 model. In *Radon: Proceedings of the twenty-fourth annual meeting of the National Council on Radiation Protection and Measurements.* Ed. N. H. Harley, 115–26. Washington, D.C., 30–31 March.

Lees, R. E. M.; Steele, R.; and Roberts, J. H. 1987. A case-control study of lung cancer relative to domestic radon exposure. *Int. J. Epidemiol.* 16:7–12.

Letourneau, E. G., et al. 1983. *Lung cancer mortality and indoor radon concentrations in 18 Canadian cities: Proceedings of the sixteenth midyear topical meeting of the Health Physics Society.* Albuquerque, N.M. National Technical Information Service CONF-830101, distribution category UC-41.

Logue, J., and Fox, J. 1985. Health hazards associated with elevated levels of indoor radon: 1985. Pennsylvania. *MMWR* 34(43):657–58.

Lubin, J. H. 1988. Methods for the analysis of radon-exposed populations. *Yale J. Biol. Med.* 61:195–214.

Lubin, J. H., and Boice, J. D. 1989. Estimating Rn-induced lung cancer in the U.S. *Health Phys.,* 57:417–27.

McDowell, E. M., and Trump, B. F. 1983. Histogenesis of preneoplastic and neoplastic lesions in tracheobronchial epithelium. In *Survey and synthesis of pathology research,* 235–79. Basel: S. Karger.

Murray, J. F. 1986. *The normal lung.* Philadelphia: W. B. Saunders.

National Council on Radiation Protection and Measurements. 1984a. *Exposure from the uranium series with emphasis on radon and its daughters.* Bethesda, Md.: NCRP Report no. 77.

National Council on Radiation Protection and Measurements. 1984b. *Evaluation of occupational and environmental exposure to radon and radon daughters in the United States.* Bethesda, Md.: NCRP Report no. 78.

National Institute for Occupational Safety and Health. 1987. *Radon progeny in underground mines: A recommended standard for occupational exposure.* Washington, D.C.: Government Printing Office. DHHS Publication no. NIOSH/88-101.

National Research Council (committee on the biological effects of ionizing radiation) 1988. *Health risks of radon and other internally deposited alpha-emitters: BEIR IV.* Washington, D.C.: National Academy Press.

Nazaroff, W. W., and Nero, A. V., Jr., eds. 1988. *Radon and its decay products in indoor air.* New York: John Wiley & Sons.

Nazaroff, W. W.; Moed, B. A.; and Sextro, R. G. 1988. Soil as a source of indoor radon: Generation, migration, and entry. In *Radon and its decay products in indoor air.* Ed. W. W. Nazaroff and A. V. Nero, Jr., 57–112. New York: John Wiley & Sons.

Nazaroff, W. W., et al. 1988. Radon entry via potable water. In *Radon and its decay products in indoor air.* Ed. W. W. Nazaroff and A. V. Nero, Jr., 131–57. New York: John Wiley & Sons.

Nero, A. V., Jr. 1988. Radon and its decay products in indoor air: An overview. In *Radon and its decay products in indoor air.* Ed. W. W. Nazaroff and A. V. Nero, Jr., 1–53. New York: John Wiley & Sons.

Nero, A. V., and Nazaroff, W. W. 1984. Characterizing the source of radon indoors. *Radiat. Prot. Dosim.* 7:23–39.

Nero, A. V., et al. 1986. Distribution of airborne radon-222 concentrations in U.S. homes. *Science* 234:992–97.

Nero, A. V.; Revzan, K. L.; and Sextro, R. G. 1987. Appraisal of the *U.S. data on indoor radon concentrations.* Presented at the fourth international symposium of the natural radiation environment, 30–31 December, Lisbon, Berkeley, Calif.: Lawrence Berkeley Laboratories. Report LBL 243-45.

New Jersey State Department of Health. 1989. *A case-control study of radon and lung cancer among New Jersey women:* Technical report, phase 1.

Nuclear Energy Agency (Organization for Economic Cooperation and Development). 1983. *Dosimetry aspects of exposure to radon and thoron daughter products.* Washington, D.C.: OECD.

Pershagen, G.; Damber, L.; and Falk, R. 1984. Exposure to radon in dwellings and lung cancer: A pilot study. In *Indoor air, Vol. 2: Radon, passive smoking, particulates and housing epidemiology.* Ed. B. Berglund, T. Lindvall, and J. Sundell, 73–78. Stockholm: Swedish Council for Building Research.

Phillips, C. R.; Khan, A.; and Leung, H. M. Y. 1988. The nature and determination of the unattached fraction of radon and thoron progeny. In *Radon and its decay products in indoor air.* Ed. W. W. Nazaroff and A. V. Nero, Jr., 203–56. New York: John Wiley & Sons.

Puskin, J. S., and Nelson, C. B. 1989. EPA's perspective on risks from residential radon exposure. *J. Air Pollut. Control Assoc.* 39:915–20.

Samet, J. M. 1989. Radon and lung cancer. *J. Natl. Cancer Inst.* 81:745–57.

Samet, J. M., and Hornung, R. W. 1990. Review of radon and lung cancer risk. *Risk Analysis* 1:65–75.

Samet, J. M., and Nero, A. V., Jr. 1989. Indoor radon and lung cancer. *N. Engl. J. Med.* 320:591–94.

Samet, J. M., et al. 1989. Radon progeny exposure and lung cancer risk in New Mexico uranium miners: A case-control study. *Health Phys.,* 56:415–21.

Simpson, S. G., and Comstock, G. W. 1983. Lung cancer and housing characteristics. *Arch. Environ. Health* 38:248–51.

Stranden, E. 1988. Building materials as a source of indoor radon. In *Radon and its decay products in indoor air.* Ed. W. W. Nazaroff and A. V. Nero, Jr., 113–30. New York: John Wiley & Sons.

Svensson, C.; Eklund, G.; and Pershagen, G. 1987. Indoor exposure to radon from the ground and bronchial cancer in women. *Int. Arch. Occup. Environ. Health* 59:123–31.

Svensson, C.; Pershagen, G.; and Klominek, J. 1989. Lung cancer in women and type of dwelling in relation to radon exposure. *Cancer Res.* 49:1861–65.

U.S. Department of Health and Human Services. 1982. *The health consequences of smoking: Cancer. A report of the surgeon general.* Washington, D.C.: Government Printing Office. DHHS Publication no. PHS 82-50179.

U.S. Department of Health and Human Services. 1984. *The health consequences of smoking: Chronic obstructive lung disease. A report of the surgeon general.* Washington, D.C.: Public Health Service, Office of Smoking and Health, Government Printing Office. DHHS Publication no. PHS 84-50525.

U.S. Environmental Protection Agency. 1986. *A citizen's guide to radon: What it is and what to do about it.* Washington, D.C.: Government Printing Office. DHHS Publication no. OPA/86/004.

U.S. Environmental Protection Agency. 1987. *Radon reference manual.* Washington, D.C.: Office of Radiation Programs, U.S. Environmental Protection Agency. Publication no. EPA/520/1-87-20.

Whittemore, A. S., and McMillan, A. 1983. Lung cancer mortality among U.S. uranium miners: A reappraisal. *J. Natl. Cancer Inst.* 71:489–99.

World Health Organization (International Agency for Research on Cancer). 1986. *IARC monographs on the evaluation of the carcinogenic risk of chemicals to humans: Tobacco smoking,* Vol. 38. Lyon, France: IARC.

# III. CONTROL AND LEGAL ASPECTS

# 16

# CONTROL STRATEGIES

Jerry F. Ludwig, Ph.D.
William Turner, M.S.

For centuries, air quality and thermal conditions in buildings have been recognized as important determinants of health and comfort. Unfortunately, in times of escalating fuel costs, energy is often saved by reducing ventilation to inadequate levels, and air quality and thermal comfort may become conflicting goals. This chapter addresses thermal comfort and indoor air quality in the context of relevant aspects of building design and construction, the consequences for air quality of changing use and operation of a building, and methods for air cleaning.

## HISTORY OF VENTILATION AND THERMAL COMFORT CONTROL

The art and industry of comfort conditioning (heating, ventilating, and air conditioning) have evolved falteringly and gradually over hundreds of years. Its history includes such illustrious names as Leonardo da Vinci (Ingles 1952), Galileo (Ingles 1952), Benjamin Franklin (Franklin 1906), Florence Nightingale, Dr. John Billings (Billings 1893), Thomas Tredgold (Woolrich 1947), Dr. John Gorre, and the man often referred to as *the father of air conditioning*, Willis H. Carrier (Ingles 1952). Comfort conditioning first became widely used in the United States during the early 1920s in motion picture theaters. Several hundred theaters were comfort conditioned by the end of that decade (Ingles 1952), and since then, comfort conditioning and ventilation have become a major consideration in many countries, usually as a building code or lease requirement, for all buildings designed for human occupancy.

Presently, systems for comfort conditioning typically represent about 10 percent of the first cost of the average commercial-institutional building built in the United States (verbal communication). Commercial-institutional buildings represented 7 percent of the total energy consumption in the United States in 1986 (U.S. Department of Energy 1988), of which the majority was used for comfort conditioning. These figures indicate the substantial cost of comfort conditioning and the potential interactions between the design and operation of heating, ventilating, and air conditioning (HVAC) systems and energy costs.

In the years that immediately followed the oil embargo of 1973, public concerns about the cost of energy resources increased greatly, and attempts were made to reduce the energy cost of comfort conditioning. One approach was to identify and plug energy leaks in building HVAC systems. Since the energy cost of heating the outdoor air brought into a building for ventilation is a significant operating expense and is readily identifiable in budgets, it was often intensely scrutinized. The American Society of Heating, Refrigerating and Air-Conditioning Engineers (ASHRAE) specified the use of minimum permissible ventilation rates in buildings in its publication *Energy Conservation in Buildings* (ASHRAE *Standard 90-75*) (Janssen 1987). However, in many documented cases, a building operator compromised the quality of air provided to the building occupants (and the energy efficiency of the HVAC system) by reducing significantly the amount of outdoor air brought into the building via the building's HVAC system. For a time, thermal comfort in some commercial and institutional buildings was compromised by a thermostat set-back program mandated by the U.S. government.

To estimate energy cost savings by such practices, the effect of increasing the ventilation rate from 5 to 20 cfm per person on the annual energy consumption and construction costs of a building was modeled for a prototype 600,000-square foot, thirty-eight-story office building (Eto and Meyer 1988). Using DOE–2.1C, a computer model, the effect of the change was simulated from climate and energy cost data for ten cities in the United States and three in Canada. The modeling showed that the annual energy operating costs of the buildings were increased less than 5 percent with the higher ventilation rate. However, this increment was expressed as a percentage of total costs, which included energy used for many purposes other than comfort conditioning. Construction costs for the HVAC system to handle the higher minimum outside ventilation rates were estimated to increase total building construction costs by less than 0.5 percent.

Before the oil embargo of 1973, energy was inexpensive and often regarded by the general public as having negligible cost. Consequently, HVAC systems were designed for low construction costs, with little or no consideration given to energy consumption. In the 1980s, greater consideration was given to both the initial capital outlay and the operating expenses. However, even at the greater energy costs of the present, the expense of providing comfortable indoor air quality in an office building is still a minor proportion of the total operating expenses, which include salaries, health care, and other costs of maintaining a business (Woods and Crawford 1989).

The problems caused by reducing the amount of outdoor air brought indoors have been worsened by modern construction practices. To control thermal heat loss through the building envelope, air leakage (infiltration) was often decreased. The practice of controlling infiltration by construction methods, widespread in residential construction, has now become increasingly common in commercial construction. New construction materials, which tend to increase the concentrations of a variety of organic chemicals, may be used to reduce infiltration. These chemicals are present in products used as mastics, adhesives, and sealers. The use of composite materials, which also contain volatile compounds, has become increasingly common in the interior of buildings. Thus, indoor air quality problems have been worsened by the contemporary combination of more pollution sources and less dilution of air.

## EVOLUTION OF CONTROL STRATEGIES FOR INDOOR AIR QUALITY AND THERMAL COMFORT

Building designs are diverse, and buildings often serve purposes unanticipated in the original design. Some buildings are constructed under restrictions of government bidding procedures or are developed to meet a functional demand of local economics (e.g., offices and apartments). In addition, building designs tend to reflect the availability of local construction materials, labor resources, and energy costs. Often, considerations related to the HVAC system which extend beyond the required minimal codes are subjugated to concerns other than air quality.

As building design and construction techniques have changed to conform with available resources and style, building HVAC systems have also evolved. This section describes some of the types of HVAC systems which have been used typically in commercial-institutional buildings in the United States since the beginning of the twentieth century (Haines 1987; ASHRAE 1987). Emphasis is placed on changes that were made in HVAC system designs consequent to the 1973 oil embargo and the effects that these changes have had on indoor air quality and thermal comfort.

The HVAC system in a commercial-institutional building is usually the primary means for meeting thermal comfort requirements. It is also relied upon to dilute the concentrations of occupant-generated bioeffluents and other pollutants. Conventional design has resulted in several types of HVAC systems. Once the amount of outdoor air required for the building has been determined, usually by local or state building codes, a system for supplying this air to the occupied space is designed. For residential structures, natural infiltration of air has generally been the source of outdoor air, although newer homes may have specific systems. In general, for commercial, industrial, and institutional buildings, outdoor air is deliberately drawn into the HVAC system in a manner similar to the system schematically illustrated in Figure 16.1.

The requirements for ventilation air vary with the intended use of the space. Certain types of areas, such as laboratories, animal care facilities, hospital operating rooms, and special manufacturing areas, may require the use of 100 percent outdoor air, which must be conditioned for comfort. However, in most commercial buildings, for saving energy and reducing capital costs of HVAC equipment, the supply air from the HVAC units has proportionally more recirculated air than

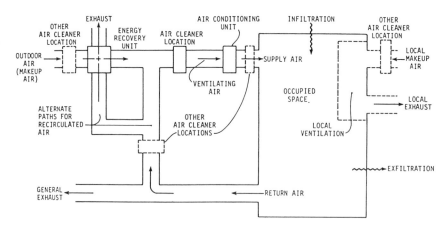

Figure 16.1. General ventilation system. *Source:* ASHRAE Standard 62-1989. By permission.

ventilation (outside) air. Typically, only a minimal amount of outdoor air is introduced into the space to dilute internally generated contaminants.

The simplest method of controlling the volume of outdoor air supplied to the space is to open a "minimum outside air" damper whenever the HVAC system is operated in a "building-occupied" mode. This type of outdoor air control is simple to understand, maintain, and operate (Figure 16.1) (ASHRAE 1989b), and the thermal conditions of the outdoor air in many climates are such that less heating or cooling of the incoming air is required than for the recirculated air from the space. Two types of outdoor air volume control strategies which minimize heating or cooling requirements are currently used. These two strategies are commonly referred to as *economizer cycles*. One strategy controls the proportion of outdoor air and return air to achieve the desired supply air condition based solely on temperature conditions of the two airstreams whereas the second bases the proportions of outdoor air and return air on the "enthalpy" conditions of the two airstreams. These control strategies operate identically, with the exception that the enthalpy control strategy considers the total heat value (i.e., temperature and humidity) of both the return air and outdoor air whereas the sensible control strategy considers only the dry-bulb temperature of the two airstreams.

To minimize capital cost, HVAC systems are often designed with one unit to control the thermal comfort conditions in many spaces in the building, even though requirements may vary among the spaces. Other HVAC systems employ control strategies to achieve thermal comfort conditions in all zones simultaneously. The following paragraphs describe some of the more widely used of these HVAC design strategies, with emphasis on the advantages and disadvantages of each.

*Dual-duct HVAC systems*, as the name implies, are multizone systems with two ducts (one hot, the other cold) and with mixing dampers (boxes) located near the zone. This type of system is generally used for smaller zones and responds to load perturbations faster than other types of systems. These systems also ensure that a consistent amount of supply air is delivered at all times.

*Single-duct variable-volume systems* provide control with only a single duct. The supply air in many of these systems is maintained at a temperature that varies according to the season. The individual zone thermostats vary the quantity of air supplied to the zone to maintain the desired temperature conditions. Change from *cooling* to *heating* alters the set point of the supply air thermostat and reverses the action of the zone thermostat. For example, on *cooling*, the zone thermostat modulates the open air damper toward minimum closure as the zone temperature decreases; the change to *heating* causes the opposite sequence to take place. With this system, however, it is not possible to heat some zones and simultaneously cool others, and overcooling or not cooling sufficiently can be a problem with heterogeneous areas. Single-duct variable-volume systems may be a problem in buildings with differential radiant heating loads. If minimum damper position detents (stops) are not installed on the zone damper to prevent complete closing, air quality may be compromised in zones with low cooling loads.

*Dual-duct variable-volume systems*, as the name implies, are multizone systems with two ducts (one hot, the other cold) that have mixing dampers (boxes) located near each zone. To maintain the desired temperature conditions, the individual zone thermostats vary the quantity of air supplied to the zone by changing the position of a supply air damper near the zone supply diffuser(s). Unlike the single-duct variable-volume system, this system is capable of heating some zones while simultaneously cooling others. Because of the capital cost of this system, it is seldom designed as part of new construction and is usually introduced as a conversion of a simple dual-duct system to a variable-volume system for the purpose of lowering operating costs in perimeter areas of a building.

*Terminal reheat systems* provide control with a single duct. The air supply temperature is essentially constant, or reset slightly, at a value suitable for comfort all year round. Reheat coils for each zone are controlled by zone thermostats to satisfy zone temperature requirements, thus providing more flexibility than variable-volume systems. The terminal reheat system can provide simultaneous heating of some zones and cooling of other zones. Terminal reheat systems cost somewhat more to install than variable-volume systems, and depending upon the design, they consume more energy. Some of the operating cost disadvantages of the terminal reheat systems may be overcome by combining terminal reheat with variable-volume systems.

*Fan-coil systems* are essentially small single-zone air-handling units with a fan, filter, and an oversized coil that may be used for both hot and chilled water. Some more sophisticated but more expensive units are divided into heating and cooling sections. If outside air is not ducted to the fan-coil unit, it must be provided to the occupants through some other means.

*Induction-coil systems* depend upon a central source of temperature-controlled high-pressure air which induces a secondary flow of air across the unit coil. The induction coil is supplied with hot or chilled water through a two-, three-, or four-pipe system. Thus, it is necessary to control the primary air supply temperature furnished by the central air unit and control the flow of hot or chilled water to the coil according to the heating or cooling demand in the induction-coil zone.

## "STATE OF THE ART" CONTROL STRATEGIES FOR INDOOR AIR QUALITY AND THERMAL COMFORT

The usual approach in designing for acceptable indoor air quality within a conditioned space has been based on the mass balance technique. Assuming that the ventilation air and the air of a conditioned space are completely and instantaneously mixed, a general equation for the concentration of an indoor air pollutant (Constance 1970; Drivas, Simmonds, and Shair 1972; Esman 1978; Ishizu 1980; Maldonado 1982; Maldonado and Woods 1983; Offerman et al. 1983; Sandburg 1981, 1983; Skaret 1982; Skaret and Mathisen 1983; Turk 1963, 1968; Woods and Crawford 1989) can be expressed as

$$V \frac{dC}{dt} = G + Q_s C_s - Q_e C - Q_r E_r C \qquad (1)$$

where

$C$  represents the contaminant concentration;

$V \frac{dC}{dt}$  represents the change in the mass of a contaminant in a volume with respect to time (g/s);

$G$  represents the generation rate of the contaminant (g/s);

$Q_s C_s$  represents the rate at which a contaminant is entering into a space in the supply air (g/s). $Q_s$ is the volume flow rate in volumes per time, and $C_s$ is the external concentration in mass per volume;

$Q_e C$  represents the rate at which a contaminant is removed from a space by the exhaust air (g/s). $Q_e$ is the exhaust air volume flow rate in volumes per time. $C$ is concentration in mass per volume;

$Q_r E_r C$  represents the removal rate of a contaminant from a space by filtration techniques (or other loss mechanisms) (g/s). $E_r$ is the filter removal efficiency (unitless). $Q_r$ is the volume flow rate through a filter, device, or ductwork that removes some mass (volume per time). $C$ is defined above.

In this equation, four key parameters control the concentration of indoor air pollutants: source strength, air entering, air exhausting, and removal in the space. Thus, four approaches are evident for reducing concentrations of indoor pollutants: (a) source control (reduce $G$, the contaminant generation rate); (b) dilution ventilation (reduce $Q_s C_s$, dilute the polluted air with cleaner air); (c) local exhaust (increase $Q_e C$, i.e., exhaust the polluted air); and (d) air cleaning (increase $Q_r E_r C$, i.e., remove the pollutants from the air in the space using contaminant filtration techniques). Each control technique is discussed in the following sections.

Solving Equation 1 for steady-state conditions (i.e., $V \cdot dC/dt = 0$) and assuming that $G$, $Q_s$, $Q_e$, $E_r$, and $C_s$ are constant gives the following result (Woods and Crawford 1989):

$$C = \frac{G + Q_s C_s}{Q_e + Q_r E_r} = \frac{A}{B} \qquad (2)$$

where

$A = G + Q_s C_s$    the combination of air contaminants entering the control volume by internal generation and from outside;

$B = Q_e + Q_r E_r$    the combination of contaminant removal by exhausting and filtration.

Examination of this expression shows that once a contaminant enters the control volume either by internal generation or by being brought in with air from outside the control volume (i.e., $A$, the source term, is greater than zero), complete elimination of occupant exposure to the contaminant requires that $B$, the removal term, increase to infinity (Figure 16.2).

Although this expression points to the obvious solution of removing the pollution source as the best way to reduce pollution concentration within a confined environment, removal may not always be practical or possible.

Pollution sources in buildings may be the building materials, the furnishings or decorating materials, consumer products used within the building, and various processes such as photocopying. Achievement of a source-free environment is impossible. Some pollution sources can be used at the discretion of building occupants; however, the occupants have no control over the building materials specified by the designer or builder. Only recently have manufacturers begun producing low-emission materials, such as adhesives and paints, for finishing or decorating the interiors (Harriman Associates staff, personal communication 1989).

Some home builders now attempt to reduce the amount of toxic or hazardous materials used in construction (Small 1983; Bierman-Little, personal communication 1988). These builders have focused on the use of building materials known to contain fewer potentially irritating compounds, such as paints and interior finishes not emitting volatile organic compounds and insulation materials that do not contain irritating fibers. This approach incurs additional construction costs. Unfortunately, only limited information is available concerning the pollutant source strengths of building materials. However, guidelines for building products and consumer product substitution have been published recently (Fossel 1987; Natural Resource Council of Maine 1987).

Some large companies have limited the type of finish materials used when remodeling inhabited commercial buildings, avoiding the use of solvent-based paints, adhesives, or epoxy finishes (verbal communication). A few companies also have attempted to limit the use of materials emitting toxic compounds in new

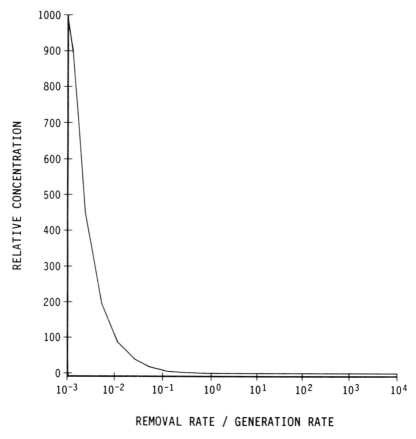

Figure 16.2. Concentration versus removal rate/generation rate for a ventilation system operating in steady-state conditions.

commercial office buildings (Wetherall, personal communication 1988). This approach to source control has not been used widely in commercial buildings because information on pollutant source strengths of building materials is limited and because commercial office buildings are typically ventilated at higher rates than residences.

SOURCE MODIFICATION

Some exposures can be reduced through source modification when the source cannot be totally eliminated. The source strength can be changed chemically or physically by using sealers, reducing the frequency of use, or altering other characteristics of the space, for example, moisture. Also, the exposure can be reduced by relocation or redistribution of the source.

For example, restricting smoking to specific locations reduces the number of areas directly impacted by environmental tobacco smoke (ETS). The approach of concentrating smokers in fewer locations may change the magnitude of personal exposures to ETS but does not produce a smoke-free environment. If the designated smoking area is served by an HVAC system that recirculates the return air to other locations in the building, areas that are intended to be smoke free, ETS exposures still occur. Many modern buildings may recirculate 50–85 percent of the air; the newer commercial aircraft (Boeing 757 and 767 models) recirculate up to 50 percent of the cabin air (National Research Council [NRC] 1986). Simply separating smokers and nonsmokers within the same air space may reduce, but does not eliminate, exposure of nonsmokers to ETS (U.S. Department of Health and Human Services [DHHS] 1986; Bearg and Turner 1987).

DILUTION BY GENERAL VENTILATION

Dilution ventilation refers to ventilation with uncontaminated air to reduce the concentration of contaminants in a room or building for the purpose of health hazard or nuisance control (American Conference of Governmental Industrial Hygienists [ACGIH] 1984). This method of control continues to be used widely in commercial office buildings, schools, institutions, multifamily housing, and modern homes. Dilution provides a comfortable environment with lower levels of potentially odoriferous and irritating compounds. General ventilation is often supplemented with local exhaust.

Historically, ASHRAE ventilation guidelines have been based on the dilution approach, with "clean" outdoor air used to dilute stale indoor air to acceptable odor levels. The work by Yaglou was particularly prominent (Yaglou, Ripley, and Coggins 1936; Yaglou and Witheridge 1937). More recently, the minimum ventilation recommendations for outside air supply set out in ASHRAE *Standard 62-1989* (ASHRAE 1989b) were based on several criteria, including odors, in addition to expected pollutant source strengths and occupant comfort requirements.

Researchers have sought recently to use a mass balance approach to specify the amount of ventilation air needed to provide acceptable pollutant concentrations for pollutants of known source emission rates. One problem with this approach is the actuality of the assumption of perfect mixing.

The mass balance equation (Equation 1) for predicting pollutant concentration in the space as a function of time is solved for the non-steady-state case (i.e., $V \cdot dC/dt \neq 0$) by integration. Assuming that $G$, $Q_s$, $Q_e$, $Q_r$, $E_r$, and $C_s$ are all constant over these integration limits, the following result is obtained.

$$C = \frac{G + Q_s C_s}{Q_e + Q_r E_r} = \frac{A}{B} \, [1 - e^{[(-(Q_e + Q_r E_r)/V) \cdot t]}] + [1 - e^{(-(Q_e + Q_r E_r)/V)}] \qquad (3)$$

Although this analytical model accounts for all sources and sinks within the control volume, it has been shown that in many cases this model either underpredicts or overpredicts the actual concentration of pollutants. The poor fit of the model can usually be attributed to imperfect mixing. Figure 16.3 illustrates qualitatively the design techniques that should be either employed or avoided to facilitate "good mixing" of dilution air in a ventilated space. The quantitative differences between measurements and modeled results are reflected in a "mixing" or "ventilation efficiency" factor.

At least two different mixing factors (Drivas, Simmonds, and Shair 1972; Ishizu 1980) and nine different ventilation efficiency factors (Skaret and Mathisen 1983; Maldonado and Woods 1983; Offerman et al. 1983; Sandburg 1981, 1983) have been proposed and applied. All of these parameters emphasize that mixing and ventilation efficiencies are important with respect to controlling indoor air pollutants. These parameters represent a complex process and vary with geometry, thermal parameters, and meteorologic conditions at the time of measurement.

One long-used approach for determining required amounts of outside air for dilution ventilation has been based upon "acceptable" odor levels. This approach involves determining what ventilation rates would be required for visitors entering an area not to object to the odor. This approach was first used in a test chamber by Yaglou and developed further by Cain and Leaderer.

Cain and co-workers (1983) evaluated odors associated with ETS (see Chapter 6). They reported that ventilation rates up to 30 cfm outside air per smoking occupant were not sufficient to achieve a 75–80 percent acceptance of the odor by visitors to the space, which was the criterion for adequacy of ventilation. They concluded that a ventilation rate as high as 100 cfm per smoking occupant might be necessary to meet the criterion of acceptability in situations in which smoking takes place more or less continuously. Cain and co-workers also reported that surfaces in an enclosed room seem to be important sinks for tobacco smoke indoors and that absorbed particles may carry condensed volatiles that could evaporate gradually, thereby imparting a lingering odor. To prevent this contamination of surfaces in a smoking area, Bearg and Turner (1987) recommended local exhaust ventilation as the preferred method of control.

The concept of odor acceptance has been used to evaluate the air quality of buildings. Using an odor panel as a subjective instrument, Fanger (1987) defined the olf (abbreviation for olfaction unit) as the emission rate of bioeffluents from a standard sedentary person in thermal comfort. The curve shown in Figure 16.4 was based on comprehensive studies of more than one thousand sedentary male and female occupants judged by approximately two hundred male and female judges.

Fanger used this subjective instrument to quantify pollution sources in twenty offices and assembly halls in Copenhagen. Each space was visited three times; (a) when the space was unoccupied and unventilated, to quantify pollution sources from materials in the space; (b) when the space was unoccupied and ventilated, to quantify the combined pollution sources in the space and ventilation system; and (c) when the space was normally occupied and ventilated, to quantify the combined effects of the occupants and pollution sources in the space and ventilation system. Each judge was asked to determine whether the air quality was acceptable or not and to evaluate odor intensity. Figure 16.5 illustrates the results obtained

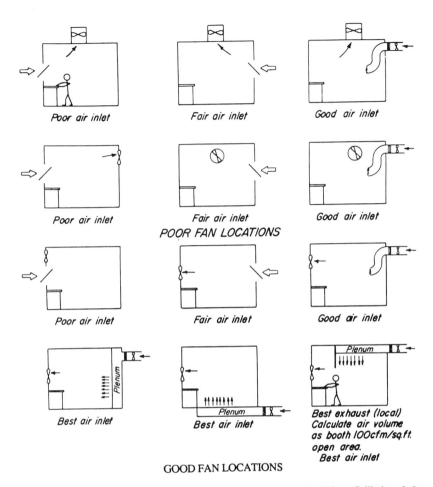

Poor air inlet        Fair air inlet        Good air inlet

Poor air inlet        Fair air inlet        Good air inlet

**POOR FAN LOCATIONS**

Poor air inlet        Fair air inlet        Good air inlet

Best air inlet        Best air inlet        Best exhaust (local)
Calculate air volume
as booth $100cfm/sq.ft.$
open area.
Best air inlet

**GOOD FAN LOCATIONS**

Figure 16.3. General techniques to avoid or employ to facilitate good mixing of dilution air in a ventilated space. Some general rules of dilution ventilation should be followed in order to facilitate good mixing of dilution air in the ventilated zone. The top six designs are examples of poor exhaust air duct placement. The exhaust port is above or behind the work surface (which is the point of contaminant release), causing smoke, fumes, or gases emitted at the workbench to be drawn into the worker's breathing zone. The bottom six diagrams all have the exhaust ports located in the work area. In this location, the exhaust port will provide local exhaust for the work bench in addition to the general room air exhaust. Also demonstrated by this figure are correct and incorrect inlet air locations. Poor inlet air locations either short-circuit directly to the exhaust or push the contaminants from the bench (source) into the room; fair inlet locations do not mix the workbench emissions with room supply air; the best air inlet uses a plenum to distribute makeup air over a large area. *Source:* ACGIH (1984).

from this investigation. Surprisingly, Fanger found that people were the source for only about 25 percent of the odor generation. The materials and ducting (HVAC) system were very important odor sources, each contributing about 40 percent of the perceived odor strength. Generalizing from Fanger's studies, it should not be

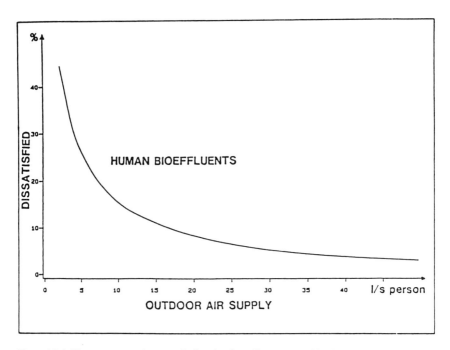

Figure 16.4. The percentage of persons finding the air quality unacceptable when entering a space with a given ventilation rate. *Source:* Fanger (1987), reprinted with permission.

surprising that ventilation standards designed to dilute "people odors" are, in many cases, found to be insufficient.

LOCAL EXHAUST VENTILATION

An advantage of local exhaust ventilation over dilution ventilation is that proper placement of exhaust registers and supply grilles can achieve plug-flow (one directional airflow) through the space. This type of air movement provides the maximum air contaminant removal for a given airflow and is effective in energy conservation and in meeting the requirements of multiple-use spaces. For example, the most efficient way to ventilate a space in which pollutants are emitted in thermally buoyant plumes (i.e., cigarette smoke) is to locate the supply air diffusers in the lower regions of the space and the exhaust registers near the ceiling. This type of exhaust situation has been described in detail by the Norwegian Technical Institute (Skaret 1982) and recently recommended in ASHRAE *Standard 62-1989* (ASHRAE 1989b) as "increasing ventilation efficiency." Exhaust strategies based on the natural tendencies of some air pollutants to stratify vertically in the space have yielded successful results in smoking lounges, print rooms, computer rooms, and industrial facilities. It is also an appropriate strategy for kitchens, where combustion emissions and/or cooking-generated odors rise in buoyant air.

## QUANTIFIED POLLUTION SOURCES

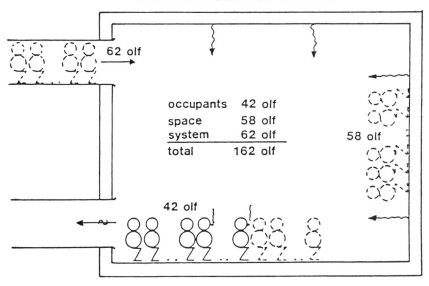

| occupants | 42 olf |
| space | 58 olf |
| system | 62 olf |
| total | 162 olf |

Figure 16.5. Mean values of pollution sources quantified in twenty offices and assembly halls in Copenhagen. The spaces had a mean size of 2,210 m² and an average of seventeen occupants. As an average, five of the occupants were smokers, each polluting six olf. This makes the seventeen occupants pollute forty-two olf. There were large differences in the pollution sources from space to space. *Source:* Fanger (1987), reprinted with permission.

Local exhaust is frequently utilized in residences and commercial buildings and in industrial applications. The goal of good local exhaust ventilation design is to minimize the air volume required and to maximize the collection efficiency. The exhausting of air also requires that quantities of makeup air (approximately equal in volume to that exhausted) be supplied to the room or zone from which the contaminants are being exhausted. Aside from the complete elimination of activities causing emissions, this approach has the greatest potential for achieving environments with low concentrations of contaminants. Certain principles should be followed in using local exhaust (verbal communication with IBM corporate safety officer and with mechanics staff at Harriman Associates):

1. The area should be properly designed to isolate the contaminant to be exhausted.
2. The area also needs to be isolated from the rest of the recirculating air-handling system to prevent the transport of the air contaminants to other locations in the building.
3. The location of both the exhaust register and the makeup supply air and the adjoining rooms' pressure relationships are also important for the correct operation of an exhaust system. It is important that the supply and exhaust be

Table 16.1  Portable Air Cleaner Descriptions and Results

| Device Type | Device Number | Device Description | Retail Costs[a] ($) Device | Filter | Speed | Power (watts) | Flow Rate (m³ h⁻¹) | Ratio (m³ h⁻¹/watt) | Efficiency[b] (%) | ECR[c] (m³ h⁻¹) |
|---|---|---|---|---|---|---|---|---|---|---|
| Panel filters | PF1 | Foam filter | 30 | 4 | High | 20 | 17 | 0.9 | 0 ± 1 | 0 ± 2 |
| | PF2 | Electret filter | 40 | 5 | High | 27 | 49 | 1.8 | 11 ± 1 | 5 ± 2 |
| | PF3 | Electret filter | 35 | 6 | High | 18 | 36 | 2.0 | 16 ± 3 | 5 ± 2 |
| | PF4 | Negative corona | 150 | 12 | Medium | 28 | 29 | 1.0 | 39 ± 11 | 12 ± 3 |
| Extended surface filters | ES1 | Electret filter and negative ion generator | 295 | 16 | High | 32 | 112 | 3.5 | 86 ± 9 | 97 ± 3 |
| Electrostatic | ES2 | HEPA filter | 395 | 77 | Medium | 67 | 267 | 4.0 | 115 ± 17 | 306 ± 14 |
| | EP1 | Two-stage flat plate, positive corona | 370 | 15 (carbon) | Medium | 109 | 366 | 3.4 | 57 ± 11 | 207 ± 32 |
| | EP2 | Two-stage flat plate, positive corona | 395 | 15 (carbon) | Medium | 77 | 340 | 4.4 | 58 ± 6 | 197 ± 9 |
| Ion generators | IG1 | Residential model, negative corona, positive collector | 80 | None | | 2 | 0 | | | 2 ± 2 |
| | IG2 | Commercial model, negative corona, no collector | 120 | None | | 3 | 0 | | | 51 ± 2 |
| Circulating fan | CF1 | Oscillating fan, two units | 52 each | None | High | 44 each | 3,060[d] each | 69.6 | 0 ± 1 | 2 ± 2 |

Source: Offerman et al. (1985), reprinted with permission.

[a] Retail costs obtained from manufacturers or local distributors (prices as of mid-1983).
[b] Efficiency calculated as the observed effective cleaning rate divided by the measured airflow rate (±90% confidence limits).
[c] Effective cleaning rate calculated as the flow rate of particle-free air required to produce the observed decay rate in cigarette smoke.
[d] Flow rate as reported by the manufacturer.

located so as to minimize any short-circuiting of the supply air directly to the exhaust air (Turner and Bearg 1987).

4. The exhaust fan for the system should also be located outside or as close to the outside as possible so that the ductwork transporting the air contaminants is under negative pressure in the building. If the ductwork is not leak tight and is under positive pressure, leakage of air contaminants may occur.

5. The exhaust discharge must be designed to avoid reentrainment of the exhausted material. Guidelines for the correct design of exhaust systems are presented in the ACGIH *Industrial Ventilation Handbook* (ACGIH 1988; ASHRAE 1989a).

AIR CLEANING

Air cleaning refers to the use of equipment to remove undesirable contaminants from air. The air cleaning device may be designed as part of the HVAC system or as an isolated installation near the site of contaminant generation. Air cleaning equipment designed to remove particles from the air stream typically includes a medium efficiency filter to remove larger particles and either a final filter (high efficiency particulate air [HEPA] filter) or electrostatic precipitators, which can remove the smaller respirable particles. Most particle removal systems have not been designed to also remove the volatile, semivolatile, or gaseous components of an airstream (Bearg and Turner 1987).

Air cleaners for control of particulate matter are available as both in-duct devices and as portable unducted devices (Offerman et al. 1985; Consumer Reports 1985; Godish 1989). In-duct devices are designed to be integrated with the forced-air HVAC system, whereas portable air cleaners are designed primarily for cleaning the air in one room. In-duct devices have been available for the past thirty years. During that time, their performance has been assessed (Silverman and Dennis 1956, 1959), and performance evaluation standards have been devised (ASHRAE 1976). Since about 1982, a variety of portable air cleaners has appeared on the market. Prices of these portable devices range from $10 to $500 (Godish 1989). Little information on performance, other than general claims by the manufacturer, is available. The results of published studies of portable air cleaners indicate a wide range of performance (Whitby, Anderson, and Rubow 1983; New Shelter 1982; Offerman et al. 1985); Table 16.1 shows the results of one such study (Offerman et al. 1985).

Removal of particles from air by mechanical filtration is accomplished by passing air through a fibrous medium. The deposition mechanisms of impaction, interception, and diffusion predominate for different conditions of particle size and air velocity. Figure 16.6 illustrates the relationship between filter efficiency and particle size for a typical fibrous filter. Three basic kinds of fibrous media filters are available for indoor air cleaning: dry, viscous impingement, and charged-media filters.

Dry-type panel filters have high porosities and low efficiencies. Their typical application is as a dust stop or coarse roughing filter to protect mechanical equip-

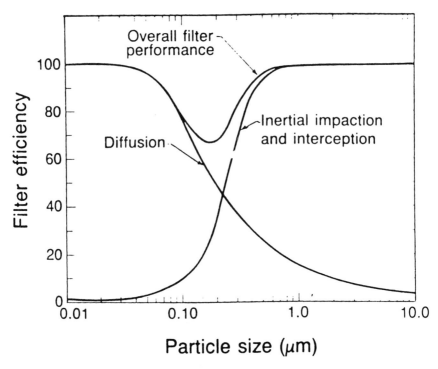

Figure 16.6. Particle removal efficiency as a function of particle size for a typical fibrous filter. *Source:* Reprinted with permission from *Atmospheric Environment* 19, Offerman F. J. et al., Control of respirable particles in indoor air with portable air cleaners. Copyright 1985, Pergamon Press PLC.

ment in HVAC systems and home furnaces or as prefilters for higher efficiency filters. Dry-type panel filters collect large particles by impaction and interception. The media of dry panel filters are commonly open-cell foams, nonwoven textile cloth, or paperlike mats of glass or cellulose fibers.

Viscous media panel filters are comprised of coarse fibers coated by a viscous, oily material to which particles adhere as they impact or impinge on the filter media. Like dry-type panel filters, these filters have low efficiencies for the particle range common to indoor air but are very efficient in collecting fabric dust or lint.

Extended surface dry-type filters are those in which the fiber thickness or density is increased to increase collection efficiency. To offset the resulting increased resistance to airflow, the surface area of the filter is increased, principally by pleating the filter medium. Extended surface filters are available in a variety of designs and performance levels. They vary in media thickness and density, fiber size, media materials, number of pleats per unit area, and filter depth. The filter medium typically is in the form of a random fiber orientation mat or blanket. Common media fibers include cellulose, bonded glass, wool felt, and synthetics.

The most efficient of the extended media filters commonly available is the HEPA filter. HEPA filters are characterized by efficiencies in excess of 99.97 percent at a minimum particle diameter of 0.3 $\mu$m. HEPA filters, originally designed for the nuclear power industry, are widely used in industrial and military clean rooms and have been incorporated recently into portable room air cleaners (Offerman et al. 1985; Godish 1989, Jorgensen, 1983).

Electrostatic precipitators remove particles from the air by electrostatic forces. Three basic designs are available: low-voltage, two-stage, charged-media non-ionizing, and charged-media ionizing precipitators.

The two-stage low-voltage electrostatic precipitators (often referred to as electronic air cleaners) are used widely in residential, commercial, and office buildings. The units are packaged either as freestanding modular units that are suspended from the ceiling or mounted on the wall or as in-duct units installed in residential heating/cooling systems or, in large buildings, placed in the HVAC system. Electronic air cleaner operation is based on the principle that particles moving in an airstream can be electrically charged and subsequently collected on plates of opposite charge. The electronic air cleaner draws particle-laden air past a series of ionizing wires that produce positive ions. The ions attach to the particles and make them positively charged. The air then passes through channels that consist of a series of alternate positively and negatively charged collection plates. The negatively charged plates attract and hold the positively charged particles which lose their positive charge and take on the negative charge of the plate.

Typical ionization potentials are 12 kV whereas the collection plates commonly carry a 6-kV potential difference between plates. During the ionization process, the corona discharge near the ionizing wire produces ozone. To minimize ozone production, most ionizing plate devices use positive coronas since this polarity produces less ozone. The efficiency of the collection plates gradually decreases as the plates become coated with particles, and the accumulated particles reduce the strength of the electrostatic forces. Plates must then be cleaned to remove their accumulated particle load, typically by washing with hot water. Electronic air cleaners installed in large HVAC systems often are equipped with cleaning subsystems for this purpose.

Charged media nonionizing air cleaners combine characteristics of both electronic air cleaners and dry filters. These units consist of a dielectric filtering medium made of a mat of glass fiber, cellulose, or some similar material supported on a grid of alternatively charged or grounded members. A strong electrostatic field is formed through the dielectric filter medium. As particles approach the charged filter medium, they are polarized and drawn to it. Since this filter is a media filter, resistance to airflow increases as the filter becomes soiled. The filter therefore has a limited life before it must be replaced.

Charged media ionizing air cleaners pass the particle-laden airstream through a corona discharge ionizer that charges the particles. Particles are then collected on a charged-media filter.

The removal of gaseous contaminants from air can be achieved by the application of a variety of well-known principles, including adsorption, chemisorption, catalytic oxidation or reduction, and absorption. Adsorption is a chemical/physical phenomenon in which gases, vapors, or liquids coming into contact with a surface adhere to it. This adherence results from the same physical forces that hold atoms, ions, and molecules together in a solid state. Although adsorption is a chemical/physical phenomenon, no chemical reaction takes place. Heat is released and is approximately equal to that liberated when the adsorbed gas or vapor undergoes condensation.

Although adsorption occurs on a variety of solid surfaces, only a few materials have properties suitable for air cleaning: activated carbons, molecular sieves, zeolites, porous clay minerals, silica gel, and activated alumina. These materials have high surface area to volume ratios and surfaces typically comprised of vast labyrinths of submicroscopic pores and channels.

*Chemisorption* refers to chemical reactions taking place on the large internal surface area of sorbents. These surfaces are often coated or impregnated with chemicals that will selectively react with or chemisorb molecules from a gas stream.

Some adsorption materials remove gases/vapors by catalyzing their conversion to other less objectionable forms. For instance, activated carbon catalyzes ozone to oxygen. Activated carbon has also been shown to speed other reactions. The activated carbon is frequently impregnated with catalysts for specific applications.

*Absorption* refers to a chemical reaction that occurs between an absorbing medium and contaminant gases in air. In industrial applications, a variety of contaminant gases (including sulfur dioxide and hydrochloride) are removed from waste gas streams by absorbing them in water or in a reactive liquid reagent or slurry.

Because of the complex nature of indoor air pollutant mixtures and the selectivity of gaseous filtration techniques, filtration for removal of gaseous contaminants has been used less widely than particulate filtration. Studies of the air cleaning effectiveness of adsorption/chemisorption systems have been very limited and often based on subjective criteria (Jorgensen 1983; Godish 1989).

The performance of air cleaning equipment in a space can be predicted relatively easily with information to characterize the pollutant and its source strength. For example, consider a home of 270 m³ (9,600 ft³) in which ETS is controlled to acceptable levels by natural infiltration at 2.0 air changes per hour (ACH). If the homeowner weatherizes the home, reducing the infiltration rate to 0.5 ACH, and smoking habits do not change, the level of ETS is increased fourfold. If the homeowner purchases a device of 85 percent efficiency to remove the ETS, the device needs to be capable of cleaning 1.75 ACH or 475 m³/hour (280 cfm). In order for this air cleaner to be most effective, it should be positioned in the room in which the most smoking activity occurs. Likewise, to control air pollution within a single room, the appropriate air cleaner can be chosen using the guidance given by the mass balance equation shown in Equation 2. Assuming that the amount of pollutant removed by exhausting air ($Q_e$) from the space is reduced, an air cleaner with the appropriate flow $(Q_r)$ and $(E_r)$ quotient can be used to compensate for the reduction of air exchange.

## RADON AND OTHER SOIL GASES

The control of radon in indoor environments poses unique problems. The major cause of elevated levels of radon in homes, schools, and commercial buildings is the transport of soil gases from the earth under or around a building into the structure through pressure-driven flow (Figure 16.7). Consequently, the most effective control strategy in residences for radon gas (and other soil gases) originating from the soil is to combine sealing with active reduction of the pressure outside the foundation walls or under the floor. This approach actively prevents the flow of the gas into the structure (Nazaroff and Nero 1984; Nazaroff et al. 1987; D'Ottavio and Dietz 1987; Ericson and Schmied 1984; Brennan and Turner 1986; Turner and Brennan 1985; Turner et al. 1988; Piersol and Fugler 1987). The same principle has been applied in residences for control of volatile organic compounds, termiticides, and gases from landfill decomposition (Jurinski 1984; van de Wiel and Bloemen 1987; Lillie and Barnes 1987; Qazi 1987; Jaquith, McDavit, and Reinert 1987). Other techniques that have been utilized in homes include building pressur-

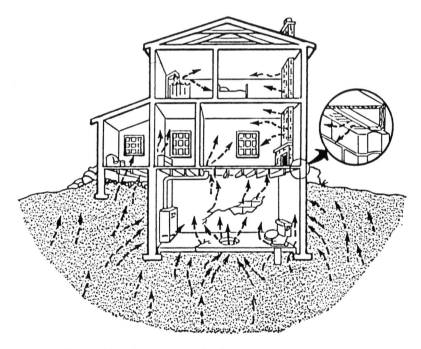

Figure 16.7. Radon entry routes into homes. *Source:* U.S. EPA (1988).

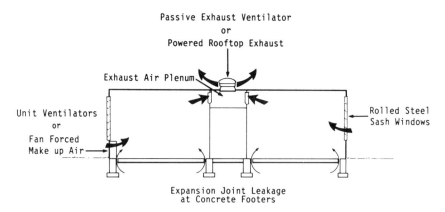

Figure 16.8. Radon entry into buildings under negative pressure.

ization, soil pressurization, specialized building ventilation (i.e., basement exhaust and first floor supply), and air cleaning devices.

Recent data collected for schools and commercial buildings suggest that in many cases, proper design and operation of the ventilation system will prevent soil gases from entering a building. However, this control strategy will only work when the ventilation system is in operation and the building is occupied (Turner and co-workers, personal communication 1990). One of the major causes of negative pressure in a structure is exhaust-only ventilation or a ventilation system that is not supplied with sufficient makeup air (Figure 16.8).

Techniques for constructing radon-resistant residences have been researched and published by the Environmental Protection Agency (EPA) (U.S. EPA 1987, 1988). Techniques for constructing radon-resistant schools and commercial buildings have been suggested, and draft guidelines for this type of building are expected to be available from the EPA by the end of 1990. Engineering firms and designers are now reported to be incorporating features into building designs to reduce the likelihood of soil gas problems (personal communication).

## STRATEGIES FOR POLLUTANT CONTROL

Strategies for pollution control are numerous and depend upon the pollutant present. Table 16.2 lists the more common pollutants by source and presents a summary of the control options that are available for each source.

## OPPORTUNITIES FOR IMPROVING BUILDING CONTROL SYSTEMS

Avoidance of contaminants that may be generated or emitted in the occupied space is the most effective method of control. Architects and interior designers are only now becoming aware of the impact on indoor air quality of their choices of

Table 16.2  Strategies for Pollutant Control

| Typical Source | Pollutant | Equipment and Material Selection | Ventilation Design | Occupant Involvement |
|---|---|---|---|---|
| Earth and rock beneath home (entering through cracks and holes in the foundation) | Radon and daughters; organic vapors from contaminated ground water | Vapor barrier around foundation; good dampproofing; seal cracks and holes, traps in floor drains, 100% basement seal, and subslab ventilation | Vent crawlspace, vent sumphole to exterior, vent under slab, vent basement, or whole house vent | Vent as near to source as possible (subslab, basement, or whole house); seal cracks and holes; maintain seals and fans; move building; replace backfill |
| Well water | Radon | Install suitable charcoal scrubber aerator system | Vent bath and laundry | Maintain scrubber or aerator |
| Insulation in building and on pipes | Asbestos | Do not use; coat existing asbestos with a sealant; enclose and isolate area | Not applicable | Do not disturb, unless a professional; educate service and maintenance personnel; respiratory protection for some activities |
| Urea-formaldehyde foam insulation, glues, particleboard, fiberglass insulation; furniture, paneling, masking, plywood | Formaldehyde | Use low-emission materials; seal source materials from living space | Vent house, particularly when new or when work has recently been done | Maintain covering or fan equipment |
| Dust mites, molds, fungus, bacteria, virus, animal dander | Biologic microorganisms | Moisture control with good insulation in building shell, good foundation, dampproofing, proper intake duct design (no condensation) | Provide adequate ventilation to bath and kitchen crawl-spaces to maintain inside relative humidity of 35–50% | Clean filters in air handlers, exhaust excess moisture, maintainence and cleaning of potential sources such as humidifiers, drain pans in HVAC and refrigerators |

(continued)

Table 16.2  (*Continued*)

| Typical Source | Pollutant | Equipment and Material Selection | Ventilation Design | Occupant Involvement |
|---|---|---|---|---|
| Hairsprays, paints, cleansers, glues, fabric softeners, pesticides, perfumes, deodorizers, carpet cleaners, art and hobby supplies | Organic vapors | Substitute waterbase or non-volatile substances; label instructions and contents clearly | Ventilate specific source areas (e.g., laundry, shop) (cross-ventilation) | Read labels, use safest products and follow directions; substitute products with less volatile solvents |
| Unvented heaters, kerosene or gas | $NO_2$, $SO_2$, CO, particles | Do not use in inhabited space; provide outside combustion air | | Consider vented units; added insulation as replacement; keep units tuned and maintained |
| Wood stoves, fireplaces | Particles, aldehydes, aromatics | Proper chimney and combustion air; airtight design catalyst | Supply correct combustion | Wood stoves with an updraft |
| Cigarettes, cigars | Particles, nicotine, gases | Not applicable | Exhaust smoke | Provide separate zones; develop no-smoking policies; provide incentives for cessation |
| Gas stoves, pilots, burners | CO, $NO_2$ | Pilotless ignition; "tune" appliance | Ventilating hood, room exhaust fan | Use range fan or room fan; do not use range for space heating |
| Outside air: loading docks, attached or underground garages, reentrained exhaust, neighboring sources | Particles, gases, odors | Proper separation and design of exhaust and intake vents; maintain positive pressure in building; provide separation of zones within structure | Separate zone ventilation of source areas | Maintain equipment in good working condition; do not permit trucks to idle at loading docks |

building materials, furnishings, and wall and floor coverings. Whenever possible, low-emission materials should always be specified for use within the interior envelope of a building. Manufacturers of building materials, furnishings, and surface treatments also need to realize that they should be concerned with emissions from their materials and products. These emissions should be identified and quantified. Studies should also be conducted to quantify the emissions of materials as they age and to learn whether products can be cured so that most of the pollutant has been emitted by the time the product is installed in a building.

Buildings currently incapable of meeting the increased minimum ventilation rates should be modified to meet these requirements. In some cases in which the current HVAC system is already operating at heating or cooling capacity, the installation of heat recovery ventilation systems may be an attractive way to minimize the capital cost of the system retrofit.

Systems exist currently for filtering recirculated and contaminated outdoor air. As filtration is practiced more widely, the experience gained and the economy of scale may make these systems more appealing to building owners.

Some HVAC control manufacturers are pursuing sensor technology to measure surrogate indoor air contaminants such as carbon dioxide. Using a monitoring technique, the outdoor air dampers might be modulated to control the level of the surrogate contaminant. These devices may provide opportunities to make the building somewhat more responsive to changing occupancy conditions and yet conserve energy used to condition ventilation air from outdoors.

Architects and engineers need to inform building owners and managers of the design assumptions of building control strategies. The architect or engineer should provide guidance to the building owner concerning the consequences of building remodeling and/or system changes on the functioning of control strategies. ASHRAE *Public Review Draft GPC 1P: Guideline for Commissioning of HVAC Systems* (ASHRAE 1988) has been written to address these concerns.

Better communications between the building owner and the architect/engineer would also be helpful for purposes of planning the occupancy patterns of the building. Building occupants may unknowingly violate the control strategies developed by the architect/engineer when remodeling the space.

*SUMMARY*

Much research is currently directed toward the subject of indoor air quality and its control, and new information is being published constantly. In this chapter we have attempted to present some of the problems of air pollution control and control systems and the state of the art equipment and strategies available to deal with those problems.

Present public awareness of the possible hazards of poor indoor air quality, coupled with the high cost of the energy required to maintain acceptable air quality and comfort levels in buildings, make it incumbent upon everyone concerned with building construction, maintenance, management, or ownership to study the subject of indoor air pollution and its control. The quality of indoor air can be monitored; polluting substances can be avoided; and air-conditioning systems can be updated or converted if they become inefficient or inadequate. The price of failure to do any one of these things can be high in terms of money or of health.

## REFERENCES

American Conference of Governmental Industrial Hygienists (committee on industrial ventilation). 1984. *Industrial ventilation: A manual of recommended practice,* 18th ed. Lansing, Mich.: ACGIH.

American Conference of Governmental Industrial Hygienists (committee on industrial ventilation). 1988. *Industrial ventilation: A manual of recommended practice,* 19th ed. Lansing, Mich.: ACGIH.

American Society of Heating, Refrigerating, and Air-Conditioning Engineers. 1976. *Standard 52-76: Method of testing air-cleaning devices used in general ventilation for removing particulate matter.* Atlanta, Ga.: ASHRAE.

American Society of Heating, Refrigerating, and Air-Conditioning Engineers. 1987. Automatic control. In *ASHRAE Handbook.* Atlanta, Ga.: HVAC systems and applications, ASHRAE.

American Society of Heating, Refrigerating, and Air-Conditioning Engineers. 1988. *Public Review Draft GPC 1P. Guideline for commissioning of HVAC systems.* Atlanta, Ga.: ASHRAE.

American Society of Heating, Refrigerating, and Air-Conditioning Engineers. 1989a. Air flow around buildings. In *ASHRAE Handbook.* Atlanta, Ga.: ASHRAE.

American Society of Heating, Refrigerating, and Air-Conditioning Engineers. 1989b. *Standard 62-1989: Ventilation for acceptable indoor air quality.* Atlanta, Ga.: ASHRAE.

Bearg, D. W. 1987. *Achieving tobacco smoke-free environments: The problems and some solutions.* Atlanta, Ga.: ASHRAE.

Bearg, D. W., and Turner, W. A. 1985. Building assessment techniques for indoor air quality evaluations. In *Proceedings of the APCA international speciality conference on indoor air quality in cold climates: Hazards and Abatement Measures,* 29 April–1 May, Ottawa, Canada.

Bearg, D. W., and Turner, W. A. 1987. Achieving tobacco smoke-free environments: The problem and some solutions. Paper presented at ASHRAE IAQ '87, May, Washington, D.C.

Billings, J. S. 1893. *Ventilation and heating.* New York: The Engineering Record.

Brennan, T., and Turner, W. A. 1986. Defeating radon. *Solar Age Mag.* 11:33–37.

Cain, W. S., et al. 1983. Ventilation requirements in buildings: Control of occupancy odor and tobacco smoke odor. *Atmos. Environ.* 17:1183–97.

Constance, J. D. 1970. Mixing factor is guide to ventilation. *Power* 114(2):56–57.

Consumer Reports. 1985. Air cleaners. *Consumer Rep.* 50:7–11.

D'Ottavio, T. W., and Dietz, R. N. 1987. Radon source rate measurements using multiple perfluorocarbon tracers. In *Indoor air '87: Proceedings of the fourth international conference on indoor air quality and climate.* Ed. B. Seifert et al., Vol. 2, 388–92. Berlin: Institute for Water, Soil, and Air Hygiene.

Drivas, P. J.; Simmonds, P. G.; and Shair, F. H. 1972. Experimental characterization of ventilation systems in buildings. *Environ. Sci. Technol.* 6:609–14.

Ericson, S., and Schmied, H. 1984. Modified technology in new constructions, and cost effective remedial action in existing structures, to prevent infiltration of soil gas carrying radon. In *Proceedings of the third international conference on indoor air quality and climate.* Ed. B. Berglund, T. Lindvall, and J. Sundell, Vol. 2. Stockholm: Swedish Council for Building Research.

Esman, N. A. 1978. Characterization of contaminant concentrations in enclosed spaces. *Environ. Sci. Technol.* 12:337–39.

Eto, J. H., and Meyer, C. 1988. The HVAC costs of increased fresh air ventilation rates in office buildings. *ASHRAE Trans.* 94, Part 2:331–45.

Fanger, P. O. 1987. A solution to the sick-building mystery. In *Indoor air '87: Proceedings of the fourth international conference on indoor air quality and climate.* Ed. B. Seifert et al., Vol. 4, 49–56. Berlin: Institute for Water, Soil, and Air Hygiene.

Fossel, P. 1987. Sick home blues. *Harrowsmith* 11:46–55.

Franklin, B. 1906. Pennsylvania fireplaces. Reprinted in *Am. Soc. Heat. Vent. Eng. Trans.* 12.

Godish, T. 1989. *Indoor air pollution control.* Chelsea, Mich.: Lewis Publishers.

Haines, R. 1987. *Control systems for heating, ventilating, and air conditioning.* New York: Van Nostrand Reinhold Company.

Ingles, M. 1952. *Willis Haviland Carrier: Father of air conditioning.* Garden City, N.Y.: Country Life Press.

Ishizu, Y. 1980. General equation for the estimation of indoor pollution. *Am. Chem. Soc. Environ. Sci. Technol.* 14(10):1254–57.

Janssen, J. E. 1987. Ventilation for acceptable indoor air quality. In *Proceedings from IFMA '87, eighth annual international facility management conference and exposition,* 1–4 November. Dallas, Tex.

Jaquith, D. A.; McDavit, W. M.; and Reinert, J. C. 1987. Monitoring of air levels of termiticides in homes in the United States. In *Indoor air '87: Proceedings of the fourth international conference on indoor air quality and climate.* Ed. B. Seifert et al., Vol. 1, 230–34. Berlin: Institute for Water, Soil, and Air Hygiene.

Jorgensen, R., ed. 1983. *Air cleaning from fan engineering: An engineer's handbook on fans and their application,* 29.1–46. Buffalo, N.Y.: Buffalo Forge Company.

Jurinski, N. B. 1984. The evaluation of chlordane and heptachlor vapor concentrations within buildings treated for insect pest control. In *Proceedings of the third international conference on indoor air quality and climate.* Ed. B. Berglund, T. Lindvall, and J. Sundell, Vol. 4, 51–56. Stockholm, Sweden: Swedish Council for Building Research.

Lillie, T. H., and Barnes, E. S. 1987. Airborne termiticide levels in houses on United States Air Force installations. In *Indoor air '87: Proceedings of the fourth international conference on indoor air quality and climate.* Ed. B. Seifert et al., Vol. 1, 200–204. Berlin: Institute for Water, Soil, and Air Hygiene.

Maldonado, E. A. B. 1982. A method to characterize air exchange in residences for evaluation of indoor air quality. Ph.D. dissertation. Ames: Iowa State University.

Maldonado, E. A. B., and Woods, J. E. 1983. Ventilation efficiency as a means of characterizing air distribution in a building for indoor air quality evaluation. *ASHRAE Trans.* 89, Part 2b:496–506.

National Research Council. 1986. *The airline cabin environment: Air quality and safety.* Washington, D.C.: National Academy Press.

National Resource Council of Maine. 1987. *Tips on toxics: Suggested safe substitutes.* Augusta, Maine: NRC.

Nazaroff, W. W., and Nero, A. V. 1984. Transport of radon from soil into residences. In *Proceedings of the third international conference on indoor air quality and climate.* Ed. B. Berglund, T. Lindvall, and J. Sundell, Vol. 2, 15–20. Stockholm, Sweden: Swedish Council for Building Research.

Nazaroff, W. W., et al. 1987. Experiments on pollutant transport from soil into residential basements by pressure-driven airflow. *Environ. Sci. Technol.* 21(5):459–66.

New Shelter. 1982. *A test of small air cleaners.* Rodale Press, New Shelter, July/August: 49–57.

Offerman, F. J., et al. 1983. Ventilation efficiencies of wall-or-window-mounted residential air-to-air heat exchangers. *ASHRAE Trans.* 89, Part 2b:507–29.

Offerman, F. J., et al. 1985. Control of respirable particles in indoor air with portable air cleaners. *Atmos. Environ.* 19:1761–71.

Piersol, P., and Fugler, D. 1987. *Development and evaluation of soil gas sampling techniques for the research division, policy development and research sector. Final Report, P-5340/FG.* Ontario, Canada: Ontario Research Foundation, Canada Mortgage and Housing Corporation, and Gratner Lee Associates.

Qazi, A. H. 1987. Termiticides in indoor environments. In *Indoor air '87: Proceedings of the fourth international conference on indoor air quality and climate.* Ed. B. Seifert et al., Vol. 1. Berlin: Institute for Water, Soil, and Air Hygiene.

Sandburg, M. 1981. What is ventilation efficiency? *Build. Environ.* 16:123–35.

Sandburg, M. 1983. Ventilation efficiency as a guide to design. *ASHRAE Trans.* 89, Part 2:455–79.

Silverman, L., and Dennis, R. 1956. Removal of air-borne particulates and allergens by a portable electrostatic precipitator. *Air Cond. Heat. Ventil.* 53:75–80.

Silverman, L., and Dennis, R. 1959. Pollen removal by air filters. *Air Cond. Heat. Ventil.* 56:61–66.

Skaret, E. 1982. *Ventilation by stratification and displacement.* Trondheim, Norway: Norwegian Institute of Technology, Division of Heating and Ventilating. Publication no. N-7034.

Skaret, E., and Mathisen, H. M. 1983. Ventilation efficiency: A guide to efficient ventilation. *ASHRAE Trans.* 89, Part 2:480–95.

Small, B. 1983. *Indoor air pollution and housing: Technology.* Bookwood, Ontario, Canada: Loc IAO, Technology and Health Foundation.

Turk, A. 1963. Measurement of odorous vapors in test chambers: Theoretical considerations. *ASHRAE J.* October: 55–58.

Turk, A. 1968. *Concentrations of odorous vapors in test chambers: Basic principles of sensory evaluation;* 79–83. Philadelphia: American Society for Testing and Materials, Publication no. ASTM STP 433.

Turner, W. A., and Brennan, T. 1985. Radon's threat can be subdued. *Solar Age Mag.* 19–22.

Turner, W. A., and Bearg, D. W. 1987. Delivering "designed" cfm of outside air to the occupants, problems and solutions. Paper presented at ASHRAE IAQ '87, May, Washington, D.C.

Turner, W. A.; Bearg, D. W.; and Spengler, J. D. 1986. Indoor air quality evaluations, procedures and results. Presented at ASHRAE, IAQ-86: Managing Indoor Air for Health and Energy Conservation, 20–23 April, Atlanta, Ga.

Turner, W. A.; Bearg, D. W.; and Spengler, J. D. 1989. Diagnostic aspects of sick building syndrome: Comprehensive IAQ/HVAC system diagnostics for buildings with elevated IAQ complaint levels. Measurements of toxic and related air pollutants. In *Proceedings of the U.S. EPA/AWMA international symposium,* May, Raleigh, N.C.

Turner, W. A., et al. 1988. Defeating soil gas transport into residential and commercial structures. In *Proceedings of the EEBA, Energy Efficient Building Conference and Exposition,* 28–29 April, Portland, Maine.

U.S. Department of Energy. 1988. *Annual energy review.* Washington, D.C.: Energy Information Administration. Publication no. 0384(88).

U.S. Department of Health and Human Services. 1986. *The health consequences of involuntary smoking: A report of the surgeon general.* Washington, D.C.: Government Printing Office. DHHS Publication no. (CDC) 87/8398.

U.S. Environmental Protection Agency. 1987. *Radon reduction in new construction: An interim guide.* Washington, D.C.: Government Printing Office. Publication no. OPA/87/009.

U.S. Environmental Protection Agency. 1988. *Radon reduction techniques for detached houses: Technical guidance.* Research Triangle Park, N.C., Government Printing Office. Publication no. EPA/625/5-87/019.

van de Wiel, H., and Bloemen, H. 1987. The relation between soil pollution and indoor air pollution with volatile organic compounds. In *Indoor air '87: Proceedings of the fourth international conference on indoor air quality and climate.* Ed. B. Seifert et al., Vol. 1, 122–25. Berlin: Institute for Water, Soil, and Air Hygiene.

Whitby, K. T.; Anderson, G. R.; and Rubow, K. L. 1983. Dynamic method for evaluating room size air purifiers. *ASHRAE Trans.* 89:172–82.

Wilson, D. J. 1983. A design procedure for estimated air intake contamination from nearby exhaust events. *ASHRAE Trans.* 89:683–90.

Woods, J. E., and Crawford, R. R. 1989. Cost avoidance and productivity in owning and operating buildings. *Occupational Medicine: State of the Art Reviews,* Vol. 4, No. 4, 753–70. Philadelphia: Hanley & Belfus.

Woolrich, W. R. 1947. Mechanical refrigeration: It's America's birthright. Part II: *Refrig. Eng.* March/April:305–8.

Yaglou, C. P., and Witheridge, W. N. 1937. Ventilation requirements, part 2: *ASHVE Trans.* 43:423–36.

Yaglou, C. P.; Riley, E. C.; and Coggins, D. I. 1936. Ventilation requirements. *ASHVE Trans.* 42:133–62.

# 17

# LEGAL ASPECTS OF INDOOR AIR POLLUTION

Laurence S. Kirsch, M.S., J.D.

Increased knowledge about the possible dangers of indoor air pollution has created a different type of danger for a broad spectrum of the business community: the threat of massive lawsuits. Complaints from office workers concerning fatigue, headaches, respiratory and skin irritation, and stress in particular indoor environments have been reported for years but often have resulted in nothing more than ostracism and, perhaps, a referral to a psychiatrist.

Emerging information about the "sick-building syndrome" and the increased public awareness that has resulted from increased media attention have changed that picture markedly. Armed with new data that appear to show health effects from passive cigarette smoke, formaldehyde, radon, asbestos, and other substances, as well as from "tight buildings" themselves (buildings with inadequate ventilation), plaintiffs who believe that they have been injured by the air inside their homes or offices are beginning to take the offensive. They are lobbying on the local, state, and federal levels for protective legislation, and in the absence of such legislation, they are suing for both damages to their health and damages to their property.

These cases are complex not only in the nature of the technical proof that must be developed and presented, but also in the number of parties involved. In cases in which plaintiffs cannot readily identify one particular defendant that can be held responsible for their injuries, some plaintiffs have opted to sue every possible defendant in sight. One such case involved approximately two hundred named and unnamed defendants (*Buckley* v. *Kruger-Benson-Ziemer*).

The building industry faces particular risk. Suits have been filed against architects, builders, contractors, building product manufacturers, and realtors. The possible scope of liability extends further, however, to building owners, building sellers, and, in the commercial context, employers. Even utilities may find themselves in court because of their role in encouraging tighter building envelopes.

The first section of this chapter reviews the liability potential for workplace indoor air pollution by highlighting the legal bases that have been employed, that are now being employed, and that may be employed in the future in indoor pollution litigation against parties such as architects, contractors, and product manufacturers. The second section raises certain problems posed by these lawsuits for plaintiffs and defendants alike. The third section discusses the status of lawsuits that have been brought concerning indoor air pollution and the sick-building syndrome.

## CAUSES OF ACTIONS IN INDOOR POLLUTION LITIGATION

Six basic legal theories create rights upon which individuals injured by indoor air pollution often sue for recompense. Knowledge of the legal theories, which overlap substantially, is important because different theories may permit recovery against different defendants. A seventh catch-all category of miscellaneous legal theories is included to illustrate some less-used possibilities for claiming legal liability.

### CONTRACTUAL OBLIGATIONS/EXPRESSED WARRANTIES

Expressed warranties are positive representations made by the seller of a product to the purchaser. They can arise in any transaction between any two parties and can appear in sales contracts, labels, advertising, or samples. In one case relevant to this discussion (*Bradley* v. *Brucker*), a seller of a house was aware that a buyer had a lung condition that made him sensitive to moisture. The seller warranted in the purchase agreement that the basement would be dry except for condensation. But within four months of the house purchase, water appeared in the basement. The court found a breach of the expressed warranty. A similar case (*Alfieri* v. *Cabot Corp.*) involved a label on a bag of charcoal representing that the charcoal was "[ideal] for cooking, in or out of doors." The charcoal was used to cook steaks outdoors, but the smoldering grill was later brought inside a cabin. One person died from carbon monoxide poisoning, and another became ill. The charcoal company was held liable, based in part on the expressed warranty. Breach of written warranty claims are common in formaldehyde exposure cases, particularly those involving mobile homes (e.g., *Mobile America Sales Corp.* v. *Smith*).

Liability for breach of an expressed warranty, where such a breach can be proved, is attractive for plaintiffs because of its simplicity. Liability depends not on any particular knowledge of fault by the seller, but only on the falsity of the representation.

Employers may seek to rely on expressed warranties in suing companies who have supplied products that pollute the workplace, in breach of affirmative representations. Cases in which injured individuals file lawsuits involving breaches of expressed warranties, however, are more likely to arise in the residential than in the commercial context. In the residential setting, the injured individual is more likely to be the person to whom the warranty was extended. In the work environment, employees have more limited control over their surroundings. They are probably not involved in purchasing decisions concerning the work environment and, therefore, would not have been the direct recipients of expressed warranties. An employee might have to argue that he or she was the intended third-party beneficiary of an expressed warranty made by a seller of a dangerous building product to the employer. Such a showing might not be difficult where employees use dangerous products labeled by a manufacturer for the employees' safety.

CONTRACTUAL OBLIGATIONS/IMPLIED WARRANTIES

Even where the seller of goods makes no expressed warranties, the courts imply certain fundamental warranties. For example, goods are implicitly warranted to be fit for the ordinary purposes for which they are used. A plaintiff who suffered respiratory injury from the release of irritating fumes while using a bathroom cleaner prevailed in a suit against the manufacturer because the product was not fit for ordinary use (*Shirley* v. *The Drackett Products Co.*).

Any product that creates noxious indoor pollutants may be argued to be unfit for its ordinary use. A kerosene heater that, in its normal operation, asphyxiates the occupants of a room clearly would not be fit for its ordinary use. Similarly, if urea-formaldehyde foam insulation or particleboard releases formaldehyde gas into a building, rendering the indoor air dangerous, the product may breach its implied warranty. Nonetheless, courts are still wrestling with the precise bounds of the implied warranty protection. In particular, courts have taken divergent views concerning liability for the reactions of individuals particularly sensitive to certain chemicals. In a case involving exposure to formaldehyde leading to severe and permanent asthma, a plaintiff was required to show that a reasonably foreseeable and appreciable number of users who are exposed to the product would suffer some ill effect, but the plaintiff was not required to show that other users would suffer a reaction as severe as that experienced by the plaintiff (*Tiderman* v. *Fleetwood Homes of Washington*).

Using a theory counteracting traditional notions of *caveat emptor*, courts have decided that buildings themselves carry implied warranties: warranties of fitness for human habitation (see *Elderkin* v. *Gaster*; *Waggoner* v. *Midwestern Development*; *Jones* v. *Gatewood*; *Davis and DeLaTorre* 1984). Such warranties usually run from the original builder or vendor of the building, and in many states, the warranty is not limited to the first purchaser. In one case, for example, the third buyers of a house were awarded damages from a builder when they discovered strong formaldehyde odors from the original carpet and padding installed in the building. The odors made the house uninhabitable, breaching the warranty of habitability (*Blagg* v. *Fred Hunt Co.*).

It is uncertain, however, whether implied warranties of habitability apply to commercial as well as residential property. In at least some jurisdictions, the services of architects and engineers are subject to their own implied warranties. The courts often deem that architects and engineers warrant, by implication, that the plans and specifications they produce will yield a structure reasonably fit for its

380   Laurence S. Kirsch

intended purpose (e.g., *Bloomsburg Mills* v. *Sordoni Construction Co.*). A structure with unhealthy levels of indoor contaminants may breach this implied warranty, subjecting architects and engineers to possible liability. In some states, such as California, the implied warranty of fitness for human habitation has been extended to landlord-tenant relationships. Tenants are now able to sue for injuries caused by unfit housing owned by landlords. Some states impose this obligation by statute. See, for example, Minn. Stat. 504.18(1)(a). In such states, injured employees may be able to sue their employer's landlord, alleging a breach of the implied warranty of habitability by the commercial landlord. Buildings that do not provide for adequate ventilation or that contain products emitting hazardous fumes may subject their owners to liability. Some states, however, require a showing that the landlord had knowledge of the condition before awarding judgment for the plaintiffs (e.g., *Meyer* v. *Parkin*).

NEGLIGENCE

Negligence is probably the most familiar basis for liability and is perhaps the most broadly applicable. Negligence is simply a failure to exercise due care, defined as the degree of care that would be exercised by a "reasonable person." Individuals may be found negligent in the performance of services or in the manufacture of products. An architect might be deemed negligent in designing a building without adequate ventilation or by specifying the use of unsafe products in the building; an insulation contractor might be negligent if the mixing of urea-formaldehyde insulation was improper and resulted in the release of formaldehyde gas; the manufacturer of a kerosene heater may be negligent in failing to provide adequate warnings that the heater should be used only in well-ventilated areas.

In some situations, certain individuals can be held responsible for the negligence of others. For example, a homeowner has recovered against a builder for the asphyxiation of her husband from carbon monoxide leaking from a gas heater that was incorrectly installed in the house by a subcontractor (*Dow* v. *Holly Mfg. Co.*).

For both plaintiffs and defendants, however, negligence actions have severe drawbacks. The plaintiff must show that the defendant's conduct was unreasonable. The obvious difficulty is in determining the necessary measures that constitute "due care." Negligence actions are inherently unpredictable. Different judges or juries faced with similar facts may arrive at different conclusions. These ambiguities place possible defendants in a cloud of uncertainty; they cannot know what is expected of them because the standards always shift. Will building owners or utilities be held liable to later purchasers for negligently weatherizing their structures so tightly that indoor pollutants are not able to escape? Will realtors be held negligent for failing to test and disclose levels of indoor pollutants?

As knowledge about indoor air pollution increases, building professionals will increasingly be required to consider the consequences of their actions on the indoor environment. The precise contours of the emerging obligation can be drawn only by future litigation. Negligence actions also force the parties to deal with defenses such as contributory negligence and assumption of risk.

Strict liability applies to liability for defective products. Strict liability does not depend on "fault," as does negligence. This theory of liability shifts the focus of legal inquiry from conduct of the manufacturer to the product itself. In some cases, courts have taken strict liability a step further, holding a manufacturer liable for defects that were scientifically unknowable at the time of the product's manufacture. A product can be defective either because of its manufacture or its design. For example, urea-formaldehyde foam insulation that offgases formaldehyde vapors because the constituent chemicals were not mixed in the proper proportions may be considered to have a manufacturing defect. On the other hand, a mobile home that contains dangerous components or that does not permit sufficient ventilation may be deemed defectively designed (*Heritage* v. *Pioneer Brokerage & Sales*). If a product cannot be made safe, the manufacturer must provide adequate warnings that would render it safe for use. A manufacturer of a gas heater, for example, was held liable in a case in which it failed to provide adequate warnings concerning the proper height of the chimney, and a person who used the heater without a proper chimney died from asphyxiation (*Wallinger* v. *Martin Stamping and Stove Co.*).

Defendants in strict liability cases have frequently relied upon a "state-of-the-art" defense, arguing that they had insufficient knowledge for liability to be appropriate. In a 1987 decision, the Supreme Court of Hawaii held that a defendant's knowledge is irrelevant in a strict liability case. The court decided that since strict liability causes of action are based upon the inherently dangerous nature of the product, the state-of-the-art defense is precluded. Thus, a manufacturer can be held liable to plaintiffs for injuries brought about by a defective product even when there was no knowledge of danger at the time of production (*Johnson* v. *Raybestos-Manhattan, Inc.*). Courts in at least two other states have handed down similar decisions (*Beshada* v. *Johns-Manville Products Corp.*; *Carrecter* v. *Colson Equipment Co.*).

Recovery under a strict liability theory is not limited to the purchaser of the product. Anyone injured by a defective product, including employees in the work environment, can sue. The relative ease of recovery under a strict liability theory makes product liability suits attractive to plaintiffs; they are dreaded by defendants. The key limitation of strict liability in the indoor environment is that it applies only to products. In some but not all jurisdictions, a building itself is a product subject to strict products liability. Although strict liability was at first extended only to mass-produced buildings (*Kriegler* v. *Eichler Homes*), it has been applied more recently to non-mass-produced buildings as well (*McDonald* v. *Mianecki*). In such jurisdictions, plaintiffs may seek to employ strict liability in suits against the builders of commercial buildings now known to have unhealthy indoor air. A necessary corollary of the strict liability theory is that it can be used only against the manufacturer of the product or the builder of a building. It probably cannot constitute the basis for suits against architects, realtors, or utilities.

States impose a different set of obligations on the sellers of property. In general, a seller and the seller's real estate agent must not misrepresent any important fact about the property being sold. Innocent as well as knowing misrepresentations may trigger liability (*Spargnapani* v. *Wright*). Moreover, silence is often insufficient. Sellers are usually obligated to disclose serious latent defects in the property sold, whether or not the buyer asks about them (*Quashnock* v. *Frost*; *Maples* v. *Porath* [termite infestation]; *Cooper* v. *Jevne* [substandard construction]; *Weintraub* v. *Krobatsch* [roaches]. But see *Diaz* v. *Keyes Co.* (1962), in which there was no obligation to disclose. Nor can sellers make statements recklessly. For example, even a general statement that "everything's fine" with the property can give rise to liability when that statement is made in reckless disregard of the truth (*Hammond* v. *Matthes*).

Employers may sue the prior owners of business property (or their agents) for misrepresentation or fraud in the purchase of land. It is likely that similar suits could be filed against landlords by employers that lease their property. Whether injured employees could successfully sue based on misrepresentations made to their employers, however, is somewhat more speculative.

A 1987 federal district court decision illustrates how a misrepresentation/fraud theory can be applied to an indoor air pollution situation (*Barth* v. *Firestone Tire and Rubber Co.*). An employee sued his employer for exposure to a variety of industrial toxins. The plaintiff's attorneys argued that the claim fell outside the exclusivity provisions of the state's workers' compensation system. The attorneys alleged that the employer fraudulently concealed its knowledge of the injury and denied and disguised the use of dangerous substances in order to avoid regulation. Although the court rejected the plaintiff's willful assault theory, it was convinced by the argument of fraudulent concealment.

In *Bardura* v. *Orkin* (1987), a chlordane poisoning case, the plaintiffs alleged that the company had used unfair or deceptive means to persuade the plaintiffs to purchase pest control services for a termite problem that did not exist. The jury returned a verdict for the plaintiffs.

### LANDOWNER OR LAND OCCUPIER LIABILITY

Owners or occupiers of land have an obligation to protect their business invitees on the land. This obligation extends not only to dangers actually known to the owner or occupier, but also to defects discoverable through the exercise of reasonable care (e.g., *F.W. Woolworth Co.* v. *Williams*). For example, if a customer of a business is injured by indoor air pollution while on the business premises, the business would be liable if it knew or should have known of the danger. Whether the business owned the premises or leased them would not affect its liability.

Whether the landlord of property leased to a business remains liable for the condition of the property is a separate question. Although lessors of land traditionally did not owe any obligations to their lessees, the traditional rules have been changed by the application of implied warranties of habitability to the lessor-lessee relationship. Even under the more traditional doctrine, landlords are obligated to disclose concealed dangerous conditions unknown to the lessee. Moreover, landlords remain liable for parts of the premises that remain under their control, such as hallways or lobbies (Prosser 1971).

Thus, employees injured by indoor air pollution may be able to sue the owners of the business premises in which they work, assuming that the property is owned by someone other than the employer. Moreover, employees may attempt suits directly against the employer. Although workers' compensation schemes normally bar such direct suits, employees have attempted to circumvent the bar by alleging that the employer acted intentionally (*Blankenship* v. *Cincinnati Milacron Chemicals*) or by employing the dual capacity doctrine based on the employer's obligations as an owner or occupier of the property (*Duprey* v. *Shane*; *Panagos* v. *North Detroit General Hospital*). Such suits are more likely to prevail when the business premises are open to the general public.

Commercial leases and sale contracts often contain provisions disclaiming any obligations by the landlord or buyer. Yet other provisions require that the tenant or buyer indemnify the current owner for any liability relating to the property. Although courts have not hesitated to invalidate, based on unconscionability, disclaimer provisions when applied to homeowners who were not aware of the meaning of these provisions, the courts would probably not interfere when more sophisticated commercial concerns agree to disclaimers (U.C.C. Section 2–719, 1977, unconscionability of limitations on consequential damages for personal injury). Nonetheless, disclaimers might serve only to prevent suits by the employer against its landlord and might not affect suits by other injured individuals. Indemnification provisions, similarly, would not affect the liability of the landlord but might give the landlord certain rights to sue the tenant—the employer—to recover any judgments paid to injured employees. The permissibility of such a claim is generally governed by workers' compensation statutes because the claim would make the employer liable for the injuries of its employees (Weisgall 1977). Commercial leases also typically require both parties to maintain insurance, and such insurance may cover all or part of the loss.

MISCELLANEOUS LEGAL THEORIES

Some employees have brought suit alleging that their sensitivity to indoor air pollution is a handicap that entitles them to protected status. The court in *Vickers* v. *Veterans Administration* (1982) agreed that an employee who was "unusually sensitive to tobacco smoke" was handicapped within the meaning of the Vocational Rehabilitation Act. The court further held, however, that since the Veterans Administration had made reasonable accommodation efforts, no discrimination had occurred.

Assault and battery is another legal theory of liability plaintiffs can use to try to obtain redress for their injuries from indoor air pollution. Such a claim was made by an employee (*McCracken* v. *Sloan*) who was subjected to cigar smoke. The court held, however, that consent to such ordinary contacts is assumed.

Other possible claims for plaintiffs in indoor air pollution cases include nuisance, infliction of emotional distress, conspiracy, and equitable remedies.

## BARRIERS FOR PLAINTIFFS AND DEFENDANTS
## IN INDOOR AIR LITIGATION

Litigants seeking compensation for personal injury or property damages face all of the barriers normally attendant to parties of toxic tort actions. Both plaintiffs and defendants face substantial difficulties involving the investigation, proof, and presentation of highly complex technical issues at the frontiers of scientific knowledge. In addition, the parties face other theoretical and practical hurdles that will be discussed below.

### BARRIERS FOR PLAINTIFFS

*Statutes of Limitations*   Long latency periods for the manifestations of some diseases often bring plaintiffs' claims into conflict with applicable statutes of limitation that require suits to be filed within a certain time of the injury. The critical distinction with which the courts have wrestled is whether the time period starts to run from the exposure to a hazardous substance or from the date of discovery of the injury.

In the last couple of years, some states have changed their statutes of limitation for toxic tort litigation so that plaintiffs have a better chance of having their claims heard. For instance, New York has adopted the "discovery" rule, which starts the clock when the plaintiffs knew or should have known of their injury (L 1986, Ch. 682, 4).

Questions as to whether the statute of limitations has run can become quite complex. In *Vincent* v. *A.C. & S., Inc.* (1987), the U.S. Court of Appeals for the Fifth Circuit had to decide whether a settlement between the plaintiff and several asbestos manufacturers constituted a "voluntary dismissal" that would time-bar the plaintiff from amending the complaint to add claims against other manufacturers. Although Louisiana has a one-year statute of limitations, under state law it is interrupted by a suit on the same cause of action and it resumes once the suit is no longer pending unless the suit is "voluntarily dismissed" by the plaintiff. The court ruled that the settlement was not a voluntary dismissal. In *Huff* v. *Fibreboard Corp.* (1987), a widow filed suit within two months of her husband's death from asbestosis in 1979. The U.S. Court of Appeals for the Tenth Circuit ruled that the husband should have known of his condition as of 1975, when he visited a doctor about lung problems. The court held that the widow's claim was time-barred by Oklahoma's two-year statute of limitations.

*Proof of Causation of the Alleged Injury*   Plaintiffs must prove that the injury they claim to be suffering was inflicted by the cause alleged. The ease with which such showings can be made varies with the particular source of injury: proof of a causal relationship between asbestos exposure and asbestosis or mesothelioma is far simpler than proof of a relationship between tightly insulated houses and radon exposure, and in turn, between radon exposure and lung cancer. Similarly, proof that nose or throat irritation was caused by formaldehyde vapors or passive cigarette smoke may be difficult.

In order to provide medical causation, plaintiffs may have to rely on toxicity data from studies conducted on the dangerous substance in question. Laypeople on a jury may have difficulty understanding information of such a technical and scientific nature. Sometimes the plaintiff may have to rely on a novel theory of injury. Expert testimony in support of such a theory is particularly susceptible to being offset by expert testimony that the theory is unproven or unaccepted by some in the medical community. Testimony in support of a novel theory of causation may even be barred if the court decides that the scientific community has not generally accepted the theory. Proof of causation is complicated further by the fact that an illness can frequently be caused by multiple factors.

As scientific knowledge grows and as additional cases are litigated, the burden of proving causality may ease. Already, various proposals have been made to ease this burden by shifting presumptions in favor of the plaintiff once the plaintiff makes a limited threshold showing of injury (Trauberman 1983). Another development that will benefit plaintiffs is the practice of awarding medical monitoring costs when there may be future health effects (e.g., *Barth* v. *Firestone Tire and Rubber Co.*).

Given the large number of parties potentially responsible for high levels of indoor pollution in a building, a plaintiff may have difficulty showing that any individual defendant should be liable. For example, courts will have to decide who should bear the burden of injuries from high levels of combustion pollutants in a well-insulated structure: the manufacturers of the gas stove and furnace, the architect who designed the tightly insulated building, the builder who built it, or the owner of the structure who directed that the building be energy efficient. Each party, from a technical standpoint, is in some way responsible for the ambient levels present in the building.

*Proof of a Nexus between Cause of Injury and the Defendant*   Employees who can manage to sue within the applicable statute of limitations period and show that their injuries were caused by exposure to a certain hazardous substance must nonetheless show that the particular defendants they are suing should be held liable for that exposure. In the asbestos personal injury cases now overloading the nation's courts, for example, shipyard workers have often been exposed to the asbestos of numerous different manufacturers. These workers, not knowing which manufacturers' asbestos caused their injuries, typically sue all of the companies, and the courts have been required to find ways to apportion liability. Some courts have held that all manufacturers should be "jointly and severally liable" for the entire injury (*Borel* v. *Fibreboard Paper Products Corp.*). Some courts have chosen to apportion liability according to the individual companies' market shares (*Sindell* v. *Abbott Laboratories*). Yet other courts have discussed an "enterprise liability" scheme, involving a broad application of joint and several liability on all manufacturers involved coupled with a loosened causation requirement (*Hall* v. *E.I. DuPont de Nemours and Co.*). It remains to be seen whether any of these theories is extended and applied to indoor pollution litigation.

*Practical Barriers*   Toxic tort litigation is costly and unpredictable. The high transaction costs of litigating personal injury cases and the lengthy delays before receipt of final compensation, assuming that compensation is awarded, discourage trials for all but the most severe injuries.

One of the primary practical barriers to plaintiffs in indoor air pollution litigation apparently is the identification of the appropriate defendant. In the context of most occupational injuries, the manufacturer of a particular product can usually be identified and held responsible for the injury. The simplicity of suing for product liability often leads employees injured in the workplace to sue the manufacturer of the product that injured them. In some indoor air pollution cases, plaintiffs can also sue a manufacturer, such as the manufacturer of formaldehyde insulation, the manufacturer of a defective ventilation system, or the manufacturer of a defective heater.

Not all indoor air pollutants, however, result from a manufactured product. Radon, for example, is a natural element present in the soil, water, and air. In seeking compensation for injuries from such pollutants, therefore, the identification of the appropriate defendant or defendants for a claim may be more difficult. Nonetheless, creative legal minds can construct new chains of causation that point the finger of liability at some solvent party. For example, a plaintiff can sue the company that weatherized the building so tightly that radon could not escape, the architect who designed the building with inadequate ventilation, or the contractor who laid the foundation with the crack that allowed the radon to seep into the building. Each of these chains of causation must be factually justified, and as the cause becomes more remote, the chance of recovery becomes smaller. Of course, in those jurisdictions in which a building is considered a product subject to strict liability law, a plaintiff could allege that a building with excessive interior concentrations of radon is itself a defective product for which its builder should be strictly liable.

Employees who suffer from indoor air pollution in the workplace may file a workers' compensation claim. An injured worker may also decide to institute a suit against a third party. Most states have workers' compensation systems that forbid any lawsuit against the employer. In such a situation the employee will often sue one or more third parties in order to overcome the workers' compensation exclusivity provision. The third-party defendant (frequently the building owner or operator) can then bring the employer into the suit by various methods, including filing a cross-claim. Third-party suits are often attractive because the plaintiff is not subjected to the law ceilings on recovery imposed by workers' compensation schemes. In addition to the larger compensatory damages available, injured plaintiffs may also be awarded punitive damages (in excess of the actual injuries sustained). Each of these advantages translates into distinct disadvantages for the defendants in common lawsuits, who may be subjected to large jury verdicts for conduct that cannot be characterized as blameworthy and for injuries partially caused by the employee's or employer's own negligence.

A claim of intentional conduct on the part of the employer is another method employees are using to take their claims out of the exclusive province of some workers' compensation schemes. To make the requisite showing, an employee may not hope to prove that the employer intended to harm the employee, but only that the employer intended to expose the employee to dangerous substances. Some courts, however, have required a showing that the employer intended to harm the employee (*Prescott* v. *United States*; *Evans* v. *Allentown Portland Cement Co.*; *Castlebury* v. *Frost-Johnson Lumber*).

The dual capacity doctrine has been used as a device to enable an employee to sue the employer in an indoor air pollution situation. When the employer is acting in some capacity in addition to that of an employer, the employee can name the employer as a defendant in that other capacity. An example would be an employee suing the landlord or the manufacturer of the harmful product who also happens to be the employer.

Employees have also succeeded in suing their employers directly by alleging a fraudulent concealment of a hazardous condition in the workplace. For example, in *Johns-Manville Products Corp.* v. *Superior Court of Contra Costa County* (1980), the California Supreme Court ruled that an employee could sue his employer based on an allegation that the employer had fraudulently concealed its knowledge that the employee was suffering from a disease caused by the ingestion of asbestos and had fraudulently concealed the hazardous nature of the asbestos to which the employee was exposed. Courts have not uniformly adopted this exception, however. Other courts still hold that allegations of fraudulent concealment do not take the claim out of the exclusive workers' compensation system (*Kofron* v. *Amoco Chemicals Corp.*).

BARRIERS FOR DEFENDANTS

Defendants face barriers at least as substantial as those faced by plaintiffs in indoor air liability suits. Defendants can be subject to baseless nuisance suits that are brought solely for the purpose of coercing a settlement. Faced with such a suit, a defendant has the unpleasant choice of paying funds in order to settle a claim that has no foundation, thereby making itself a possible target for future baseless claims, or of bearing the substantial costs of defending the case. The cost of defending nonfrivolous claims is considerable as well. In the workplace environment, lawsuits by employees who claim they have been injured by the building in which they work can also have an effect on the morale of other employees. Once one employee makes such a claim, other employees are likely to question whether certain symptoms of theirs might be related to the workplace as well. If not addressed appropriately, a claim of sick-building syndrome raised by one employee can soon engulf an employer in a multitude of claims and grievances. That all of these claims may have no relationship to the building is difficult for the employer to establish.

## STATUS OF INDOOR AIR LIABILITY SUITS

Notwithstanding the barriers to recovery, suits that can be characterized as indoor air pollution liability suits are multiplying. A discussion follows of the current state of legal actions in the area of indoor air pollution.

### FORMALDEHYDE

Suits for personal injuries or property damage relating to exposure to formaldehyde, typically either from urea-formaldehyde foam insulation or from particleboard in mobile homes, have burgeoned during and after the Consumer Products Safety Commission investigation and eventual ban on urea-formaldehyde foam insulation in 1982. (The ban was overturned by the U.S. Court of Appeals for the Fifth Circuit in *Gulf South Insulation* v. *Consumer Product Safety Commission*).

More than two thousand formaldehyde-related lawsuits have been filed in the United States, and many more suits have been filed in Canada. At least three of these suits have led to jury verdicts in excess of $500,000. Numerous out-of-court settlements have also involved six-figure sums. Formaldehyde suits have named as defendants—in addition to the manufacturers of the formaldehyde—architects, builders, building contracting companies, building product manufacturers, and realtors.

Several cases are proceeding as class action lawsuits on behalf of numerous parties, but a number of courts have refused to certify formaldehyde cases for class action procedures because the differences among the cases can be greater than their similarities, necessitating an individualized approach (*Caruso* v. *Celsius Insulation Resources*; *Brummett* v. *Skyline Corp.*; *Kegley* v. *Borden, Inc.*; *Delaney* v. *Borden, Inc.*).

As of the end of 1987, formaldehyde litigation was declining. A number of factors can be cited as significant causes of this decline. First of all, after the 1982 ban on urea-formaldehyde foam insulation, its use virtually ceased. Second, for the last five to ten years formaldehyde product emissions have been significantly reduced by the industry's adoption of various corrective measures. Third, the extent of victims' injuries is usually relatively minor and nonspecific. Fourth, formaldehyde plaintiffs have the usual difficulty of trying to establish causation. Fifth, there has been a decrease in both publicity and public awareness about health risks associated with formaldehyde. Other indoor air pollutants, such as radon and chlordane, have become the story of the day. Sixth, many producers, distributors, and installers of formaldehyde which might be named as defendants have filed for bankruptcy. Finally, most urea formaldehyde foam insulation cases that have been brought to trial have resulted in defense verdicts.

At least one family living in a house contaminated with high levels of radon gas sued a company that operated a nearby uranium mine that produced the mill tailings placed in and around the foundation of their house. The court agreed that the plaintiffs were entitled to a trial on whether the presence of the radon had forcibly evicted them from their house, agreeing that the defendant's actions may have "constituted a denial of physical access to the property." The court also permitted claims for punitive damages and for chromosomal damage that had occurred as a result of the radon exposure (*Brafford* v. *Susquehanna Corp.*). The litigants settled the case, terms of the accord are confidential.

Other suits have also been filed on behalf of plaintiffs owning houses built on uranium mill tailings. At least one other radon lawsuit is being contemplated on behalf of an owner of a house that has elevated radon levels not attributable to mill tailings. That homeowner was forced to expend substantial sums of money to isolate the source of and reduce high radon concentrations in his energy-efficient house. This lawsuit would be directed principally against a ventilating contractor who installed a defective ventilating system that permitted radon from soil to enter the house's air supply.

A panel of arbitrators recently decided a radon suit that involved a real estate transaction. The contract included an escape clause that allowed the buyer to cancel the contract in the event radon levels were found to be "unsatisfactory." The buyer invoked this clause, and the seller, who had to accept a lower price as a consequence, sued the buyer for the difference. The panel of arbitrators held in the buyer's favor and said the buyer was not liable for the decrease in value that resulted from the knowledge of radon levels.

## CHLORDANE AND OTHER PESTICIDES

Numerous suits have been filed involving the termiticide chlordane. In *Cunningham* v. *Orkin*, the plaintiffs succeeded in recovering for pain and suffering, the removal and rebuilding of the house, the contents of the house, and medical monitoring costs. The issue of punitive damages is still in dispute in this case. *Tuttle* v. *Tindol Services* resulted in a verdict of compensatory and punitive damages for the plaintiffs because of a finding that the company was negligent in applying the chemicals. The company admitted at trial that it had misapplied the termiticide.

A chlordane suit brought under a state consumer protection act alleged that the defendant mistakenly drilled holes into heat ducts and contaminated the home. The case settled for $730,000 (*Steingaszner* v. *Paramount Pest Control*).

However, in *Rabb* v. *Orkin* (1987), a South Carolina court denied a plaintiff's motion that there was sufficient evidence for a jury finding that the company was not negligent in applying the pest control chemicals to the plaintiff's home. The court ruled that the exclusion of the plaintiff's expert witness's testimony was proper where the witness would not quantify the increased health risks.

On April 21, 1988, a federal grand jury in Roanoke, Virginia, indicted Orkin

Exterminating Co. on five criminal counts of violating federal pesticide laws when its employees allegedly misapplied the pesticide Vikane, an action that the Environmental Protection Agency said resulted in the deaths of the two residents of the home in which the pesticide was applied (*U.S.* v. *Orkin Exterminating Co.*). The indictment seeks a fine of $1.7 million for alleged violations of the Federal Insecticide, Fungicide, and Rodenticide Act, which governs the labeling and use of pesticides. The specific charges alleged that the company allowed a fumigated site to be occupied before the fumigation was complete, removed a warning sign before aeration of the site was complete, failed to remove pillows and mattresses from the house, failed to use a warning agent before fumigation, and failed to use appropriate breathing apparatus in applying the pesticide. The two Orkin applicators were charged previously with involuntary manslaughter and had received suspended sentences.

TOBACCO SMOKE

Nonsmokers continue filing suit to win and enforce their rights to a smoke-free work environment. In at least one such case, a smoker intervened in a lawsuit after a co-worker won a temporary restraining order banning smoking in her work area. The smoker succeeded in frustrating the nonsmoker's attempt to obtain a preliminary injunction in the same case (*Lee* v. *Department of Public Welfare*). Judicial challenges to new state and local antismoking legislation seem inevitable.

ASBESTOS

Personal injury lawsuits by asbestos workers continue to proliferate; approximately twenty-five thousand such suits are pending nationwide. Although asbestos in buildings may pose no health problem whatsoever, suits concerning liability for the removal of asbestos have been deemed the "second wave" of asbestos litigation. Many of these "rip and replace" suits have been filed on behalf of school districts; the largest such case is a $1.4 billion class action in federal district court in Philadelphia on behalf of all public school districts and private schools nationwide (*In Re Asbestos School Litigation*). Private companies have hardly begun to sue for their costs in removing asbestos. Unlike public schools, private buildings need not be inspected for asbestos, nor has asbestos exposure in private buildings attracted as much public attention or concern. Private parties may not yet have undertaken programs for the removal of asbestos which would result in property damage suits.

At least one court has decided that the presence of asbestos in a building does not give rise to a property damage claim under an insurance policy (*U.S. Fidelity and Guaranty Co.* v. *Wilkin Insulation Co.*). In another case, hospitals were denied class action status in their suit against manufacturers to pay for the removal of asbestos (*Sisters of St. Mary et al.* v. *Aaer Sprayed Insulation et al.*).

Personal injury suits by individuals exposed to asbestos in buildings may prove to be the third wave of asbestos litigation. For example, in *Swogger* v. *Waterman Steamship Corp.* (1987), the court allowed shipowners to seek indemnification from manufacturers and distributors of asbestos put in ships. The shipowners had reached a settlement with the estate of an engineer who had died of malignant mesothelioma, allegedly caused by exposure to asbestos. In another case, a plaintiff recovered more than $500,000 from the original seller of a fireproofing material in Ohio. The company knew that the asbestos product was dangerous, but it did not warn the parties who might be harmed (*Layne* v. *GAF Corp.*). In Chicago, two widows whose husbands allegedly died from asbestos exposure each recently settled their claims with the manufacturers for close to $1 million (*Brennan* v. *Celotex*; *Wessels* v. *Celotex*). At least one court has ruled that asbestos manufacturers have a continuing duty to warn those who have been exposed to asbestos of the hazards they face, even after exposure has ended. This duty was held to be especially strong where such a warning could have reduced or removed the danger. The court in *Lockwood* v. *A.C. & S. Inc.* (1987) ruled that the plaintiff's injury might have been reduced if he had been advised to stop smoking.

Other procedural and substance aspects of asbestos cases are currently being addressed by pending litigation and court decisions.

The Illinois Supreme Court is considering the issue of whether punitive damages should be allowed for an asbestos-related illness. Such a finding would have to be based on evidence that the defendant knew that there were dangers associated with the product at the time the injury was incurred. The court is reviewing the punitive damages award handed down by the jury in *Donald Lipke* v. *Celotex* (1987). At least four states (Louisiana, Massachusetts, Nebraska, and Washington) do not allow awards for punitive damages whereas several other states (Connecticut, Michigan, and New Hampshire) limit such awards. Only a few courts have upheld punitive damages awards in asbestos cases.

In an asbestos case in which the responsible tortfeasor could not be identified, plaintiffs were unsuccessful in getting the court to adopt a theory of collective liability as a basis for relief. The plaintiff had attempted to use a market share approach to hold more than twenty defendants liable for his injury from asbestos exposure (*Case* v. *Fibreboard Corp.*). Whereas this approach has worked for the single product of diethylstilbestrol, it has been unsuccessful in cases in which asbestos-related injuries have resulted from numerous products.

The state-of-the-art defense has been precluded for defendants in two recent asbestos decisions. In *In Re Asbestos Litigation*, the U.S. Court of Appeals for the Third Circuit agreed with New Jersey Supreme Court decisions that had abolished such a defense in asbestos personal injury suits (829 F. 2d 1233, 3rd Cir. 1987) (see also *Johnson* v. *Raybestos-Manhattan* [1987]).

There has been a difference of opinion between courts in Pennsylvania and Illinois as to whether the diagnosis of alleged asbestosis and subsequent diagnosis of alleged asbestos-related cancer constitute two separate causes of action with reference to the statute of limitations. The court in *Roush* v. *GAF Corp.* (1987) ruled that these two diagnoses were the basis for only a single cause of action. In *VaSalle* v. *Celotex Corp.* (1987), the court held that asbestosis and asbestos-related cancer were two distinct diseases, and, therefore, each gives rise to its own cause of action. Thus, the suit for asbestos-related cancer was not time-barred by a two-year statute of limitations even though a diagnosis of asbestosis had been made three years earlier.

In a twist on the usual theme of legal claims, a former asbestos manufacturer that had been paying asbestos injury claims filed suit in a federal district court in Kansas claiming that many of these claims were fraudulent. The manufacturer named lawyers, medical experts, and the workers as defendants. The suit was filed under the federal Racketeer Influenced and Concept Organizations Act and claimed that physical exams of workers were either inadequate or false and that the doctors were not qualified (*Raymark Industries, Inc.* v. *Stemple*).

SICK-BUILDING SYNDROME AND MISCELLANEOUS INDOOR AIR POLLUTION CASES

Plaintiffs unable to identify particular pollutants that are responsible for their alleged injuries have begun to file court suits and workers' compensation claims alleging that they suffer from sick-building syndrome and, therefore, are entitled to recovery from the named defendants.

Perhaps the first of these cases is *Buckley* v. *Kruger-Benson-Ziemer* (1987). In *Buckley*, the plaintiff sued approximately two hundred named and unnamed defendants for his personal injuries, allegedly sustained after he was exposed to indoor pollutants in his tightly enclosed workspace. The defendants included the builder of the building, along with its architect, engineer, and ventilation contractor; and the manufacturers, sellers, and installers of numerous products used in the building. The case was settled before trial for an estimated $622,500.

In August 1986, Alaska state employees filed personal injury claims against the architect, contractors, and owner of an office building alleging illness from microbiologic contaminants (*Henley* v. *The Blomfield Co.*). The problem caused by the contaminants allegedly was so severe that one employee collapsed at his desk, and the building was finally evacuated. The cause of the problem was traced to the air-conditioning system, which was itself contaminated with a variety of fungi. The plaintiffs are claiming that the defendants are liable under strict liability, negligence, recklessness, and theories of breach of explicit and implicit warranties of fitness.

A couple in Massachusetts has filed suit against Charles L. Elliot Co., Elliot's insurer, and the couple's home insurer to recover damages resulting from oil gushing into and vaporizing in the couple's home. As a result of this incident the couple had to vacate their house. They also allege damages from illness, emotional harm, loss of personal property, and the medically necessitated quitting of a job.

In *Stillman* v. *South Florida Savings and Loan*, indoor air issues have emerged in a counterclaim. Upon discovering alleged indoor air pollution problems in a building it was occupying, South Florida Savings and Loan vacated its premises. Stillman sued the savings and loan company for rent due and other costs. The bank counterclaimed, alleging that the landlord did not provide a safe working environment, pointing to a failure to maintain a proper air-conditioning system.

Workers' compensation claims involving indoor pollution have emerged as well. For example, David Lindahl, while working in the Department of Energy housed in the James Madison Memorial Building on Capitol Hill, contracted Legionnaire's disease. He filed a workers' compensation claim but was denied recovery because of failure to prove a causal connection between working in that building and contracting the disease, according to *Washingtonian* Magazine.

Workers' compensation claims based on indoor air pollution do not always fail, however, as evidenced by *Ava Goldman v. Broward County Board of County Commissioners*. In this case, the defendant agreed to compensate the plaintiff shortly before court proceedings began. The plaintiff claimed she had been exposed to pathogenic molds, and tests showed that there was a high level of fungus *Aspergillus niger* in the office's air.

One case that is likely to receive more attention in the future is *Vermont v. Staco* (1988). In this case Vermont used the liability provisions of the federal superfund law to recover the costs of cleaning up workers' homes that were allegedly contaminated with hazardous substances from a worksite. The company produced mercury thermometers, and employees supposedly transported some of this hazardous substance to their homes as a result of the plant's alleged inadequate industrial hygiene practices. The basis of liability, according to the state and the court, is that the small quantities of the chemical that left the plant on the workers' clothing qualified as a release of a hazardous substance. This ruling marks a significant expansion of traditional superfund liability.

## SUMMARY

Complaints filed alleging that plaintiffs suffer from sick buildings frequently name any and all parties associated with the construction and operation of the buildings in question, including architects, contractors, engineers, manufacturers, sellers, distributors, and installers. The theories of legal liability relied upon will often include strict liability, negligent liability, and any other liability claims available to the plaintiff. As a result, litigation over indoor pollution is likely to continue and expand. This trend raises questions about the best way to resolve indoor air pollution issues. The trend may be unfortunate for defendants and plaintiffs alike. It may be unfortunate for defendants because most of the defendants who will find themselves in court over sick-building problems cannot truly be considered responsible for these problems. Nonetheless, they will be required to bear the cost of litigating or perhaps settling these claims. Increased resort to litigation may be unfortunate for plaintiffs who might have legitimate claims because of the delays, uncertainties, and high costs of litigation. Whatever the merits of concerns for indoor pollution issues, these concerns may best be resolved in forums other than local courthouses across the country.

# REFERENCES

Alfieri v. Cabot Corp., 17 App.Div.2d 455, 235 N.Y.S.2d 753 (1962), aff'd, 13 N.Y.2d 1027, 245 N.Y.S.2d 600, 195 N.E.2d 310 (1963).

Asbestos Litigation, 829 F.2d 1233 (3d Cir. 1987).

Asbestos School Litigation, No. 83-0268 (E.D. Pa. 1984).

Bardura v. Orkin, 664 F.Supp. 1218 (N.D. Ill. 1987).

Barth v. Firestone Tire and Rubber Co., 661 F.Supp. 193 (N.D. Calif. 1987).

Barth v. Firestone Tire and Rubber Co., 661 F.Supp. 193, 196, 203-205 (N.D. Calif. 1987).

Beshada v. Johns-Manville Products Corp., 90 N.J. 191, 447 A.2d 539 (1982).

Blagg v. Fred Hunt Co., 272 Ark. 179 (1981).

Blankenship v. Cincinnati Milacron Chemicals, 69 Ohio St.2d 608, 433 N.E.2d 572 (1982).

Bloomsburg Mills v. Sordoni Construction Co., 401 Pa. 358, 164 A.2d 201 (1960).

Borel v. Fibreboard Paper Products Corp., 493 F.2d 1076 (5th Cir. 1974).

Bradley v. Brucker, 69 PA. MONT. COUNTY L. RPTR. 38 (1952).

Brafford v. Susquehanna Corp., 586 F.Supp. 14 (D. Colo. 1984).

Brennan v. Celotex, Cook Cty. Cir. Ct., No. 81 L22907.

Brummett v. Skyline Corp., No. C81-01013-L (B) (W.D. Ky. June 3, 1985).

Buckley v. Kruger-Benson-Ziemer, No. 143393 (Super. Ct. Santa Barbara Cty., Calif., 1987).

Carrecter v. Colson Equipment Co., 499 A.2d 326, 330-31 (Pa. Super. 1985).

Caruso v. Celsius Insulation Resources, 101 F.R.D. 530 (M.D. Pa. 1984).

Case v. Fibreboard Corp., 743 P2d 1062, Sup. Ct. Okla., No. 67749, Sept. 22, 1987.

Castlebury v. Frost-Johnson Lumber, 238 S.W. 141, 143 (Tex. Civ. App. 1926).

Cooper v. Jevne, 56 Cal. App.3d 860, 128 CALIF. RPTR. 724 (1976).

Cunningham v. Orkin, CA5, No. 86-3444.

Davis and DeLaTorre. *A Fresh Look at Premises Liability as Affected by the Warranty of Habitability,* 59 WASH. L. REV. 141 (1984).

Delaney v. Borden, Inc., 99 F.R.D. 44 (E.D. Pa. 1983).

Diaz v. Keyes Co., 143 So.2d 554 (Fla. App. 1962).

Dow v. Holly Mfg. Co., 49 Calif.2d 720, 321 P.2d 736 (1958).

Duprey v. Shane, 241 P.2d 78 (Calif. App. 1951), aff'd, 39 Calif.2d 781, 249 P.2d 8 (1952).

Elderkin v. Gaster, 447 Pa. 118, 288 A.2d 771 (1972).

Evans v. Allentown Portland Cement Co., 433 Pa. 595, 525 A.2d 646 (1969).

Goldman v. Broward County Board of County Commissioners, Claim No. 287-48-1830. Broward County Office of Deputy Commissioner, Florida Department of Labor and Employment Security, stipulation signed Feb. 3, 1988.

Gulf South Insulation v. Consumer Product Safety Commission, 701 F.2d 1137 (5th Cir. 1983).

Hall v. E. I. DuPont de Nemours and Co., 345 F.Supp. 353 (E.D.N.Y. 1972).

Hammond v. Matthes, 109 Mich. App. 352, 311 N.W.2d 357 (1981).

Henley v. The Blomfield Co., No. 3AN-86-10483 (3d Jud. Dist. Anchorage, Alaska).

Heritage v. Pioneer Brokerage and Sales, 604 P.2d 1059 (Alaska 1979).

Huff v. Fibreboard Corp., 836 F.2d 473 (10th Cir. 1987).

Johns-Manville Products Corp. v. Superior Court of Contra Costa County, 27 Calif.3d 465, 165 CALIF. RPTR. 858, 612 P.2d 948 (1980).

Johnson v. Raybestos-Manhattan, Inc., 740 P.2d 548 (Haw. 1987).

Jones v. Gatewood, 381 P.2d 158 (Okla. 1963); Annot., 25 A.L.R.3d 383 (1969).

Kegley v. Borden, Inc., No. 82-2-03317-5 (Wash. Sup. Ct., Spokane, Sept. 27, 1983).

Kofron v. Amoco Chemicals Corp., 441 A.2d 226 (Del. 1982).

Kriegler v. Eichler Homes, 269 Calif. App.2d 224, 74 CALIF. RPTR. 749 (1969).

Layne v. GAF Corp., No. 84-074194 (Ct. of Common Pleas, Cuyahoga Cty., Ohio, Oct. 6, 1987).

Lee v. Department of Public Welfare, No. 15385 (Mass. Bristol Cty. Super. 1983).

Lipke v. Celotex, 505 NE2d 1213, Ill. Sup. Ct., No. 65014, March 10, 1987.

Lockwood v. A.C. & S. Inc., Wash. Sup. Ct., No. 53061-1, Oct. 15, 1987, 744 P2d 605.

Maples v. Porath, 638 S.W.2d 337 (Mo. App. 1982).

McCracken v. Sloan, 40 N.C. 214, 252 S.E.2d 250 (1979).

McDonald v. Mianecki, 79 N.J. 275, 398 A.2d 1283 (1979).

Meyer v. Parkin, 350 N.W.2d 435 (Minn. 1984).

Mobile America Sales Corp. v. Smith, slip op. (Tex. 1st Ct. App., Sept. 13, 1984).

Panagos v. North Detroit General Hospital, 35 Mich. App. 554, 192 N.W.2d 542 (1971).

Prescott v. United States, 523 F.Supp. 918 (D. Nev. 1981).

Prosser, W. *The Law of Torts* 63 (4th. ed., 1971).

Quashnock v. Frost, 445 A.2d 121 (Pa. Sup. 1982).

Rabb v. Orkin, 677 F.Supp. 424, D.C.S.C. Nos. 6:87-0174-3 and 6:86-1879-3, Oct. 30, 1987.

Raymark Industries, Inc. v. Stemple, D. Kan., No. 88-1014.

Roush v. GAF Corp., C.A. No. 84-1315 (W. Pa., Oct. 21, 1987).

Shirley v. The Drackett Products Co., 26 Mich. App. 644, 182 N.W.2d 762 (1970).

Sindell v. Abbott Laboratories, 26 Calif.3d 588, 163 CALIF. RPTR. 132, 607 P.2d 924 (1979).

Sisters of St. Mary et al. v. Aaer Sprayed Insulation et al., Cir. Ct., Dane Cty., No. 85CV5952, Dec. 17, 1987.

Spargnapani v. Wright, 110 A.2d 82 (D.C. 1954).

Steingaszner v. Paramount Pest Control, Va. Cir. Ct., Alexandria, No. 9955, Apr. 26, 1987.

Stillman v. South Florida Savings and Loan, No. 87-07013 (Fla. Cir. Ct. 17th Jud. Dist.).

Swogger v. Waterman Steamship Corp., 518 N.Y.S.2d 715, Index No. 13163/79 (N.Y. Co. July 8, 1987).

Tiderman v. Fleetwood Homes of Washington, 102 Wash.2d 344, 684 P.2d 1302 (1984).

Trauberman. *Statutory Reform of "Toxic Torts": Relieving Legal, Scientific and Economic Burdens on the Chemical Victim.* 7 HARV. ENVTL. L. REV. 177 (1983).

Tuttle v. Tindol Services, Ga. Sup. Ct. (Fulton Cty.).

U.S. v. Orkin Exterminating Co., W.D. Va., No. 88-00040, Apr. 21, 1988.

U.S. Fidelity and Guaranty Co. v. Wilkin Insulation Co., 84 CH 11676 (Cir. Ct. Cook Cty., 1987).

VaSalle v. Celotex Corp., 515 N.E.2d 684, No. 86-1683 (Ill. App. Ct., Sept. 24, 1987).

Vermont v. Staco, 86-190 (D. Vt., Jan. 6, 1988).

Vickers v. Veterans Administration, 549 F.Supp. 85 (W.D. Wash. 1982).

Vincent v. A.C. & S., Inc., 833 F.2d 553 (5th Cir. 1987).

Waggoner v. Midwestern Development, 154 N.W.2d 803 (S.D. 1967).

Wallinger v. Martin Stamping and Stove Co., 93 Ill. App.2d 437, 436 N.E.2d 755 (1968).

Weintraub v. Krobatsch, 65 N.J. 445, 317 A.2d 68 (1974).

Weisgall. *Product Liability in the Workplace: The Effect of Workers' Compensation on the Rights and Liabilities of Third Parties*. WIS. L. REV. 1035 (1977).

Wessels v. Celotex, Cook Cty. Cir. Ct., No. 81 L26094.

Woolworth Co. v. Williams, 41 F.2d 970 (D.C. Cir. 1930).

# INDEX

Synergism, cigarette smoke-radon interaction, 337
System evaluation, 86

Temperature
    effective, 19–20
    inside vs. outside, airflow, 74–76
Temporal constraints, environmental screening, 88–89
Tenax, VOC sampling, 255–56
Terpenes, 253, 262–63
Tetrachloroethylene, 5, 253, 261–62
Therapy, carbon monoxide poisoning, 196
Thermophilic actinomycetes, hypersensitivity pneumonitis, 294
Third-party suits, 387
Time patterns, exposure, 111–13
Time scale, environmental screening, 88–89
Time-activity patterns, 114, 116–17, 118–19, 133
Tissue hypoxia, carbon monoxide poisoning, 195–96
Tissue solubility, nitrogen dioxide, 171
Tobacco combustion, sources and concentrations, 34, 41–45
Tobacco smoke, 135–37, 391. *See also* Environmental tobacco smoke
Toluene, air quality standards, 5
Tracer gas techniques, 71–73
Transportation environments, tobacco smoke pollution, 134
1,1,1-Trichloroethane, 253, 262
Trichloroethylene, 5, 253
Tuberculosis, indoor air transmission, 278, 280

U.S. homes, radon concentrations, 326–29
Uranium-238, 323
Urban exposures, 38–39, 191–93, 336
Urea-formaldehyde foam insulation (UFFI), 48–50, 223–24, 225, 238–39, 244–45
Urea-formaldehyde resins, 224–25, 226
Urine, rodent allergen, 291–92

Vascular disease patients, exercise tolerance, carbon monoxide, 201
Vehicular emissions, 8–11, 40–41
Ventilation
    assessment methods, 71–73
    ETS control, 159–60
    thermal comfort control, historical perspective, 351–53
    windows and doors, 69–70
Ventilation air, purposes, 17–18
Ventilation efficiency factors, 360
Ventilation equipment and appliances, 76–77

Ventilation rates, carbon monoxide, 192
Ventilation requirements, 353–54
Ventilation standards, 16–19, 153, 154–55
Ventilation systems
    airborne infection, 275, 276, 277, 280–81
    sick-building syndrome, 310–11
Vertebrates, disease reservoirs, 274–75
Viability, disease agent, airborne infection rate, 278
Vinyl chloride, health effects, 260
Viral challenge, respiratory, nitrogen dioxide, 171
Virulence, disease agent, airborne infection rate, 279
Viruses, airborne infection, 273–81
Volatile organic compounds (VOCs), 252–72. *See also* Formaldehyde
    air quality standards, 5
    body concentrations, 264
    concentrations, indoor vs. outdoor, 268–59
    exposure reduction, 264–65
    exposure sources and sinks, 253, 254–55
    exposure studies, 258–63
    identification and characterization, 253–54
    indoor air, 259–63
    population exposure assessment, 124–25
    sampling and measurement, 95, 96, 97, 103, 255–57
    sick-building syndrome, 313–15
    sources and concentrations, 34, 46–51

Warranties
    expressed, liability, 379–80
    implied, liability, 380–81
Water, 260–61, 274–75, 325
Water heaters, emissions, 172, 192, 193
Wheeze, children, ETS, 139
Wind effects, 76
Wood burning, 40
Wood preservatives, indoor levels, 263
Wood products, formaldehyde, 48
Wood smoke, 209–22
    health effects, 213–19
    respiratory symptoms in children, 218–19
    sources of exposure, 211–12, 219
Wood stoves, emissions, 209–12
Wooden houses, radon, 336
Work-related health complaints, outbreaks, 306–7, 308
Workers' compensation claims, 384, 387, 393–94
Workforce characteristics, sick-building syndrome, 313

Designed by Chris Harris
Composed by The Composing Room of Michigan, Inc.
in Times Roman text and display.
Printed on 60-lb. Finch Opaque
by Edwards Brothers Incorporated.